Electronic Health Records

Second Edition

WITHDRAWN
UTSA LIBRARIES

RENEWALS 458-4574
DATE DUE

GAYLORD			PRI

D1019247

WITHDRAWN
LIBRARIES

Electronic

Health

Records

A Guide for Clinicians
and Administrators

Second Edition

JEROME H. CARTER, MD, FACP

ACP PRESS
AMERICAN COLLEGE OF PHYSICIANS   PHILADELPHIA

Associate Publisher and Manager, Books Publishing: Tom Hartman
Production Supervisor: Allan S. Kleinberg
Senior Editor: Karen C. Nolan
Editorial Coordinator: Angela Gabella
Cover Design: Lisa Torrieri
Index: Kathleen Patterson

Copyright © 2008 by the American College of Physicians. All rights reserved. No part of this book may be reproduced in any form by any means (electronic, mechanical, xerographic, or other) or held in any information storage and retrieval systems without written permission from the publisher.

Printed in the United States of America
Printing/binding by Versa Press
Composition by Atlis Graphics

Publisher's Note: Although a number of EHR vendors and products are mentioned within the text of this book, and some chapter authors are formally affiliated with an EHR vendor, this in no way implies an endorsement of the products or vendors by the editor or the American College of Physicians.

Library of Congress Cataloging-in-Publication Data

Electronic health records : a guide for clinicians and administrators / editor, Jerome H. Carter.—2nd ed.
     p. ; cm.
   Rev. ed. of: Electronic medical records. c2001.
   Includes bibliographical references and index.
   ISBN 978-1-930513-97-6
   1. Medical records—Data processing.   I. Carter, Jerome, 1955- II. Electronic medical records.
   [DNLM: 1. Medical Records Systems, Computerized.   2. Forms and Records Control—methods.   WX 173 E373 2008]

R864.A42 2008
610.285—dc22

Library
University of Texas
at San Antonio

08 09 10 11 12 / 10 9 8 7 6 5 4 3 2 1

Dedication

This is to all those people who have made my life possible:

LaSalle and Viola Carter, my parents for inspiring me

Janice, my wife, for her love and support

Janie Herbert, the best mother-in-law ever

And my daughter Joy, whose name says it all.

Visit <u>www.acponline.org/ehr</u> for more information on electronic health records.

Contributors

Jeroan J. Allison, MD, MS
Professor of Medicine, Divisions of
General Internal Medicine and
Preventive Medicine
Assistant Dean for Continuing
Medical Education
University of Alabama at
Birmingham
Birmingham, AL

Lyle Berkowitz, MD
Clinical Associate Professor of
Medicine
Feinberg School of Medicine
Northwestern University
Medical Director of Clinical
Information Systems
Northwestern Memorial Physicians
Group (NMPG)
Chicago, IL

Stephen E. Brossette, MD, PhD
Vice President
Cardinal Health
Birmingham, AL

Jerome H. Carter, MD, FACP
CEO
NT&M Informatics, Inc.
Adjunct Clinical Associate Professor
of Medical Education
Morehouse School of Medicine
Atlanta, GA

Sarah T. Corley, MD, FACP
Chief Medical Officer
NextGen Healthcare Information
Systems, Inc.
Horsham, PA

Daniel C. Davis, Jr., MD, FACP
CEO, Interactive Care Technologies
Honolulu
Assistant Chief Department of
Medicine
Queen's Medical Center
Honolulu
Clinical Associate Professor of
Medicine
John A Burns School of Medicine
University of Hawaii
Honolulu, HI

Erica L. Drazen, ScD, BS
Vice President
First Consulting Group
Lexington, MA

Thomas K. Houston, MD, MPH
Associate Professor of Medicine
University of Alabama at
Birmingham
Birmingham, AL

John J. Janas III, MD
CEO, Clinical Content
Consultants
Concord, NH

Merida L. Johns, PhD
President, Holistic Solutions
Visiting Professor
College of St. Scholastica
Woodstock, IL

Terri Thompson Mallett, Esquire
Administrative Law Judge
District of Columbia Government
Washington, DC

Naveen Maram, MD, MSHI, MPH
Medical Vocabulary Engineer
Intermountain Healthcare
Salt Lake City, UT

Daniel R. Masys, MD
Professor and Chair
Dept. of Biomedical Informatics
Vanderbilt University School of
    Medicine
Nashville, TN

**Blackford Middleton, MD, MPH,
    MSc, FACP**
Assistant Professor of Medicine
Harvard Medical School
Associate Physician
Brigham & Women's Hospital
Boston, MA
Partners HealthCare System
Wellesley, MA

Suchit Mishra, MSEE
Security Researcher
Adobe Systems Inc.
San Jose, CA

**Matthew Morgan, MD, MSc,
    FRCP(C)**
Courtyard Group Ltd;
Faculty of Medicine University of
    Toronto
University Health Network
Toronto, Ontario, Canada

**Jerome A. Osheroff, MD, FACP,
    FACMI**
Chief Clinical Informatics Officer
Thomson Healthcare
Adjunct Assistant Professor of
    Medicine
University of Pennsylvania Health
    System
Cherry Hill, NJ

Ashwin B. Philar, MSEE
McKesson Senior Software Engineer
San Francisco, CA

Caroline Samuels, MD
Core Teaching Faculty
Howard University Medical Center
Washington, DC
Teaching Faculty, Internal Medicine
Prince George's Hospital Center
Bethesda, MD

Bruce Slater, MD, MPH
Associate Professor (CHS) of
    Medicine and of Biostatistics and
    Medical Informatics
School of Medicine and Public Health
University of Wisconsin
Medical Director of Computerized
    Decision Support
University of Wisconsin Hospital
    and Clinics
Madison, WI

Thomas C. Tinstman, MD
Independent Consultant and
    Senior Advisor
Health Technology Center
San Francisco, CA

**Feliciano B. Yu, Jr., MD, MSHI,
    MSPH, CPHIMS**
Assistant Professor, Department
    of Pediatrics
University of Alabama School of
    Medicine at Birmingham
Medical Informaticist
Children's Health System
    Information Technology
    Division
Birmingham, AL

Preface to the Second Edition

Much has changed in the world of electronic health records (EHRs) since the first edition. What is perhaps the most important event occurred in the summer of 2003 when the Department of Health and Human Services asked the Institute of Medicine to provide specific guidance in helping to understand what capabilities an EHR should have in order to support patient care. The outcome of that request was the document "Key Capabilities of an Electronic Health Record System". This document was then used by HL-7 to create a functional model for EHRs that then became the basis for the criteria used for certifying EHR products by the Certification Commission for Health Information Technology (CCHIT). EHRs are increasingly seen as the key technology in addressing concerns in patient safety, quality of care, and cost reduction. This viewpoint is reflected by the 2005 creation of the federal-level Office of the National Coordinator for Health Information Technology (ONCHIT), which is charged with overseeing the widespread adoption of health information technology. Many states, with California and Massachusetts being excellent examples, are actively pursuing EHR adoption. Thus, EHRs, which were little more than a curiosity when this book was conceived in 1999, have become mainstream products and a major part of health care delivery.

On a more personal note, when the first edition of this book was published in 2001, I was Director of Informatics at the 1917 Patient Care and Research Clinic, University of Alabama-Birmingham. In that role I led a four-year effort to design and implement an EHR. That effort was completed successfully in September 2004, and the 1917 Computer-Based Patient Record is now in active use supporting HIV/AIDS clinical activities. (Those who wish to know more about the 1917 CPR may download a presentation at www.mshug.org/docs/techforumRedmond2007/Carter_J_Willig_J_8_21_HPT.pdf).

While the EHR was in the design phase, the 1917 Clinic became part of a consortium of medical centers working to build a national HIV/AIDS outcomes research network, CFAR Network of Integrated Clinical Systems (C-NICS), an effort that brought to the forefront the complex issues of data exchange, privacy/confidentiality and security. The content of this book has been directly affected by these experiences and the ascendancy of EHRs in public policy and the marketplace. These influences have resulted in new chapters on decision support, informatics data standards, project management, implementation planning, practice analysis, workflow analysis, and common security problems.

Changes to the Second Edition

The main goal of this book is to provide practical information and guidance to those interested in implementing an EHR. We have retained the overall organization from the first edition in which the book is divided into two major parts. Part One consists of 13 chapters that are best thought of as in-depth tutorials that address major technical and policy issues such as hardware, database systems, informatics standards, decision-support, and security and confidentiality. When applicable, references/resources for further reading are provided.

Part Two has a completely different approach. It is designed as a "Workbook". Here the goal is to offer practical advice on the actual steps involved in selecting and implementing an EHR. In response to the many questions received regarding the best way to select an EHR product, Part Two is now divided into separate "Selection" and "Implementation" sections. We have strived to better explain how to select the best EHR for your office by offering a method with clearly defined steps and outcomes based on the authors' real-world experiences.

New in the implementation section are chapters on workflow and project management because experience has shown that these two areas cause the most trouble during implementation. Security is another area often overlooked and for that reason we have added a second chapter focusing on security best practices.

We recognize that readers hail from a wide variety of practice environments, and we have endeavored to address their varied needs as best we could without making the text too long or suffering a loss of focus. We have adapted the chapters that discuss practice analysis, product selection, security, and team building with consideration for the limited resources that exist in small practices.

How to Use This Book

It is expected that readers will come to this work with quite different backgrounds, and to that end the following suggestions are offered based upon the knowledge of the reader and the type of resources that are at his or her disposal.

Clinician/Administrator in a Small Group

Often in small groups or solo practices the clinician or administrator has little technical knowledge and access to limited resources. A major consulting firm is out of the question, and the technical person involved may be the retailer who sold you the practice management system (or possibly a relative who "knows a lot about computers"). The cost of failure will be high in terms of dollars and morale. If you fall into this group, caution is the keyword. Read Chapter 1 to get a feel for what an EHR is and what basic EHR designs are available. Next, move on to Chapter 11 and finally Part Two, the workbook chapters. These chapters contain the bulk of what you will need to know to understand your needs, interact with vendors, select a product, and plan your implementation. Using this approach, chapters in Part One may be used as a reference when there is a need for additional information. Do not allow your desire to do "something" make you do something that you later regret.

Clinicians/Administrators Who are Members of "Selection Committees"

Usually a selection committee implies a fair-sized practice or a more diverse setting (e.g., hospital, multi-specialty group). Since there are so many backgrounds and skill sets represented on these committees, effective communication is often a real problem. Words and concepts are tossed about that are not understood by all members. If your understanding of technical issues is minimal, then start with Chapters 1-6. If product selection is the main focus of the committee, move on to the "Selection" section of the workbook. The process chapters (Chapters 7 and 8) in Part One will also be enlightening.

Clinicians/Administrators who are Members of an Implementation Group

Because organizations vary widely in how they name committees, the advice given here assumes that a product has been selected. During implementation the main issue is how to fit the organization to the product in terms of features, functions, and workflow. The most useful chapters in Part One are likely to be those that deal with informatics standards and business and clinical processes: Chapters 1, 6-9, 11, and the Implementation section of the workbook.

Quality Improvement Initiatives

Patient safety and quality improvement are two of the major drivers behind the current interest in EHRs. However, even though EHRs may be quite effective in patient safety and quality efforts, the benefits are not necessarily automatic. Specific features and functions are required in EHRs to support anything beyond basic quality/safety initiatives. Review Chapters 7-10 for a discussion of EHR-related process and quality improvement issues. Next, move on to Chapter 6, Informatics Standards, and finish with workbook chapters that address product features, workflow, and process analysis (Chapters 16, 17, 21, and 23).

Medical Directors

The implementation of an EHR may be either a godsend or the worst thing that has ever happened in your professional life. As the spokesman for the medical staff, your opinion counts tremendously and therefore should be well informed. Very likely you have access to technical staff and consultants. Unfortunately, they may have a vested interested in influencing your opinion. Part One has the information you need to understand the terms and concepts that will be discussed repeatedly in your meetings, demonstrations, and site visits. If quality improvement is a major reason for EHR implementation, you should give Chapters 1, and 6-10 particular scrutiny. If a clinical data repository is being considered, add Chapter 4 to your must-read list. If your major concern is selecting and implementing an EHR, read the workbook (Chapters 14-25) and refer to the Part One chapters to fill in knowledge gaps.

CEO/CIO and Other High Level Administrators

All of the issues covered in the book are important to you. However, because many jobs will be delegated to those with appropriate expertise, the information that you require is likely to be at a fairly high conceptual level. Consequently, Chapters 1, 11 and 12 will probably be most useful. In addition, the chapters in the Workbook that discuss contracts, RFPs, and project management (18, 19, and 22) should be informative.

Technical Personnel with Little EHR Knowledge

Your major challenges will be understanding how EHRs differ from other types of software and dealing with the new group of clinical users that you will inherit with the EHR. Chapters 1, 4, 6, 7, 8, 11, 12, and 13 should be useful.

Final Remarks

Privacy, security, and the legal aspects of EHRs are important topics that most people find less than interesting reading. However, these are very important topics, and everyone should read these chapters. Supplement your reading with other materials from the reference listings and the resources in Appendix B. You will be surprised at how quickly once incomprehensible technical articles and discussions begin to make perfectly good sense.

Acknowledgements

I would like to thank the editorial staff of American College of Physicians, Thomas Hartman, Angela Gabella, Karen Nolan, and Marla Sussman, who helped in so many ways to improve the content and readability of the book, as well as to produce a beautiful design. Once again the College's informatics staff helped with the glossary: Thom Kuhn, Steve Spadt, Margo Williams, and Maria Rudolph.

Taking an EHR from an idea to a fully implemented system is a once-in-a-lifetime experience. I would like to thank those brave souls at the 1917 Clinic at the University of Alabama-Birmingham who believed in the project and supported me: Michael Saag, Executive Director of the clinic and current Director, Division of Infectious Diseases, for making the entire effort possible, and the rest of the administrators at the clinic, especially Jim Raper, Karen Savage, and Michael Kilby for their help and support.

Building and deploying an EHR takes many hands and I could not have done it without dedicated and brilliant assistants: Ashwin Philar, software engineer; Suchit Mishra, systems and security; Naveen Maram and Pradnya Warnekar, vocabulary/terminology specialists; Robin Hood, HIPAA guru; Davendra Sohal, workflow and support; and Ray O'Neil, end-user support. I would also like to thank James Willig and Manojkumar Patil for their on-going efforts to update and expand the system since my departure.

I was very pleasantly surprised by the enthusiasm expressed by my fellow authors when they were informed that a second edition was underway. The dedication to quality and patience with my critiques demonstrated by all has made my task as editor much easier. I am grateful for your efforts and honored by your commitment to produce the best possible text.

Finally I would like to thank everyone who sent thoughtful comments and suggestions for changes to the second edition. I hope that you are pleased with the outcome. As always I would love to hear from you, and should you be so moved stop by www.computingforclinicians.com.

Jerome H Carter, MD, FACP
Atlanta, Georgia
January 2008

Preface to the First Edition

The inspiration for this book came from the many clinicians whom I have encountered over the past four years who found themselves in the frustrating position of wanting to implement an electronic medical record (EMR) system and having no idea where to start the process. Invariably, their first words to me after the usual pleasantries were "Which system should I buy?" My response always began with "That depends . . ." and the ensuing brief discussion was rarely sufficient to answer their query.

This book is an attempt to answer the many questions that arise when implementing an EMR system. As an aid to the reader, the book is divided into two parts. In Part One the reader will find in-depth discussions of technologies, issues, and processes. When applicable, references for further reading are provided. However, this should in no way be understood to imply that Part One is an academic work with little practical value. It offers the background information required to understand the important EMR issues that arise as one journeys from initial curiosity to final implementation. Think of Part One as providing the "what" and "why" of EMR-related technologies and issues.

Part Two has a completely different approach. It is designed as a Workbook. Here the goal is to offer practical advice on the actual steps involved in implementing an EMR system. The information provided in its chapters is thoroughly infused with the "hands-on" experience of the authors. Though Part Two offers useful advice for readers in all practice environments, it should be particularly useful to those in a solo practice or small group and to others who cannot afford to retain the services of major consulting firms or do not have access to a good deal of on-site technical expertise. Part Two covers the everyday issues of negotiating a contract, evaluating products, understanding practice needs, and planning.

How To Use This Book

Electronic Medical Records for Clinicians and Administrators contains a good deal of information, much of it quite technical—all of it necessary to achieve a working knowledge of the important issues faced when moving from paper to an EMR. It is expected that readers will come to this work with quite different backgrounds, and to that end the following suggestions are offered based upon the knowledge of the reader and the type of resources that are at his or her disposal. The following groups should encompass the majority of readers.

Clinician/Administrator with Little Technical Knowledge and Access to Limited Resources

Often in small groups or solo practices the clinician or administrator has little technical knowledge and access to limited resources. A major consulting firm is out of the question, and the technical person involved may be the retailer who sold you the practice management system (or possibly a relative who "knows a lot about computers"). The cost of failure will be high in terms of dollars and morale. If you fall into this group, caution is the keyword. Take time to read Chapters 1–3, 5–7, 10–12, and all of the Workbook (Part Two). These chapters offer insight into the issues most pressing for those in your situation. Once you have become familiar with the concepts and issues that they discuss, then go back and finish the remaining chapters. Do not take lightly the admonitions offered in the Workbook. Most of all, do not allow your desire to do "something" make you do something that you come to regret.

Clinicians/Administrators who are Members of "Selection Committees"

Usually a selection committee implies a fair-sized practice or a more diverse setting (e.g., hospital, multi-specialty group). In such cases technical personnel and consultants are often available, both of whom can be very helpful during product selection and implementation. If you are a member of this group, you will likely have little direct say over the most important issues. Your role becomes that of protecting the interests of those you represent (unless of course you are the committee chairman!). Your understanding of the key issues is extremely important. If you have a fairly good grasp of technical matters, then issues related to work-flow, practice environment, and general operations should guide your reading. Chapters 6–12 will probably be most helpful initially, with Chapters 1–5 acting as an occasional reference. The Workbook will be useful in helping you prepare your colleagues for the changes that lie ahead.

Medical Directors

The implementation of an EMR system may be either a godsend or the worse thing that has ever happened in your professional life. As the spokesman for the medical staff your opinion counts tremendously and therefore should be well-informed. Very likely you have access to technical staff and consultants. Unfortunately, they may have a vested interested in influencing your opinion. Part One has the information you need to understand the terms and concepts that will be discussed repeatedly in your meetings, demonstrations, and site visits. If quality improvement is a major reason for the implementation (e.g., order entry, guidelines), Chapters 6–10 and 16 should be given particular scrutiny. If a clinical data repository is being considered, Chapter 4 should be added to the must-read list.

CEO/CIO and Other High Level Administrators

All of the issues covered in the book are important to you. However, because many jobs will be delegated to those with appropriate expertise, the information that you require is likely to be at a fairly high conceptual level. Consequently, Chapters 8–12 will probably be most useful. In addition, the chapters in the Workbook that discuss Requests for Proposals and contracts might provide a few useful insights (see especially Chapter 18).

Technical Personnel with Little EMR Knowledge

Few health care sites have installed an EMR system, and there is no shortage of horror stories of failed implementations. Many of the failures are caused by nontechnical issues (e.g., poor planning, inadequate training). However, often the problem is a poor understanding of the technical issues associated with EMR software. For example, response times under full load, file importation, database structure, clinical vocabulary, and system integration are technical matters that can delay or doom an EMR installation. Those who may be best able to understand the potential pitfalls at an early stage are knowledgeable technical personnel. Chapters 1–5 and 16 should be of particular value to technical personnel involved in EMR projects.

Final Remarks

If you find that you do not fit into any of these groups, reading the book from beginning to end also works quite well. But do not read this book in a vacuum. Many vendors offer fully functioning demonstration programs, at little or no cost, that may be used to aid in understanding EMR features and issues. Supplement your reading with other materials; there are a number of helpful Web sites and magazines (see Appendix B). One result of the diligent reading of this book will be the mastery of the concepts and jargon associated with EMR systems. You will be surprised at how quickly once-incomprehensible technical articles and discussions begin to make perfectly good sense.

Acknowledgements

I would like to thank all those who have made this book possible. The Editorial Staff members of ACP-ASIM—Mary Ruff, David Myers, and Alicia Dillihay—have been very understanding, supportive, and patient. Former staff members of the College's Medical Informatics Department—Bob Spena, Jerry Osherhoff, Linda Sundberg, Chris Dwyer, and Steve Spadt—provided very helpful comments and suggestions.

Michael Saag, Jim Raper, Betty McCulloch, Michael Kilby, Tracey Reid, and the staff of the 1917 Research Clinic at the University of Alabama–Birmingham demonstrated exceptional patience and understanding during my many months of endless questions, interviews, meetings, and report writing. Having gone through a full-scale systems-and-requirements analysis for our home-grown EMR project, they remain cheerful and eager to continue. Thank you for your support and good humor.

Doing a book of this scope would have required more time than I alone could possibly have dedicated to such an important task. Also, the quality would not have been nearly as high without the valuable contributions of my fellow authors. I am honored to be in such good company.

Finally, I would like to thank all those who have attended my talks and seminars over the years for helping me to focus the content of the book and to understand what the important issues really are.

Jerome H. Carter, MD, FACP
February 2001

Contents

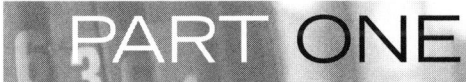

PART ONE

Electronic Health Records for Clinicians and Administrators

1

What Is the Electronic Health Record?

Jerome H. Carter, MD

Reports of using computers to support clinical data management activities date back to the late 1950s. Over the years systems have been designed that support most major activities related to health care business practices and clinical processes. The most common systems are listed below (Table 1-1).

Until recently, hospitals have led the way in the development of clinical information systems. This was owing, in part, to several factors: 1) the cost of these systems (including personnel) made information technology too expensive for smaller entities, and 2) hospitals had greater need of meeting regulatory and financial requirements. Hospital information systems (HIS) usually have, as their central component, an Admission, Discharge, and Transfer (ADT) system that manages census and patient demographic information. Billing and accounting packages are also frequently included as core components. In many community hospitals, financial and ADT systems, along with Laboratory Information Systems (LIS), comprised the complete HIS package until recently. In the past fifteen years, most hospitals, regardless of size, have begun to create information systems solutions via integration of departmental systems with the core HIS, although almost 20% still do not have electronic implementations of all major ancillary systems (1,2).

Departmental systems, especially those for pharmacy, radiology, and laboratory, have evolved from a focus on administrative tasks (scheduling, order entry, billing) to more clinically oriented functions. For example, modern pharmacy systems commonly provide drug interactions, allergy alerts, and drug monographs as part of their standard feature set. When looking at the evolution of clinical information systems, it is instructive to consider how the end-user has changed over the years. Departmental systems were designed primarily for use by workers within those departments, not health

Table 1-1

HOSPITAL INFORMATION TECHNOLOGY APPLICATIONS

System Type	Function
Master patient index	Registration and assignment of unique identifiers for all systems within a hospital or integrated delivery network.
Pharmacy information system	Medication dispensing, inventory, billing, drug information, and interactions.
Radiology information system	Scheduling, billing, and results reporting.
Picture archiving system	Storage and presentation of radiological images.
Nursing information system	Storage and collection of nursing documentation, care planning, and administrative information.
Hospital information systems	Core system manages hospital census (admission, discharge, transfer) and billing. Most often linked to departmental systems (pharmacy, laboratory, etc.).
Chart management/medical records systems	Assists in the management of paper records and aids with required statistical reporting. Used by medical records personnel.
Practice management system	Outpatient system for managing business-related information. May contain some clinical information (CPT, ICD).
Laboratory information system	Orders for lab tests and results reporting. Covers blood bank, pathology, microbiology, etc.

care providers. Thus drug interaction information was available only to pharmacists and their staffs, not directly to doctors and nurses. Clinical information systems were labeled as such because they were utilized in areas that supported clinical activities, not because they were intended for use primarily by clinicians. Of all the systems that fall under the rubric of clinical information systems, only a few are designed primarily for use by health care providers: intensive care unit systems (ICU), picture archiving and communications systems (PACS), computerized physician order entry systems (CPOE), and the EHR.

The modern era of clinical information systems is being driven by concerns of quality, patient safety, and cost, in addition to secondary business and operational issues (3). Today emphasis has shifted toward providing information systems that support providers during the process of care, resulting in the advent of CPOE systems and a much higher profile for EHRs (4).

CPOE systems provide an integrated view of orders and results (medications, radiology, laboratory) along with decision support functions (drug interactions, duplicate requests, clinical protocols, etc.) and are most often seen in hospital settings. These are complex provider-centric applications and constitute one of the fundamental building blocks of a hospital-based EHR. However, they have not yet achieved wide acceptance: fewer than 7% of American hospitals have fully functioning CPOE systems (1,5).

The EHR is the goal towards which clinical information systems have been evolving since their inception. Even so, EHR systems remain uncommon in many practice settings. Fewer than 3% of American hospitals have robust EHR systems (1), while fewer than 15% of physicians use EHRs on a regular basis (6,7).

The Electronic Health Record Concept

The growing interest in EHRs has been paralleled by an increase in the number of attempts at defining what they are. When perusing publications concerned with EHRs and associated technologies, one is quickly struck by the number of terms used to describe them. Over the years EHRs have been referred to by a number of terms: electronic medical record, electronic patient record, electronic health record, computer-stored patient record, ambulatory medical record, and computer-based medical record. Unfortunately, the definitions are conceptual and do little in the way of providing a technical, engineering, or scientific view of EHRs that could be used for either designing systems or reviewing products.

In 1991 the Institute of Medicine (IOM) published a landmark report, "The Computer-Based Patient Record: An Essential Technology for Health Care" (8), which focused attention on important EHR concepts. One of its more valuable contributions was in the area of terminology. It defines the computer-based patient record (CPR) as an "electronic patient record that resides in a system designed to support users through availability of complete and accurate data, practitioner reminders and alerts, clinical decision support systems, links to bodies of medical knowledge, and other aids" (8).

Further amplification was later provided by one of the report's editors, Richard Dick, PhD, who describes the CPR as "a representation of all of a patient's data that one would find in the paper-based record, but in a coded and structured, machined-readable form." Dick further notes that, "Clinical documentation is completed via computer and is coded within the patient's CPR. Stored data are indexed with sufficient detail to support retrieval for patient care delivery, management, and analysis" (9). Regarding the features of EHRs and EPRs, Dick writes:

> The EMR and EPR, which are in fact reasonably synonymous, are electronic, machine-readable versions of much of the data found in paper-based records, comprising both structured and unstructured patient data from disparate, computerized ancillary systems and document-imaging systems. Clinical documentation may originate in either paper records or computerized data;

however, the data are not comprehensively coded. One might consider the EMR or EPR as transitional between the paper-based record and the CPR. (9)

The perspective offered by Dick relates the CPR, EPR, and EMR along a continuum based on, among other factors, the level of granularity of stored data. A true CPR requires that every data item be uniquely coded and individually searchable; an EPR/EMR does not. EPR/EMR systems only require that the data be in electronic form.

The CPR report, while providing a conceptual framework for discussion of electronic record systems, proved to be less useful when evaluating real world products. That task fell to "Key Capabilities of EHR Systems," a report published by the Institute of Medicine in 2003 (10). Building on the work of the 1991 report, it offered a more practical definition of EHRs. The report states:

An EHR system includes: 1) longitudinal collection of electronic health information for and about persons, where health information is defined as information pertaining to the health of an individual or a health care provider to an individual; 2) immediate electronic access to person- and population-level information by authorized, and only authorized, users; 3) provision of knowledge and decision-support that enhances the quality, safety, and efficiency of patient care; and 4) support for efficient processes for health care delivery.

This definition of an EHR system encompasses all of the concepts and functionality proposed originally for the CPR; thus, we will use "EHR system" (EHR) as the official term for this text.

The 2003 report identified eight core areas for which EHR systems should provide supporting features/functions (Table 1-2) while recognizing four basic types of EHR care settings (hospitals, nursing homes, ambulatory care, community-personal health record). The functionalities identified to support

Table 1-2

CORE FUNCTIONAL AREAS IDENTIFIED BY THE 2003 IOM REPORT

- Health information and data
- Patient support
- Results management
- Electronic communication and connectivity
- Decision-support management
- Reporting and population health
- Order entry/management
- Administrative processes

these eight core areas were further expanded and developed by Health Level 7 organization (HL7) into a standard by which commercially available products could be evaluated and eventually certified by the Certification Commission for Health Information Technology (CCHIT) (11). The 2003 report acknowledges that EHR technology develops incrementally and that for a given setting or a particular product, EHR features and functions will vary over time. Therefore, many products will have advanced features in some areas while being relatively deficient in others: today's EHR products are seen as the progenitors of tomorrow's comprehensive EHR systems.

Introduction to Electronic Health Record Systems

Early efforts at building what became EHRs began in the 1960s with the COSTAR system, developed by Barnett at the Laboratory of Computer Science at Massachusetts General Hospital (12). Subsequent efforts at Duke University (13) and the Regenstrief Institute at Indiana University Medical Center (14) have all given rise to robust EHR systems that contain data for thousands of patients. While there is no formal model or standard architecture for EHR systems, these pioneering systems provided a basic model for current hospital-based and ambulatory EHR systems that has been emulated by current products.

Inpatient EHR Systems

Whereas EHR systems offer similar features and functions across care settings, they differ significantly in how that functionality is assembled.

EHR systems that support hospitals and integrated delivery systems are virtual systems created by pooling and sharing data between many component systems (15,16). Outpatient systems are usually self-contained applications in which all functions are built on top of a single, shared database. The ability of an EHR system to support advanced features such as decision support, sophisticated reporting, and coded data entry is determined by the level of integration of its component systems. Two levels of integration are common: presentation and data level (15,17,18).

System Integration

Presentation Integration

At the presentation level, users are able to view data from all connected systems through a common interface (15,17,18). The user may access a single terminal to review patient information. Systems like this are quite useful, but they are limited when users wish to do more that simple data retrieval. These systems only seem to be one coherent system because a single interface is required to interact with all of its components. Much of the enthusiasm for Intranets and Web browsers are due to their ability to support, with relative ease, presentation-level system integration (19,20).

A major downside to presentation-level integration is the lack of query capability across all systems. For example, it would not be possible to ask a question such as "find all patients with a diagnosis of congestive heart failure who are not taking an ACE inhibitor" because the patients' problem lists and medication records reside on two different computer systems. The billing system may hold the diagnosis codes, while the pharmacy system holds the medication profile. For a system to qualify as an EHR, some degree of data-level integration must be present.

Data Integration

Data integration is required for true EHR functionality and is more difficult to attain (21-23). Each component system may have its own data model and naming conventions for data elements. Data-level integration requires that all system components use a consistent scheme for coding data elements and that a mechanism be present for movement of data between systems (from components to the central system). In the case of a hospital or integrated delivery network (IDN), the central system is usually a large database called a clinical data repository (CDR) (15,16,24).

The CDR acts as the major information source for the entire EHR system (Chapter 4). The simplest CDR implementations rely solely on laboratory, radiology, pharmacy, ADT, and other standard department systems as information sources (1,2). Achieving true EHR functionality requires adding to this basic CDR environment CPOE, advanced reporting, PACS, clinical documentation, clinical decision support capability, and other provider-centric information technologies (1,2).

The goal of the CDR is to provide a common pool of data that all applications can access. The most frequently used method for populating the CDR is through the use of interfaces to link each component system. Interfaces are special software programs that move data between systems. Data that reside in component systems designed by different vendors use proprietary data models; therefore, similarly named data elements from different systems may have characteristics that prevent them from being interchangeable. Simple messaging interfaces alone cannot resolve the deeper semantic problems present by data from disparate systems (25,26). The problems that arise in reconciling terms, data elements, and data formats between component systems require additional applications, such as clinical data dictionaries, in order to provide true data-level integration. The costs and issues associated with implementating interoperability between systems, such as the lack of widely accepted data standards, create major barriers to EHR adoption for many hospitals (2,27).

Legacy systems (older systems currently in place) represent a special problem for EHR implementation for hospitals and IDNs. These older systems often cannot be easily replaced and so must become part of newer systems, thereby hampering data-level integration. In many instances, presentation-level integration is all that is possible for legacy systems.

A second approach to providing a common data pool is through the use of an integrated system that relies on a single, shared database that is used for storage by all components and applications (see Unified Database section, below).

The EHR is one instance in which ambulatory practice sites are in a much better position to implement new technologies than their often wealthier inpatient cousins. Ambulatory care sites are simpler work environments with fewer specialized information management needs. Integration issues are usually limited to practice management systems, laboratory interfaces, and office machines (e.g., EKG).

Real-World Electronic Health Record Models

Interfaced Systems: Best-of-Breed

The classic architecture for inpatient EHRs is based on the use of interfaces and is often referred to as the best-of-breed approach (so named because departmental managers bought the best component system that they could afford at the time) (28-30). Best-of-breed (Fig. 1-1) is the natural growth path to EHR functionality for most hospitals because it makes use of whatever component systems the hospital has in place. Most hospitals begin the

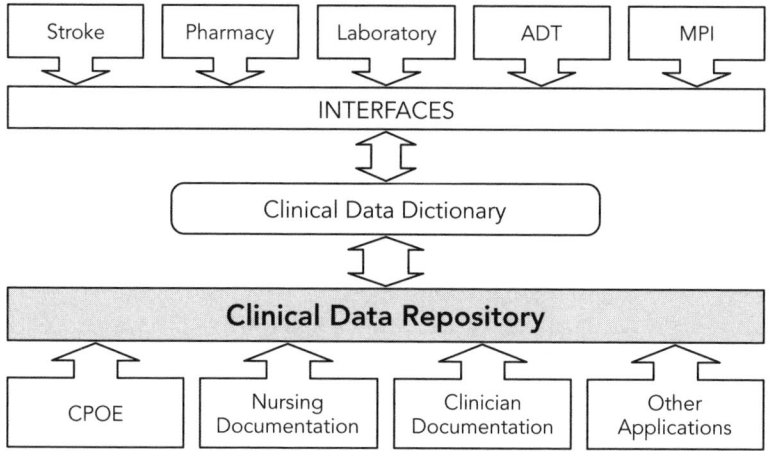

Figure 1-1 Best-of-Breed (interfaced) EHR.

journey to EHR functionality with the presence of a CDR that integrates data from departmental systems (laboratory, radiology and medication) and allows providers to access information from a single workstation (results viewing). Populating the clinical data repository, and by extension the EHR, using the best-of-breed approach results in the data integration issues discussed previously (Table 1-3). Once this foundation has been laid, advanced functionality is added over time in the form of CPOE, clinical documentation, electronic medication administration, and PACS (1,2).

Integrated Systems: Unified Database

At the other end of the spectrum are fully integrated, unified database systems (17,21,29,30). The term "unified database" will be used to denote systems that share a single underlying database to avoid confusion with the term "single source," which indicates that all systems were purchased from the same vendor. Systems from the same vendor do not necessarily share the same underlying database. Thus, single source does not automatically imply that systems are fully integrated at the data level.

Unified database systems are labeled as such because all components share a single (unified) database (Figure 1-2), eliminating the need for a separate CDR. This approach to EHR design minimizes or potentially eliminates the need for interfaces by providing true data-level integration. Unified database systems may be deployed using fewer hardware resources and simpler configurations than best-of-breed systems, making it less dif-

Table 1-3

EHR INTEGRATION MODELS

	Best-of-Breed: Interfaced	Hybrid	Unified Database: Integrated
Advantages	Build system "as-you-go". Select from best products available.	Build system "as-you-go". Fewer vendors than best-of-breed. Data integration less costly than best-of-breed. Back-up/availability better.	Single vendor. No interfaces required (or very few). Complete data integration. Back-up/availability best.
Disadvantages	Costly to get good data integration. Many interfaces required. Manage multiple vendors. Back-up/availability more difficult.	Multiple interfaces required. Manage multiple vendors.	Tied to one vendor (may have less desirable applications in some areas).

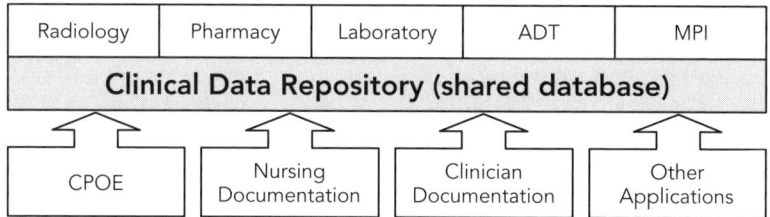

Radiology	Pharmacy	Laboratory	ADT	MPI

Clinical Data Repository (shared database)

CPOE	Nursing Documentation	Clinician Documentation	Other Applications

Figure 1-2 Unified Database (integrated) EHR.

ficult to provide high-availability deployments (less time spent with the system unavailable to users) that are easier to set up, maintain, and back up. The unified database approach to achieving EHR functionality is growing in inpatient environments, although it is the norm in physician offices (Figure 1-3).

One impediment to having a unified database EHR is that all components must be purchased from the same vendor. Because most hospitals start with a few ancillary systems and build from there, in many settings going with a unified database architecture would require getting rid of many current systems. As a result, most hospitals develop hybrid architectures that exist along a continuum between best-of-breed and unified database (see Table 1-3). The marketplace reflects the newness of the unified database product in that no vendors currently offer an inpatient EHR on a unified database platform that includes all required components.

Electronic Health Record Advanced Features and Functions

Computerized Physician Order Entry and Decision Support

Computerized physician order entry (CPOE) is an application that allows physicians to enter orders for medications, laboratory tests, procedures, and imaging studies (31,32). CPOE is usually the next major component added

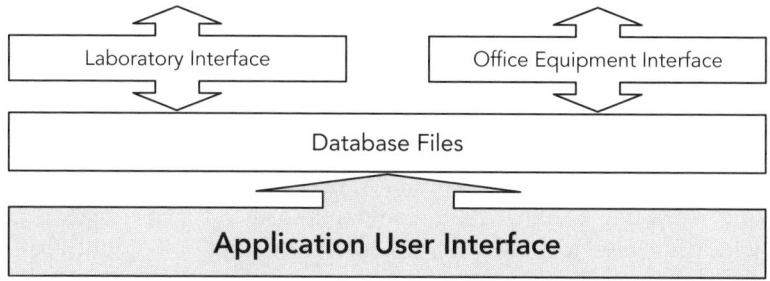

Laboratory Interface	Office Equipment Interface

Database Files

Application User Interface

Figure 1-3 Office-Based EHR.

to inpatient EHRs once the CDR is fully functional. Decision support is a key component of CPOE functionality. Basic decision support is usually implemented as alerts and reminders such as drug interactions or warnings for order duplications (e.g., ordering a chest x-ray when a current one is extant) and is usually implemented in stages. Advanced decision support features include support for protocols, advanced drug-related alerts, and aid in drug selection.

Clinical Documentation

Full charting capabilities for nurses and clinicians are a major advancement for inpatient EHRs. Documentation runs the gamut from vital signs and basic nursing assessments to advanced systems that support structured data entry for clinicians. Nursing information systems have been around for quite a while but have not always been fully integrated with other systems. Clinician documentation functionality remains uncommon in most hospitals (1,2).

Picture Archiving and Communications Systems

Radiology information systems provide access to reports of imaging studies. Gaining access to the actual image requires access to picture archiving and communications systems (PACS) functionality. PACS began as standalone applications that were available either to radiologists or to limited areas of the hospital. Through the CDR, PACS functionality is made accessible as part of the EHR. PACS may be integrated at any stage of EHR evolution (33,34).

Electronic Medication Administration Records

Ensuring that the correct patient receives the proper medication is a major safety issue. Electronic medication administration records (eMAR) applications use wrist bands with bar codes to identify patients and to check the medication to be administered against the information in pharmacy records. This helps to prevent errors related to patient identity as well as to ensure that the proper dosage and drug are administered. eMAR is often integrated with CPOE in advanced EHR environments (35,36).

Ambulatory Electronic Health Record Systems

EHR systems designed for physicians' offices represent the simplest architecture consisting of three basic components: the database management system, user interface, and external interfaces (Figure 1-3). All are contained in one (unified) database and accessed through a common interface. Care must be taken when reviewing products to avoid systems that simply replicate the functions and content of paper-based records. This design is still seen in products that rely mainly on document imaging for storage of key chart documents (e.g., progress notes, lab reports). The ultimate value of an EHR requires, as emphasized by the IOM, discrete data that can be used for analysis or by other components of the EHR to support patient care and decision-making. EHRs offering the required level of functionality are evidenced by data formats that permit laboratory results, problem lists, medication lists and other common record data to exist as coded data elements. Ambulatory EHR products have begun to differentiate themselves based on ancillary components that support advanced population health features, as well as improved data exchange/interoperability features.

Major Ancillary Components of Outpatient Systems

Disease Registries and Preventive Medicine

Taking care of patients with chronic illnesses requires managing data from a wide variety of sources over a period of years. Disease registry features that support managing a select population such as specialized recall functions, disease-based templates, flowsheets, and specialized reporting functions are becoming more common in outpatient EHRs (37,38).

Data formats that support discrete elements along with more sophisticated report writers are being added to systems due to pressures from quality concerns such as pay-for-performance programs (39). These new features encourage "systems" thinking on the part of clinicians who use these tools to review the efficacy with which they manage their patients at the population level. They provide the analyzable data required to be able to audit the practice's adherence to internal and external clinical policies and guidelines.

Two-Way Laboratory Interfaces

Downloads of laboratory results have been available for a while. Second-generation systems are now extending their external interface features with uplinks to clinical labs as well. Removal of the need for paper when ordering labs aids in practice efficiency, reduces costs, and paves the way for additional decision support functionality.

E-Prescribing

Typical EHR medication features include medication lists and prescription writers with automatic checks for allergies and drug interactions and drug information. E-prescribing promises to add new features that promote patient safety and practice efficiency. E-prescribing services may be embedded in an EHR or provided as a stand-alone product. The most important advance of e-prescribing over previous electronic prescription writing applications is the presence of a mechanism for standardized electronic data interchange (40). With an accepted standard, all EHR and e-prescribing vendors can create applications that can share and use the same data. This makes it possible to have access to formularies from third-party payers, share medication histories between providers, and securely submit prescriptions to any pharmacy that participates. These features are making their way into second-generation EHRs systems but not without a few glitches. A national study conducted in 2006 found on-going problems with e-prescribing services (41).

Electronic Health Record Supporting Technologies

Databases

Databases are the key technology underlying all EHR systems. Databases can store data in large blocks (documents or images) or as discrete items (numbers or single words). Modern database systems may hold billions of data items and manage thousands of transactions per second. A database may reside on a single computer (the server) or multiple computers. Data repositories, warehouses, and EHRs are special types of database programs (see Chapter 4). Database management systems are software programs that provide the functions required to manipulate the information stored in databases (e.g., database creation, reporting, design). The internal structure or organization of a database is referred to as a "schema." There are no standards for schema design for EHRs; consequently, EHR products built using the same database management systems may have different schemas. This creates difficulties when attempting to move from one EHR product to another. The CCHIT certification process focuses on functional issues (whether features are present and work appropriately); they do not address database-related matters.

Delivery Models

Most EHRs are deployed on computers that reside in physicians' practices and use a central computer (server) to house the main database, which is accessed using workstations (client): this is referred to as a client/server model. Using this model, practices must have access to technical expertise (e.g., systems administrators) to maintain their computer systems. Over the last 3 years, with the rise of the Internet and high-speed connections, the "application service provider" (ASP) model for EHR deployments has become more popular. In the ASP model, the EHR resides on a central computer housed by a hosting company (usually the EHR vendor) and is accessed via the Internet. The ASP model is less expensive to deploy because the practice does not have to buy a server and maintain it. The advantages of each deployment model are listed in Table 1-4.

Data Input Technologies

Data entry is a major EHR implementation issue. The traditional means of interacting with computers, the keyboard, is not the most efficient method for many EHR users. The two alternatives that have received the most attention are pen- and voice-based input.

Pen-based input relies on a device that may be used primarily like a mouse as a pointing device, or it may be used to "write" on the computer screen much like a real pen. In the latter case, what is written may be captured as "electronic ink" and look like a handwritten note or the computer may attempt to interpret what has been written (handwriting recognition) and covert it to typed text prior to storing it in the EHR. Success with handwriting recognition is limited when large amounts of data are to be entered.

Table 1-4

ASP vs Client/Server

	ASP	Client Server
Cost	Cheaper to start up Subscription: cost ongoing Maintenance included in subscription price	Large upfront expenditure Set price Maintenance is a separate fee
Hardware	Workstations with browsers	Workstation connected to server

Support Needs	For EHR system only
	Minimal need for information
	    technology support staff
		EHR and server hardware
		Requires greater information
		    technology support staff

Access Method	Broadband connection (if
	    connection is down, EHR is
	    unavailable)
	Speed may be slow due to bad
	    connection or many users
	    accessing same server
	Secure remote access from
	    anywhere
		Local access (computers are
		    directly connected)
		Server workload may affect
		    response time
		Remote access to server may
		    create security risk

Customization	Minimal customization possible	Customization possible

Security	Internet access risks
	Backups not under user control
	Vendor bankruptcy could result
	    in data loss
		Server security breachs possible
		Back-ups under user control
		Vendor bankruptcy results in
		    unsupported system but no
		    data loss

However, electronic ink is popular for drawing diagrams or other notations. The introduction of tablet PCs (computers designed to support pen-based input), which are supported by many EHR systems, are making pen-based input a workable solution (42).

Voice-recognition technology has progressed significantly over the past few years. Voice-recognition systems are now available that can handle continuous speech (no unnatural pauses between words) with relatively few errors. They are also much more affordable. Voice recognition has yet to be widely adopted as an EHR data entry mechanism. However, the technology is sufficiently mature to warrant an evaluation (43,44). In concert with templates or other structured entry formats, it can be very effective (see Chapter 3).

Networking

Local Area Networks (LAN) are groups of computers linked together to permit communication and sharing of resources. LAN technology makes computing more affordable because it permits a build-it-as-you-need-it approach to purchasing and installing both hardware and software. The main computer on a LAN is referred to as the server. Depending upon the amount of computing power required, a server may be a fast personal computer with extra memory or a special computer designed just for this purpose. In either case, a server for a small office can be purchased for a few thousand dollars.

Wireless computer capability is also changing the networking equation. Wireless networks rely on radio frequency transmissions to communicate. One great feature of using wireless technology is that users are not tied to one location. No more worrying about wiring schemes and which rooms should have terminals. The cost of wireless technology is decreasing while becoming more powerful. It is worthy of consideration when setting your networking strategy. One caveat: wireless networks may be security risks if not properly set up. Have your wireless network set up by a professional and then tested for security vulnerabilities.

Internet technologies also provide a cost-effective means for sharing applications. Applications designed for use with Internet protocols may be open to the public (Web site) or permit access only to a limited group of computers or people (intranet). Intranets are used to provide EHR applications (ASP), as well as common office applications such as word processors and spreadsheets, making intranet applications viable alternatives to LAN-based, client/server arrangements.

User Authentication

Maintaining the security of the information stored in an EHR is of the utmost importance. The standard mechanism in most EHRs for restricting access to sensitive information is passwords. Passwords can be quite effective if guarded properly. However, they can easily be forgotten or stolen. A newer approach to identifying users is via the use of biologic markers (45,46). Fingerprint and iris scanning technologies are already enjoying fairly widespread use in number of fields. Voice and face recognition systems are also available. Biometric identification is superior to passwords in two ways: they cannot be forgotten or stolen. Some laptops come with biometric access built in. The role of biometric identification for EHR security has yet to be fully determined (47).

Standardization

One of the most exciting developments in recent years is the drive to develop a set of national standards for EHRs and interoperability. HL7 published its initial EHR functional model, which contains nearly 1000 criteria organized into about 130 areas. A subset of this group is being used to define a "legal" EHR (48). The Healthcare Information Technology Standards Panel is tackling the issue of interoperability by defining formats for information exchange based on currently available standards. The work of this group may make the long-held dream of easily sharing health information between computer systems a reality (49). Only time will tell.

Summary

Over the past 40 to 50 years clinical systems have undergone significant evolution. The EHR is the ultimate goal of those who see the value of information systems in the care of patients. However, much remains to be done in the areas of data exchange/interoperability, data entry, user interfaces, database design, and security before the full benefits of EHRs can be realized.

References

1. The EMR adoption model. HIMSS Analytics. December 31, 2006. Available at http://www.himssanalytics.org/docs/EMRAM.pdf. Accessed June 25, 2007.
2. Continued Progress: Hospital use of information technology. American Hospital Association. Available at: http://www.aha.org/aha/content/2007/pdf/070227-continuedprogress.pdf. Accessed on June 25, 2007.
3. Corrigan JM, Donaldson MS, Kohn LT, et al for the Committee on Quality of Health Care in America. To err is human: building a safer health system. Washington, D.C.: National Academy Press; 2000.
4. Metzger J, Fortin J. Computerized physician order entry in community hospitals: lessons from the field. California Healthcare Foundation, First Consulting Group. 2003. Available at: www.chcf.org/documents/hospitals/CPOECommHospCorrected.pdf. Accessed on June 25, 2007.
5. CPOE Digest 2007. KLAS Enterprises. Available at: http://healthcomputing.com/Klas/Site/News/NewsLetters/2007-03/CPOE.aspx. Accessed on June 25, 2007.

6. Health information technology in the United States: The information base for progress. Available at: http://www.rwjf.org/files/publications/other/EHRReport0609.pdf. Accessed June 25, 2007.

7. Jha KA, Ferris TG, Donelan K, et al. How common are EHRs in the United States? A summary of the evidence. Health Affairs. 2006:25:w496-w507.

8. Dick RS, Steen EB, Detmer DE (Institute of Medicine). The computer-based patient record: an essential technology for health care. Revised edition. 1997.

9. Andrew W, Dick R. Venturing off the beaten path: it's time to blaze new CPR trails. Healthcare Informatics. 1997:14:36-42.

10. Institute of Medicine. Key capabilities of an EHR system: Letter report. Washington, D.C. 2003.

11. Certificate Commission for Health Information Technology. The Official site for CCHIT. Available at: http://www.cchit.org/. Accessed September 20, 2006.

12. Grossman JH, Barnett GO, Koespell TD. An automated medical record system. JAMA. 1973;263:1114-20.

13. Stead WW, Hammond WE. Computer-based medical records:the centerpiece of TMR. MD Computing. 1988;5:48-62.

14. McDonald CJ, Blevins L, Tierney WM, Martin DK. The Regenstrief medical records. MD Computing. 1988;5;34-47.

15. Vogel LH, Safran C, Perreault LE. Management of information in healthcare organizations. In Shortliffe EH, Cimino J, eds. Biomedical Informatics Computer Applications in Health Care and Biomedicine, 3rd ed. New York: Springer; 2006.

16. McCoy MJ, Bomentre BJ, Crous K. Speaking of EHRs: parsing EHR systems and the start of IT projects. J AHIMA. 2006;77:24-8.

17. Lodder H, Bakker AR, Zwetsloot JHM. Hospital information systems: technical choices. In van Bemmel JH, Musen MA, eds. Handbook of Medical Informatics. Houten, The Netherlands; 1997

18. Bleich HL, Slack WV. Designing a hospital information system: a comparison of inter-faced and integrated systems. MD Computing. 1992;9:293-6.

19. Tarczy-Hornoch P, Kwan-Gett TS, Fouche L, et al. Meeting clinician information needs by integrating access to the medical record and knowledge resources via the Web. Proc AMIA Annu Fall Symp. 1997;809-13.

20. Klimczak JC, Witten DM , Ruiz M, et al. Providing location-independent access to patient clinical narratives using Web browsers and a tiered server approach. Proc AMIA Ann Fall Symp. 1996;623-7.

21. Mohr DN, Sandberg SD. Approaches to integrating data within enterprise healthcare information systems. Proc AMIA Symp. 1999;883-6.

22. Krol M, Reich DL, Dupont J. Multi-platforms medical computer systems integration. J Med Syst. 2005;29:259-70.

23. Monteiro E. Integrating health information systems: a critical appraisal. Meth Inf Med. 2003;42:428-32.

24. Sittig DF, Pappas J, Rubalcaba P. Building and using a clinical data repository. Available at: http://www.informatics-review.com/thoughts/cdr.html. Accessed September 29, 2007.

25. Cimino JJ. From data to knowledge through concept-oriented terminologies: experience with the Medical Entities Dictionary. J Am Med Inform Assoc. 2000;7:288-97.

26. Kahn MG. Three perspectives on integrated clinical databases. Acad Med. 1997;72:281-6.

27. Overcoming barriers to EHR adoption results of survey and roundtable discussions Conducted by the Healthcare Financial Management Association. Available at: http://www.hhs.gov/healthit/ahic/materials/meeting03/ehr/HFMA_Overcoming Barriers.pdf. Accessed September 19, 2007.

28. Briggs B. The main event: best-of-breed vs. single source. Health Data Management. June, 2003;418.

29. Schuerenberg BK. Single-source strategies: one-stop shopping for health care software. Health Data Management. August, 2002;32-34,36,38,40,42.

30. Amatayakul M, Cohen MR. Construction zone: building an EHR from HIS. HMSS Conference Proceedings 2005. Available at: www.himss.org/content/files/2005proceedings/sessions/tech011.pdf. Accessed September 2007.

31. Osheroff JA, Teich JM, Middleton B, et al. A roadmap for national action on clinical decision support. J Am Med Inform Assoc. 2007;14:141-5.

32. Saving lives, reducing costs: computerized physician order entry lessons learned in community hospitals. First Consulting Group. Available at: http://www.masstech.org/ehealth/CPOE_ lessonslearned.pdf. Accessed June 25, 2007.

33. Ratib O, Swiernik M, McCoy JM. From PACS to integrated EMR. Comput Med Imaging Graph. 2003;27:207-15.

34. Munch H, Engelmann U, Schroter A, Meinzer HP. The integration of medical images with the electronic patient record and their web-based distribution. Acad Radiol. 2004;11:661-8.

35. Franklin BD, O'Grady K, Donyai P, et al. The impact of a closed-loop electronic prescribing and administration system on prescribing errors, administration errors and staff time: a before-and-after study. Qual Saf Health Care. 2007;16:279-84.

36. Paoletti RD, Suess TM, Lesko MG, et al. Using bar-code technology and medication observation methodology for safer medication administration. Am J Health Syst Pharm. 2007;64:536-43.

37. Jantos LD, Ml Holmes. IT tools for chronic disease management: How do they measure up? (2006) Available at: http://www.chcf.org/documents/chronicdisease/ITToolsForChronicDiseaseManagement.pdf. Accessed September 19, 2007.

38. Metzger J. Using computerized registries in chronic disease (2004). Available at: www.chcf.org/documents/chronicdisease/ComputerizedRegistriesInChronicDisease.pdf. Accessed September 19, 2007.

39. http://www.cms.hhs.gov/PhysicianFocusedQualInits/.

40. http://www.surescripts.com/.

41. Grossman JM, Gerland A, Reed MC, Fahlman C. Physicians' experiences using commercial e-prescribing systems health affairs. May/June 2007;26:w393-w404

42. Healthcare clinic saves money and improves quality of care with tablet PC solution. Available at: http://download.microsoft.com/documents/customerevidence/7474_Marshfield_Clinic_Case_Study_FINAL.doc. Accessed June 25, 2007.

43. Speech recognition FAQs. Available at: http://www.centerforhit.org/x1328.xml. Accessed June 25, 2007.

44. Weber J. Tomorrow's transcription tools: what new technology means for healthcare. J AHIMA. 2003;74:39-43.

45. Cappelli R, Maio D, Maltoni D, et al. Performance evaluation of fingerprint verification systems. IEEE Trans Pattern Anal Mach Intell. 2006;28:3-18.

46. George Washington University medical faculty associates deploy BIO-key biometric identification solution . Available at: http://bio-ey.com/artman/publish/article_491.shtml. Accessed June 25, 2007.

47. Fulcher J. The use of patient biometrics in accessing EHRs IJHTM, Vol. 6, No. 1, 2004.

48. www.hl7.org/ehr/.

49. http://www.ansi.org.

2

Computer Hardware and Enabling Technologies

Daniel C. Davis, Jr., MD

Nowhere is the phrase "form follows function" more important than in the selection of computer hardware for the clinical practice. Hardware selection (form) is determined by software and workflow (function). In the office computer system, the physical components of the system should be determined by the functions of the system. The physical components of the office system include the equipment (the hardware), how the hardware is linked together (the network), and the physical locations of the equipment within the office. An understanding of fundamental computing concepts and the basic parts of a computer will help determine how well different hardware components will support workflow functions in the office.

Six major topics are addressed in this chapter about computer hardware and enabling technologies:

1. Basic concepts about computer hardware

2. Hardware technologies and applications

3. Merging technologies in issues

4. Other hardware issues, privacy, and portability

5. Protecting computer equipment and data

6. Choreographing the doctor-patient-computer interaction

Basic Concepts about Computer Hardware

Computers are nothing more than sophisticated calculating machines that perform mathematical operations using a binary number system.

Understanding basic concepts about computers will help in planning the medical office computer system.

The conceptual computer has four parts:

1. Input: data that are fed to the computer

2. The computer itself, which is often called the processor

3. A program that tells the computer how to mathematically manipu-late the input

4. Output, which are data presented to the user or another computer program

Input data can be fed to the **computer** from many sources and in many forms. The input data, whether words or numbers, are translated by the computer into a machine code that the computers can understand. This code is actually a binary math system consisting of just 1's and 0's that can represent a vast array of numbers, letters, words, and concepts. A string of input data might look like "00000001" and "00000010", which are binary code for the numbers 1 and 2.

The **processor** receives the binary input data and performs mathemati-cal operations on the input data under the direction of a set of instructions called **a program**. For example, a program might instruct the processor to add "00000001" to "00000010" to get "00000011", the binary equivalent of $1 + 2 = 3$.

The computer **program** is a set of instructions, or rules, that dictate what the processor should do with the input data.

Once the processor has manipulated the input data according to the pro-gram instructions, the processor spits out the result data, which is called **output**. This output comes from the processor in the form of binary code. In our trivial example of "add 1+2", the output is "00000011". The binary output is then translated into a format useable by humans, by another pro-gram, or by another computer. In our example, "00000011" translates to the numeral 3.

Parts of the Basic Computer

The computer system in the medical office will consist of one or more per-sonal computers (PCs) connected by a network. The basic computer in this network contains six components:

1. Central Processing Unit (CPU)

2. Random Access Memory (RAM)

3. Storage memory

4. Input devices

5. Output devices

6. Connectivity devices

CPU

The processor in modern computers is often called the "Central Processing Unit" (CPU) in order to distinguish it from other processors in the computer box, such as video and audio processors (GPUs). The CPU is a computer chip that can be identified as a flat black square or rectangle, about an inch on a side, attached to the big plastic mother board inside the computer case. CPUs have evolved rapidly over the past fifty years, shrinking in size and growing in power by many orders of magnitude.

CPUs are classified by families and by speed. The large chip manufacturers use names and numbers to identify families of chips, names like Intel Pentium, Motorola's 68000 and PowerPC chips, and AMD Athlon chips. Each new generation of chip gets faster. The chips are rated by speed of the processor, which depends in part on how fast a tiny quartz crystal in the chip vibrates. This quartz crystal is called the clock and acts as a timer for the CPU. These timers vibrate several billion times per second. One billion vibrations per second is one gigahertz. The number of hertz at which the quartz crystal vibrates is called the clock speed. The faster the quartz crystal oscillates, the faster the chip can process instructions. Currently, the fastest consumer and small business computers are being shipped with CPU clock speeds of three gigahertz. In addition to clock speed, the speed of the CPU depends on how many transistors are embedded in the chip. More transistors allow the CPU to process more instructions simultaneously. Every six months or so new generations of chips are released, each new generation having more transistors and faster clock speeds. The combination of more transistors and faster clock speed in successive generations of CPUs has allowed a tremendous increase in the computing power that can be purchased for a dollar. Other factors that produce increasing CPU performance are parallel processing techniques, embedding two processors on a single-chip, and advancements in instruction management such as hyper-threading. There are many other factors that affect computer speed. Most of the medical office management and EHR software, except speech recognition, do not require extremely fast computers.

RAM

Random Access Memory (RAM) is one of two types of memory in the computer. The other type of memory is called storage memory. RAM is located in special computer chips that can be identified in your computer as rectangular dull black chips often lined up side by side either on the mother board or on a green card sticking up from the mother board. Within the RAM chip are thousands of microscopic transistors that act as tiny electrical switches that are either "on" or "off". If a transistor is in the "on" state, it is said to have a value of "1"; if the transistor is in the "off" state, it is said to have a value of "0".

How these microscopic transistors work is very interesting. A memory chip consists of a silicon sandwich that contains crisscrossing wires that are only a few molecules thick. One wire carries a current of electrons, but the current cannot flow along the wire because the wire is interrupted periodically by tiny breaks in the wire. The wire on one side of the break, called the "source" because it is the source of electrons, provides electrons that are trying to jump across the break in the wire. On the downstream side of the break, the wire is called the "drain". Electrons would like to jump across the break in the wire but cannot do so because there is a special kind of insulating silicon that fills the gap between the source end and the drain end of the wire. When no current flows across this gap, the transistor is said to be "off" and have a value of "0". Running perpendicular across the gap is another wire. If a positive current is applied to this second wire, negatively charged electrons are attracted by the positive current into the gap between the source and the drain causing the gap filling silicon to become a conductor rather than an insulator. This allows a current of electrons to flow from the source to the drain, thus turning the transistor "on". The "on" transistor is said to have a value of "1". Thus, a transistor's "on" or "off" state can represent one digit of a binary number, either "1" or "0". The value of the transistor is either "on" or "off", "1" or "0".

This binary limitation of the transistor explains why machine code uses binary math. The value of a transistor is called a "bit". Eight "bits", that is eight transistors, comprise a "byte" of information. A series of transistors can represent a series of binary numbers, which can be translated into a standard Arabic number, a letter of the alphabet, and even logical values of "true" and "false". Many thousands of transistors in the memory chip can store information that represents input data, output data, programs, and Boolean logic.

Computer chips are engineered to work with maximum length binary numbers or words. Thus, the earlier chips were "8 bit chips", meaning that the biggest binary number the chip could handle was eight binary digits long. The largest eight bit binary number is "11111111", which translates into the numeral 65,536. Newer and larger chips can handle binary numbers up to 64 bits, representing a numeral equal to 2^{64}, which is a bigger number than we should print in this book. Sometimes the CPU is said to use a "32-bit word" or "64-bit word".

A group of transistors in RAM memory can be assigned an "address", much like a street address. Specific information is stored at specific addresses within RAM so that the computer can find this information quickly.

RAM is an important determinate of how fast your computer works. When the CPU needs input data, the input must often come from storage memory, such as a disk drive. When the CPU gives output data, that data must be sent some place, such as a disk drive. Sending data to and from storage memory is one of the slowest tasks performed by the computer. Sending data to and from RAM is much faster than using a disk drive. RAM allows the computer to temporarily store input data, output data, and program instructions in a place that can be accessed much faster than the disk drives. More RAM, with faster clock speed, and larger number lengths result in a much faster computer.

RAM is measured in size as "megabytes" or "gigabytes", meaning millions or billions of bytes of memory. Current consumer and business computers are shipping with progressively larger amounts of RAM, typically 512 megabytes to four gigabytes.RAM is characterized as word size (32 bit or 64 bit words), speed, and amount supplied in the computer.

An important characteristic of RAM is that it is volatile, meaning that when the computer is turned off, the contents of the memory disappear. Some specialized computers will probably start using nonvolatile RAM in the near future. Because RAM usually does not store data after the computer is turned off, the computer needs another means of storing data permanently. Memory that stores information permanently is called storage memory.

Storage Memory

The second type of computer memory is storage memory. Because RAM memory is volatile, that is, the information in RAM disappears when the power is turned off, the computer must have a place to store information permanently. Information stored in storage memory is often the type of information that is used repeatedly, such as computer programs, input data files, and output data files. There are many forms of storage memory. Some of the common forms of storage memory are:

◆ USB memory chips

◆ Hard disks

◆ CD ROM discs

◆ DVD discs

◆ Magnetic tape

Magnetic tape is usually used for backup of servers. Floppy disks are rapidly disappearing from common use. There are several other types of storage memory that are less commonly used in the office setting. These are optical discs, memory sticks, SD cards, SmartMedia cards, CompactFlash cards, and memory PCMCIA cards. All but the hard disks are removable media; that is, the storage memory can be removed from the computer either for safe keeping or for transfer to another computer.

While floppy disks are disappearing from common use, understanding how floppy disks work helps one understand how the other storage media work. Floppy disks are thin plastic disks enclosed in a protective plastic case. The older eight inch diameter and 5 1/4 inch diameter floppy disks had protective cases that were thin and pliable; hence, the name "floppy disk." The thin plastic disk inside the floppy is coated with a very thin film of iron particles that can be magnetized. Each tiny spot on the disk can be magnetized or unmagnetized, representing a binary "1" or "0". The floppy disk is placed into a floppy drive. The drive spins the floppy disk, much like a record player, but much faster at several thousand revolutions per second. The disk drive pivots a "read-write" arm over the disk, much like the arm on a record player. At the end of the read-write arm is a tiny coil of wire, called a head, that "reads" whether each location on the floppy is magnetized or not and translates the sequential magnetic information into binary 1's and 0's that are used by the computer. The read-write head can also write to the floppy. When sequential pulses of current travel through the coil of wire in the head, a tiny magnetic field is generated. The magnetic field of the read-write head can then magnetize the iron particles at tiny discrete spots on the floppy, thus recording 1's and 0's in the form of magnetic spots onto the floppy disk.

The terms hard disk and hard drive are used interchangeably because, unlike the floppy disk, which can be removed from the floppy drive, the hard disks are fixed permanently inside the hard drive and are usually not removed. Some hard disks are accessible from the outside of the computer case and can be removed. Special removable hard disks can be removed even with the computer running; these are called "hot swappable hard drives". Hard disks are called fixed media and other storage media are called removable media. Hard disks work on the same principle as the floppy disk, using read-write heads and tiny magnetic fields to store and retrieve information on the drive. However, hard drives use rigid rather than floppy platters and use several platters and several read-write heads simultaneously. The magnetic spots on hard disks are more densely packed. These techniques allow the hard disks to store much more information than floppies. Hard disks that are currently shipping with business PCs often hold more than 250 gigabytes of information. One gigabyte equals one billion bytes of information.

Input Devices: Keyboard and Mouse

The computer gets data from the user through various input devices. The basic input devices are the keyboard and the mouse. (Variations of keyboards and pointing devices are described in the section "Peripheral Devices" later in this chapter.)

KEYBOARD

Basic input from the user comes from the computer keyboard. When the user presses a key on the computer keyboard, a tiny voltage change is generated from the mechanical action. This voltage change is translated into a unique code for the key press or combination of presses. This digital code is then sent to the computer and used as input to a program. The keys on a basic keyboard are arranged like a standard typewriter. Most keyboards also have a numeric keypad placed on the right end of the keyboard. There also are special keys that are assigned commands by individual programs or by the user. These keys are called "function keys" and are usually labeled F1 through F12. The function keys are typically located in a line across the top of the keyboard. Another group of keys, called "program keys" are used alone or in combination with the standard keys to send program commands to the computer. Some of these program keys are the "Control" key, the "Alt" key, the "Escape" key, the "Print screen" key, and the "Break" key. Different programs may assign different functions to the program keys and function keys. There are many variations on the basic keyboard design. Some of these useful variations are discussed in the Peripherals section, below.

MOUSE

The other basic input device is the "mouse". The mouse is the most commonly used "pointing device". A pointing device is a tool that allows the user to move the on-screen cursor to any place on the monitor screen and "point" to an area for input or to select a function displayed on the screen. The cursor is a symbol, such as a blinking underscore or arrow or hand, that draws the user's attention to the point on the monitor screen where input or output is being manipulated by the user. Older computer programs used a character- and line-based method of display that limited the cursor to the end of a typed line, just like an old typewriter. Modern programs use a graphical user interface, called a "GUI" and pronounced "gooey", that allows the user to move the cursor anywhere on the computer screen by manipulating a pointing device. When the user moves a pointing device, like a mouse, in a given direction, speed and distance, the cursor on the computer screen moves in the same direction, speed, and distance across the screen. The mouse is called a mouse because it is about the size of a large mouse and has a wire sticking out the backend that looks like a mouse's tail. There are many other kinds of pointing devices, but they all do principally the same thing—move the cursor around the screen. Other pointing devices are described under the Peripherals section, below.

Output Devices: The Monitor and the Printer

The computer program manipulates the input data thereby producing new output data. The output data can be presented to the user or can be sent to another program or to another computer. The devices that manage output data are called output devices. The output devices of the basic computer are the monitor and the printer.

COMPUTER MONITOR

Computer monitors come in a variety of sizes, shapes, and image quality. Monitors are also called displays, display terminals, CRTs (cathode ray tubes), VDTs (video display terminals), LCDs (liquid crystal displays), and flat screens. The most common computer monitor looks like a television. These monitors use cathode ray tubes similar to television tubes. The size of the monitor is measured by the diagonal length of the screen, measured from upper corner to the opposite lower corner. These monitors range in size from about 12 inches diagonally to 30 inches diagonally. Larger and smaller sizes are not practical for the office. The standard office monitor is 15 to 19 inches. A significant disadvantage of the standard CRT monitor is its overall size. As screen size increases, so does the front-to-back length of the CRT. A 15-inch CRT monitor may be entirely too big for a small desk in the typical examining room or at a nurse station. Monitors also are manufactured as flat panel displays like those seen in laptop computers. Most flat panel displays use LCD (liquid crystal display) technology, rather than CRT technology. The flat panel displays save desk top space, use less power, generate less heat, and are becoming less expensive. LCDs are rapidly replacing CRTs as the monitor of choice in the medical office.

The quality of the image displayed by the monitor is determined by the resolution of the monitor. Generally, higher resolution is better. Resolution is determined by the number of pixels the monitor can display, by the dot pitch of the screen, and by the number of colors the monitor can display. Occasionally one may find use for a monochrome monitor, but most modern software takes advantage of color to improve the user interface.

Pixel is a word coined from the term "picture element", which refers to the dots of light the monitor screen displays. The number of pixels that can be displayed along the horizontal axis and along the vertical axis of the screen are stated in an expression of resolution such as "640 × 480" on the low end or "1280 × 1024" on the high end. High-resolution monitors are required for better display of radiographic images. A physical characteristic of monitors is "dot pitch". Dot pitch refers to the size of the individual points of light displayed by the monitor. The smaller the dot pitch, the finer the quality of the image displayed. Currently standard office monitors are manufactured with a dot pitch of .28. Also, monitors can display a variable number of colors. The more colors the monitor displays, the higher the image quality. Image quality depends not only on the physical characteristics of the monitor but also on special image software and hardware in the computer. Dot pitch and maximum resolution are physical characteristics of the monitor. Within the hardware and software limitations of the computer, one can select the number of pixels and colors displayed by the monitor. The hardware limitations are determined by the monitor itself and by the video card capabilities. The video card connects the monitor to the computer mother board. Sometimes the video card is built into the motherboard and sometimes the video card occupies a separate slot on the motherboard, allowing the video card to be replaced or upgraded. The software limitations of the display are determined by software called a "video driver".

Which monitors one chooses for the office setting depend on which functions are important to the users. For example, if the receptionist uses a scheduling program that requires only large print on the screen, then the monitor could be a low-resolution monochrome model. And if the receptionist's work area has a lot of desk space, then a standard 15-inch CRT monitor might be adequate. A low-resolution 15-inch CRT would be a relatively inexpensive option for the receptionist. In contrast, if the physician is using a computer in a small exam room for an electronic medical record (EHR) program or for patient education with an anatomy program, then a high-resolution 15- or 17-inch flat panel display would be a better investment.

PRINTER

Printers are important output devices that are often overlooked. Despite the attraction of the "paperless office", few medical offices are truly paperless. The function of paper, its generation, flow, and disposition in the office must be understood. As with all other hardware choices, form follows function. The printer that is optimal for printing prescriptions in the exam room or at the nursing station is not likely to be the best printer for producing hundreds or thousands of multi-part billing statements or insurance claim forms. Printers are characterized by print technology, whether they handle multi-part forms, whether they feed paper by tractor or by single sheet, and how easily they handle envelopes. One must also consider printer resolution, color versus black and white, speed, cost per page, noise, and size.

Three common printer technologies are in use in the medical office today:

1. Dot matrix printers

2. Laser printers

3. Ink jet printers

Dot Matrix Printers

Dot matrix printers are the old work horses of the medical office. The dot matrix printer consists of a print head that contains a collection of small wires that poke out from the print head and strike an inked printer ribbon to deposit onto the paper a tiny bit of ink, much like the key and ribbon action of a typewriter. Dot matrix printers tend to be faster than other printer types, last longer, cost less per page printed but are much noisier and produce lower print quality. They are excellent for printing large amounts of paper, for printing multi-part forms such as statements and insurance claim forms. Dot matrix printers are usually found in the business office and are less suited for a quiet reception area or exam room.

Laser Printers

Laser printers are popular because they produce excellent print quality, are quiet, and are easy to operate. Laser printers tend to be slower than dot matrix printers and cannot handle multi-part forms like billing statements or insurance claim forms. They are excellent for printing a few on-demand charge slips in the reception area because they are quiet and because on-demand printing of charge slips is usually a low-volume function. For similar reasons, laser printers are a good choice for the exam room. Laser printers use single sheet paper. Compared to dot matrix printers of equal speed, laser printers cost more to purchase. Because the costly print mechanism must be replaced when the laser printer runs out of ink, laser printers cost more per printed page.

Ink Jet Printers

Ink jet printers are less expensive to purchase and have an intermediate cost per printed page. They tend to be slower and a little nosier than laser printers. Ink jet printers are manufactured in very small and portable sizes. They are attractive in environments where small size is more important than speed or quiet operation. Ink jet printers cannot handle multi-part forms. Ink jets use single sheet paper rather than continuous-feed paper.

The paper type required by a clinical function often influences the selection of a printer type. For example, correspondence requires high-quality, twenty-pound 8.5 × 11 cut sheet paper. A laser printer works well for correspondence. Similar heavy, expensive paper is not desirable for generating high-volume chart notes, charge tickets, or appointment schedules. Inexpensive light-weight continuous-feed tractor drive paper is a more cost-effective choice for these latter uses. Printing prescriptions with the computer presents special problems. Prescriptions are traditionally written on small 4 × 5 inch pads, a unique paper size that is used in few other office functions. One can either dedicate printers to print prescriptions on traditional prescription paper or one can print prescriptions on standard 8.5 × 11 inch paper. Printing prescriptions for controlled substances is a problem since some states require sending duplicate prescriptions to the pharmacy. Multi-part statements must be printed on heavy duty dot-matrix printers; laser and ink-jet printers cannot print on multi-part forms. Envelope and label printing present additional challenges.

Printer speed is another consideration. The difference in speed of printers, typically measured in number of pages per minute, may not seem significant until one considers office workflow. Color printing, although attractive, is slow and more costly. The three minutes it takes to print a pretty color patient handout may be too costly to the nurse when multiplied by 20 or 30 patients per day. In contrast, the fifteen seconds it takes to print a black and white patient education form on a fast laser printer may generate critical time savings in the patient-flow process.

Other factors that influence printer choice are the physical size of the printer relative to work space, the flow of foot traffic, noise generated by the printers, and paper dust.

Hardware Technologies and Applications

Types of Computer Systems

Computer systems can be classified by their complexity and size. Recent computer technology has blurred the lines between PCs, minicomputers, mainframes, client-server systems, and web-based systems.

PCs, from the term "personal computer", were formerly called microcomputers. PCs are single CPU computers that are used by one user at a time. Some newer PCs can be configured with two CPUs in order to work faster. PCs may be stand-alone machines or may be linked into a network.

Minicomputers

Microcomputers that are designed for use by more than one user at a time, typically five to one hundred users, are called minicomputers. Minicomputers may have more than one CPU. The term minicomputer was used more commonly a decade ago to distinguish the smaller minicomputers, which are slightly bigger than the standard desk-top PC, from large and very expensive mainframe computers. Minicomputers functioned like mainframes but on a smaller scale. Like mainframes, they used dumb terminals rather than PC workstations. As PC-based networks have become more powerful, the minicomputer has become less popular as a small business solution and is being replaced by servers.

Mainframes

Mainframe computers are large computers that once occupied a whole computer room. New technologies have shrunk mainframes down to refrigerator size or smaller. Mainframes are typically run by large institutions such as hospitals and insurance companies that may have hundreds or thousands of simultaneous users. Mainframes have single or multiple CPUs and typically are very fast in comparison to PCs. As with the minicomputer, more powerful PC-based networks are taking over many of the functions of the older mainframes.

Client-Server Systems

The client-server computer system is a type of computer architecture in which the end-user's PC does much of the processing function on data that are supplied by the larger central server computer. The central server computer is typically larger and faster than the client PC and can handle many users at one time. The server stores data that are used in common by the many PCs that are connected to the server. The users typically connect to the server using their PCs, which, in this configuration, are called client computers. The client computer runs client software that is designed to work closely with the server software. The idea is that the central server provides services, such as sharing of data files, printers, programs, modems, and other external connections, to the client PCs. Because most PCs do not need all of these services at one time, the services can be shared among many PCs and provide economies of scale. The economies of client-server architecture often apply even to the small medical office.

In larger installations, such as in an enterprise EHR, the servers may be housed together in a cluster or "server farm". Clustering the servers allows special architectures and programs to provide services that could not be provided by a single server in the medical office. Such services include fault tolerance, fail-over capabilities, load balancing, sophisticated backup, and other services that are necessary for mission-critical applications in enterprise EHRs and hospital information systems. The clustered servers work together seamlessly so that they seem to be acting as one computer but the system is tolerant to the failure of component server and disks. The popular Citrix architecture is often deployed in a group of servers housed in a cluster or server farm.

Web-Based Systems

The newest computer system architecture is based on internet and web technology. The software running on the PC is a "thin client" software application, commonly the web browser. In some web-based clinical applications, the client PC may need no other software than the browser. The web server sends data over the internet to the PC when requested by the PCs browser. The user modifies the data and returns the data to the central web server where the data are stored. If the client browser needs additional programs, these can be downloaded to the client browser in the form of small program applications called applets. Web-based computer systems can be confined to the office—a so-called intranet—or can be connected to the public internet outside the office. Also, the office web-based system could be connected to other remote systems through a virtual private network.

There are still many problems to be solved before web-technology becomes the principle clinical computing architecture. Many web-based applications are too slow for the busy office practice. The public Internet can fail, preventing access to the patient's EHR. There are challenging security and privacy issues. Some of the best office systems have not yet been restructured to take advantage of web technology. However, these barriers are being overcome rapidly. Within a few years many medical offices will be served primarily by web applications.

Office Workstations

"Form follows function" also applies to the choice of computer workstations for the users in your office. There are several workstation types to choose from:

◆ Full size PCs

◆ Laptops, notebooks, and sub-notebooks

◆ Network PCs

◆ Handheld computers

Most offices will choose full size PC workstations or laptops. Some clinics that are large enough to benefit from economies of scale may use thin client devices. Thin client devices are stripped down PCs that have a limited function operating system and act principally as display device for programs and data residing on a server. Handheld computers, while useful as personal information management tools, are not yet suitable as true full function workstations in the medical office network. Choice of workstation will depend on several important factors:

1. Software requirements:
   ◆ Does the software require specific workstation speed, RAM, and hard disk capacity?
   ◆ What are the specific software functions that each person will use?
   ◆ What is the optimum size and resolution of the monitor for the information that will be displayed?

2. Space and environmental requirements:
   ◆ How much space is available for the user's workstation and printer?
   ◆ Does the space required by the workstation leave enough desk or counter space for the user to work with other documents, books, or charts?
   ◆ Is there sufficient desk space to use a mouse or should space-saving alternative pointing devices be used, such as trackballs, trackpads, joy sticks, touch screens?
   ◆ Will the user be standing or sitting?
   ◆ Will heat generated by the computer equipment be an issue for workers or equipment maintenance?

- If voice recognition is to be used, will ambient noise interfere with accuracy?
- Can the user's dictation be overheard by other patients?
- Will multiple speakers be using the same voice recognition computer? If so, will the time required to load each user's speech profile interfere with patient flow?

3. Electrical power issues:
- Are there enough power outlets to accommodate each workstation and printer?
- Is there enough power capacity to run the equipment on each power circuit?
- What is the quality of the electrical power? Are there surges, spikes, and brown-outs?

4. Portable workstations:
- Are portable workstations preferred over fixed workstations?
- How will the portable workstations connect to the network—by radio wireless, infrared wireless, or hardwire cables?
- What will prevent portable workstations from being lost or stolen?
- Is the personally identifiable health information encrypted when stored on the portable so it cannot be read by someone who discovers the lost PC?
- Does the portable workstation have a keyboard with sufficient function to allow the user to input data with optimum speed?
- How long will the batteries last in the portable workstations?
- Where and how do the portables get recharged?
- If you rely on swapping out discharged batteries, where are the charged replacements stored?
- Are data lost if the batteries are changed or run down?
- Does the portable have "instant-on" capabilities so that the user can resume work at exactly the same place as when he turned the portable off? Or must the portable be rebooted every time it is turned on?

Full-Size PCs

Full-size PCs tend to have more RAM, faster CPUs, and larger hard drives. These PCs have larger cases, typically 18-24 inches in length and width and 6-8 inches in height. Some models are designed for placement on the desk top and are called desktop PCs. The combination of a standard desktop case, 15-17 inch monitor, keyboard, and mouse consumes a large part of a standard-size desk. A large desk in the physician's private office may accommodate full-size computer equipment, but these space hogs may overwhelm the small desks and counters used in the clinical areas and exam rooms. Other full-function PCs, called "tower" models, are designed to stand vertically. They fit nicely on the floor next to the desk, under the desk, or hidden in a cabinet. Two advantages of the full-size PCs are price and flexibility. Full-size PCs tend to be less expensive than PCs that have been specially engineered for space saving because full-size PCs can accommodate generic hard drives, CD ROMs, and modems. Another advantage of the full-size PCs is that they have more available expansion slots than the smaller PCs. These extra expansion slots allow the addition of upgrades and new functions such as extra modems, scanners, network interface cards, or video cameras. As computer components shrink in size, the overall dimensions of full-function PCs shrink. Some new models of desktop PCs are one third the volume of standard PCs from a few years ago.

Laptops, Notebooks, and Subnotebooks

Laptops, notebooks, and sub-notebook PCs should be considered for office workstations where saving space or portability is important. **Laptops** are portable PCs that are designed to be used sitting on your lap. They are generally the bigger of the portables and weigh about six to eight pounds but usually come with many built in features such as a full-size keyboard, a hard drive, a CD ROM, modem, and a pointing device. **Notebook PCs** are similar in design to the laptops but are somewhat smaller and lighter and may have a smaller keyboard. **Subnotebook PCs** are smaller yet: current models weigh less than three pounds. Subnotebook keyboards may be smaller than is comfortable for the average user. Screen size is smaller. In order to save size and weight, the subnotebooks may use an external floppy drive and an external CD-ROM. All of these portable devices run common PC software and standard operating systems. All of these can connect to the office network through built-in network interface cards or wireless network connection. Older portable computers may connect to the network through PCMCIA cards, all so-called PC cards. The PC cards slide into special slots on the side of the portable computer. The PC cards are credit card size devices that provide the physical wiring connection to the network. PC cards can be designed for other functions such as radio network connection, modems, extra storage memory, CD ROM, tape backups, video cameras, and digital cameras.

Network PCs

Network PC is a term that refers to PCs that are designed to work only on a network rather than as stand-alone PCs. Network PCs rely on the concept of using the central network server to store and manage most of the data used by the network PC. Even programs may be stored on the central server rather than on the PC. The main advantage of the Network PC architecture is reduction in the cost of maintaining large numbers of PCs in big networks. This cost over the life of a PC connected to the network is called "total cost of ownership". Total cost of ownership over the useful life of each standard PC on the network may be ten times the original purchase price of the PC. Network PCs are stripped down versions of the full-function PCs. The Network PC has a CPU, relatively little RAM, a keyboard, a mouse, and a monitor. Storage memory for the network PC is located on the central sever. The network PC may or may not have removable storage media or even a hard drive.

Network PCs are not in wide use among medical offices. This is due to falling prices of full-function PCs, the fact that physicians are more familiar with standard PCs, and because networks in the typical medical office are small.

Thin Client

Another option for the office workstation is to use the thin client model, as in the Citrix and Microsoft Metaframe architecture. A thin client is a very small piece of software that can run on a variety of inexpensive, stripped-down PCs or even handheld devices. The Citrix client can run on many different types of computers, thus allowing a great deal of flexibility in the choice of workstations in the medical office. This is one way of accommodating both the Apple Mac users in the same office as Windows PC users. When the user wants to run a program, he starts the Citrix client software. This software then attaches to the Citrix server, which then starts up a "virtual PC" on the server to be used by the one user. The Citrix server is often located in a remote server farm. Multiple users can attach to the same server using multiple "virtual PCs" running on the same server or server cluster. The virtual PCs running on the Citrix server can share hardware resources like RAM, hard drives, and modems. This thin client model has several advantages:

1. Allows most of the processing and software maintenance to be done at the central server

2. Allows the user to have a wide range of choices of cheap PCs

3. Decreases cost of maintaining user machines and software

4. Reduces bandwidth requirements between client and server.

Handheld Computers

While not designed as true workstations, very small handheld computers are gaining popularity among clinicians principally as personal information managers. These small computers can be held in one hand and usually fit into a shirt or coat pocket. The handheld computers run on batteries and are designed for ultimate portability. Handheld computers come in four principle forms:

1. Full-function PCs

2. Windows Mobile devices

3. Palm OS computers

4. Several other operating systems.

Full function PCs are becoming progressively smaller. The smallest full-function PCs run Windows XP and most popular Windows programs. Advantages of these little PCs are high portability, full compatibility with desktop PCs, no learning curve for the user of desk-top PCs, the same wide range of software selection available for desktop PCs, and network connectivity through on-board wireless connection or PCMCIA cards. These little machines are often held by one hand while using the other hand to type or by cradling the device in the fingers of both hands and typing with the thumbs. Their small size is their disadvantage. The display screens are small and sometimes difficult to read depending on font size and lighting conditions. Keyboards are small, making touch-typing difficult. Battery life is improving. Most of these machines have an "instant-on" function which avoids wasting time with repeated boot up cycles every time they are turned off and on.

A second variety of handheld computers are the Windows CE (WinCE) and newer **Windows Mobile** computers. These computers use a small version of the Windows operating system, which provides functions familiar to Windows users. These machines come in several sizes that range from cell phone size to palm size with very small keyboards and screens, to larger sizes with screens of ten to twelve inches and full-size keyboards. Some of these computers have touch-sensitive screens that aid in navigation. A popular Windows Mobile feature is the "instant-on" function. This function allows the Windows Mobile computer to be turned off and then turned back on, resuming work at exactly the same spot as when the machine was turned off without taking the time to reboot. This instant-on function saves several minutes that would otherwise be consumed by a boot-up process. Because the Windows Mobile machines are often carried in a pocket throughout the office and hospital, they may be turned on and off 20-30 times per day. Without the instant-on function, the user would waste 30-60 minutes per day just waiting for the computer to boot up. Newer ultra-portable devices use Linux and similar operating systems that allow the instant-on function. The screens may be backlit, making viewing in low-light situations easier. However, most handheld screens are difficult to read in full daylight. The short battery life requires that charging stations, plug-in power sources, or replacement batteries be readily available in the work site. The batteries are proprietary and are specially configured for each model.

Handheld computers running the **Palm operating system** have become very popular in the past several years, especially those that are integrated into cell phones. These devices are held in the palm of one hand. The other hand writes on the touch-sensitive screen or types on a tiny keyboard to spell out input data. A hand-writing recognition program recognizes the pen strokes and translates them into computer text. The user must learn a special method of writing in order for the computer to translate the hand-writing effectively. Like the Windows Mobile machines, the Palm computers have built-in software that serves most personal information management needs. Newer mobile devices have merged the cell phone, the personal digital assistant, and multimodal wireless connectivity. These devices can connect to the Internet and to Internet-enabled medical applications through cell phone radio and WiFi radio. Many stand-alone medical applications are available for these handheld computers. However, the cell phone computer interface is not widely applicable to EHR implementations.

Peripheral Devices

Combinations of the hardware described above comprise the basic office system. In order to make the office workflow most efficient, there are some special computer peripherals that might serve special needs in the medical office. Peripheral devices are equipment attached to the PC other than the basic monitor, keyboard, and mouse.

Keyboard Variations

Another nontraditional computer peripheral is the wireless keyboard. These keyboards attach to the PC not with a wire but with a wireless infra-red beam or a radio transmitter. Because these keyboards are not physically attached to the PC, they often have a built-in pointing device. This allows the physician more freedom in arranging the physical position of the computer, patient, and doctor in the exam room.

The wireless keyboard with integrated track-ball is particularly attractive for use in the exam room. Wireless connection between the keyboard and PC occurs through either an infrared signal or a radio signal. The infrared connections tend to be limited by line of sight in contrast to the radio-linked keyboards, which are multidirectional. A skillful clinician can place the wireless keyboard on his/her lap and type clinical notes while facing the patient and maintaining direct eye contact. With a trackball mounted on the keyboard, the clinician can avoid the distraction of fiddling with a mouse on the desk-top.

Pointing Device Variations

Several alternative pointing devices that might be useful in the medical office are track-balls, track-pads, also called touch-pads, joysticks, and touch-screens.The track-ball is a popular pointing device that works like a mouse turned upside down exposing the ball to the user. With the ball on the topside of the pointing device, the user's index finger or thumb rolls the ball to move the pointer on the screen. Track-balls can be separate from the keyboard or built into the keyboard. With the track-ball integrated in to the keyboard, the doctor can hold the keyboard in his/her lap, enter clinical findings into the EHR, and talk to the patient simultaneously. With a little practice, the computer can be integrated into the doctor-patient interaction in the exam room.

A second alternative input device is the track-pad, also called a touch pad. This is a touch-sensitive plastic pad over which one drags the finger to move the pointer on the screen. Touchpads come in several sizes, from only 1.5 inches square to 8.5 × 11 inches. Some very large touch pads can be used as drawing tablets, which allow digitization of anatomic drawings.

The joystick, a third common pointing device, is a small stick that stands up from the keyboard. These sticks are covered with a soft material that resembles a pencil erasure and are sometimes referred to as erasure heads. Large joysticks that are used for computer games have little role in the medical office.

Touch-screens allow the user to move the pointer on the screen by simply touching the screen and dragging the finger to the desired area. Touch-screens are used in wireless pad computers that allow patients to self register in the waiting room.

Each pointing device may have a special niche in the medical office depending on need. Again, form follows function.

CD and DVD Discs

The CD-ROM is a storage medium that uses laser technology to increase storage memory capacity. CD-ROM stands for "compact disc–read-only memory". CDs work like music CDs but with a computer. CD-ROMs are platters that spin rapidly in a special CD drive. The CD platter contains a foil-like material that is sandwiched between two layers of plastic. Information is stored on the CD by a sharply focused laser beam that burns tiny pits into the foil. Discs that store bits with optical technology, such as CDs and DVDs are spelled "disc" while disks that store bits with magnetic technology, such as hard disks and floppy disks, are spelled "disk". The presence or absence of a pit indicates a binary "1" or "0". Because the laser can be focused in a much smaller area than can the magnetic read-write head of a hard disk or floppy disk, the CD-ROM can store much more data in a given area. Initially, CD-ROMs were "read-only memory", meaning that the usual CD drive could not write to the CD. However, now most PCs are being shipped with inexpensive CD drives that are capable of both reading from and writing to CDs. In addition to storing a large amount of data, CDs are also removable and can serve as back-up media. A disadvantage of CDs is that moving information between the CD and the computer is slower than with hard drives, although every few months, faster and faster CD systems are released. In addition to the familiar single user CD, CD drives can be purchased in a tower configuration containing multiple CD drives. Single and multi-drive CD units can easily be placed on the office network.

DVD (digital video disc or digital versatile disc) is a removable storage medium similar to CDs but they are encoded differently and at a higher data density. Like CDs, DVDs can be read-only or read and write.

Scanners

Even when using an EHR, few offices can become truly paperless because the typical medical office receives paper communication from many sources, such as copies of old medical records, radiology reports, outside laboratory ports, correspondence, and consultations. Scanners can convert these paper documents into electronic documents that are stored in the computer and attached to the patient's EHR. The advantages and disadvantages of scanning documents are listed in Table 2-1.

There are three types of scanners commonly used in the medical office. They are distinguished from each other by how the scan head moves relative to the document being scanned. In flat-bed scanners, the document is placed flat on a piece of glass and the scan head moves past the stationary document. In a sheet-fed scanner, the document is moved past the scan head by a set of rollers much like the rollers in a typewriter or printer. Some flatbed scanners also have sheet feeders. Handheld scanners are drawn across a stationary document by the user's hand. Each scanner type has its own advantages. High-volume scanning operations use the sheet-fed scanner. While sheet-fed scanners cost more to purchase, they save on labor. Sheet-fed scanners can scan only flat documents and cannot scan books. Flat-bed scanners can scan books and other thick objects. Flat-bed scanners that have no sheet feeder require an attendant to move the original page to and from the scan bed and are labor intensive. Sheet-fed scanners can be loaded with multiple documents and require less labor. Handheld scanners are inexpensive, are slower than the other scanners, and are suitable only for occasional use in the medical office.

Scanned documents can be stored either as digital images or as text files. If documents are stored as images, the computer cannot search text content within the document. If the documents are to be stored as text files, then the documents must be scanned using an optical character-recognition (OCR) program.

Modems

Many office computer systems will have a modem that connects the office computer system to the outside world. Outside connectivity can allow for software maintenance over the telephone, access to medical records from the physician's home, or access to an internet service provider. Outside

Table 2-1

SCANNING CLINICAL DOCUMENTS INTO ELECTRONIC FORMAT

Advantages	Disadvantages
Reduction of storage space required for paper records	The scanner must be interfaced to the EMR
Fewer lost documents	The EMR must be capable of accepting scanned documents
Neater office with less paper clutter	Scanning documents can be labor intensive
Easier archive and retrieval	Indexing of documents for later retrieval can be a problem (e.g., by what data elements and key words should each document be indexed, who will do the indexing, how accurate must the indexing be?)
	If documents are not properly indexed, they may be irretrievable
	If documents are OCR'd, additional issues arise:
	1. Since no OCR system is 100% accurate, who will be responsible for proofreading and editing the OCR'd documents?
	2. If the OCR'd documents are not proofread, who will take responsibility for content errors in the scanned medical documents?
	3. Can the source document be destroyed if the clinicians using the information are not highly confident of the accuracy of the OCR'd copies?
	4. If image scanning is used, what benefits are lost by not being able to search on detailed content that is not computer searchable?

connectivity usually comes through a telephone line, broadband Internet (cable modem, DSL), or the hospital network

A telephone modem connects the office computer to remote computers by translating digital computer signals from the computer into audible analog telephone signals that are sent over standard telephone lines to distant computers. In the information technology world the telephone system is often referred to as "PSTN" (public switched telephone network) or as "POTS" (plain old telephone system).

The word modem is a contraction of "modulator-demodulator". Modems modulate (change) the digital output of the computer into analog noises that can travel over standard telephone lines much like voices. The modem on the destination computer "demodulates" (changes) the analog noises back into digital signals that the destination computer can understand. Modems are classified by the speed at which they work and by the type of line over which they operate. Standard modems currently can transmit data over a standard telephone line at 56 kilobits per second or faster. Faster telephone lines include ISDN (Integrated Digital Subscriber Network) and ADSL (Asymmetric Digital Subscriber Line), plus several new variations of ADSL, as a class called xDSL. Each type of line requires a matching type of modem. Cable modems use the cable TV system instead of telephone lines to connect computers at very high transmission speeds, up to 10 megabits per second.

Other Devices

Digital cameras can be most useful in the medical office if they are interfaced with the EHR. There needs to be an easy-to-use process to get the image into the EHR, and the EHR must be designed to accept and display digital images accurately. These cameras can be used to import photos into the electronic patient record. The digital photos can remind the staff of what a patient looks like so that the patient is recognized by sight when returning to the office. Another use of the digital camera is to record the appearance of skin lesions for the record or for consultation with a colleague. Video cameras are just beginning to appear in the medical office, principally as a tool for video house calls and video consultations.

Which peripheral devices are appropriate for the office depends primarily on the workflow and benefits expected from computerizing the office. Remember, form follows function.

Emerging Technologies and Issues

Emerging technologies will increase the usefulness of computers in the medical office. Here are a few to consider.

Voice Recognition

One of the most common computer fantasies of physicians is to bark out an order and have the computer respond instantly, with absolute accuracy, and with complete understanding, asking no questions.

The doctor, speaking rapidly, says "Computer, Mr. Smith needs a CBC, retic count, ferritin, and stools about a week after he gets the UGI. Now, Computer, begin Mr. Doe's note . . . This 45-year-old male complains of. . . ."

The computer, speaking not so robotically, says "Yes, Master", orders the tests on Mr. Smith, and begins transcribing the doctor's dictation.

While it will be many years before the office computer will do everything asked of it, computer speech recognition can be useful today in the right clinical setting. With a fast computer, good microphone, and commitment from the clinician, a speech recognition program can be a powerful adjunct to the office computing environment.

The short explanation of how speech recognition works is that the speaker's words are digitized by a sound system in the PC. The digitized speech is then compared by the speech recognition program to a previously recorded file of words and phonemes using a system of artificial intelligence that considers word frequency, word order, word associations, context, and the speaker's personal pronunciation patterns. The expert system then attempts to execute the tasks requested or to transcribe the speech into text that is displayed on the computer screen. Faster processors, more RAM, and improved speech algorithms are making speech recognition sufficiently fast and accurate to be considered for the medical office.

Speech recognition raised significant issues that may not be apparent to the inexperienced computing physician. Older speech recognition systems required the speaker to say each individual word discretely with a brief pause between words. This form of dictation, called "discrete speech recognition", is a slow and unnatural way to speak. The newer speech recognition systems allow the user to speak in a natural cadence without discrete pauses between words, so called "continuous speech recognition". Continuous speech recognition is a more natural way of dictating medical notes to the computer. Another differentiating factor among speech recognition systems is whether the system is limited to a single user or can accommodate multiple users. If the speech recognition system is able to accommodate multiple users, one needs to know how quickly the system can switch from one user to another user. If a user's voice file takes several minutes to load before he can use the system, then it will be impractical for clinicians to switch between speech recognition computers in a busy office practice. Each clinician may require a dedicated voice recognition computer.

Another issue to understand regarding speech recognition is the difference between issuing verbal commands to the computer, so-called command mode, versus automated transcription of dictated speech, so-called transcription mode. Some inexpensive speech recognition programs are limited to the command mode of speech recognition and are not suitable for transcribing clinical notes.

Another speech recognition issue is the relative value of structured data input versus free text input. Full speech recognition allows the physician to input long, rambling, unstructured free text notes. Structured versus unstructured data is an issue that affects keyboard input as well as speech recognition. However, physicians are far less likely to type large blocks of free text than they are to dictate large amounts of free text. Free text notes cannot be searched by the computer as easily as structured data can be searched. Structured clinical data are stored in a structured computer database that allows searching for specific data elements, such as medications prescribed, presence of an S3 gallop, and the date of the last diabetic eye exam. A searchable clinical database will facilitate management of your patient population.

Most EHRs have a combination of structured and unstructured data input. Some speech recognition systems allow dictation directly into the data fields of the EHR. The advantages of such a system are that it provides the speed of dictation, the cost savings of speech recognition, plus the structured database of the EHR. Some speech recognition systems will not allow dictation directly into the EHR. Rather, these systems require the user to dictate into a special text box and then to manually cut and paste the transcribed text into an EHR field. Such a cut and paste requirement will slow the busy clinician.

Three related speech recognition issues are accuracy, proofreading, and editing. Speech recognition systems are often advertised as having accuracy rates of 95% or better. However, 95% accuracy means that one out of every twenty words will be an error. Because these errors contain correctly spelled but inappropriate words, finding these word errors by proofreading after the fact is more difficult than finding spelling errors. Catching the errors on the fly during the dictation-speech recognition process is difficult because the user must juggle three mental activities at the same time. First, the user must be thinking ahead about what she is going to say. Second, the user must say what needs to be said at that very moment. Third, because the speech recognition system delays typing on the screen by a second or two, the user must also be mentally comparing what was previously said to what is being typed on the screen. Juggling several mental speech processes at once can be very disconcerting to the speaker and requires a great deal of practice. In addition, correcting the errors can be cumbersome and time consuming.

Speech recognition accuracy decreases in the presence of background noise. Some do not function well when the speaker is hoarse. Another consideration is deciding when during the patient flow process will the clinician dictate to the speech recognition system. Will it be in front of patients in the exam room as described above? Some physicians report significant benefits to dictating in the patient's presence, but many physicians are uncomfortable with the idea of patients hearing what is dictated. Will the clinician dictate between patients and, if so, is the speech recognition computer easily accessible in the immediate vicinity of the exam rooms in which the clinician is working? Will the physician require several exam rooms to be equipped with speech recognition? How will each speech recognition file on the separate computers be synchronized?

To maximize the benefit of speech recognition in the medical office, one should very carefully map out clinician workflow, commit to spending hours training the speech recognition system, training the users, and purchasing high-powered PCs, high-quality microphones, and the proper medical vocabularies.

Biometric Identification

Maintaining privacy of health information in the computer age is very important. One element of the privacy equation is knowing that the individual using the computer system is who they say they are. This problem is called "authentication" of users. Most systems are currently protected only by user-name and passwords. Passwords can be stolen, shared inappropriately, or guessed. Biometric identification systems are being used to authenticate users and patients in some sites. Biometric authentication systems take a reading of a unique biologic parameter from the user and compare the pa-rameter to a database of authenticated users. Biometric parameters that are just now emerging are fingerprint recognition, iris scanning, retinal scanning, and voice print recognition. It is quite likely that within the next few years, users of EHR systems, whether in the office, hospital, or home, will be re-quired to authenticate themselves to the computer using one of these bio-metric methods. Another method of user authentication is using proximity tags, typically an RFID (radio frequency of identification device) embedded in an ID badge. When the wearer of the RFID badge comes within a few feet of the computer, the computer becomes enabled to accept the user's pass-word. This authentication strategy sometimes is referred to as "something you have and the something you know". Another variation on the "something you have and something you know" authentication schema is to use a secu-rity token ("something you have") in combination with a password ("some-thing you know"). The security token is a small device that displays a multi-digit number that is synchronized to the central server and that changes every few seconds. The user is authenticated by entering the exact number displayed on the security token at the time of sign-on plus their password.

Machine authentication may be necessary as well as user authentication. Security breaches can occur if a hacker uses a non-secure PC to mimic a secure PC in order to access a secure network. Authentication of the de-vices logging in to the secure network can be accomplished by the use of digital certificates. A digital certificate is a specially encoded file that is is-sued to a specific computer by a certificate authority that uniquely identi-fies that specific computer. The secure server will look for the digital certificate on the device that is trying to log in. Once the device is authen-ticated, the user will be given the opportunity to authenticate himself to the server and gain access to the system. Digital certificates authenticate the de-vice or computer, but they do not authenticate the user. Usernames, pass-words, biometrics, and security tokens can authenticate the user. The combination of a device authentication and a user authentication provides the strongest security.

Telemedicine and Video Conferencing

Telemedicine is an emerging technology that may soon play a role in the medical office. Telemedicine has been eagerly awaited for decades but has met with only limited success so far due to cost, complexity, and lack of adequate reimbursement. Rapidly improving video technology, increasing bandwidth, and reimbursement of telemedicine services may enable telemedicine to become an important part of clinical care.

New Internet technologies are enabling clinicians to perform video house calls for medically fragile patients, and to remotely monitor patients' vital signs, medication compliance, and clinical conditions. Technology-enabled chronic care management may prove more effective for chronic and expensive medical conditions and in the conventional episodic office-based care model.

Conventional room video conferencing, with large TV-like monitors in auditoriums or large conference rooms, is commonly used for CME activities and medical conferences. Good-quality desktop video conferencing equipment, available for less than $1000 per PC, can allow the clinician to see colleagues or patients at the other end of the computer link. Medical images, such as radiographs, Gram stains, and digital pictures of skin lesions, can easily be attached to email or shared with colleagues using a variety of currently available telemedicine software.

The biggest barriers to wider use of telemedicine have been the cost of adequate bandwidth required for high-quality video, the cost of video conferencing equipment, and the cost of telemedicine peripheral scopes, cameras, and monitoring devices. As more bandwidth becomes available and the cost of equipment falls, clinicians, patients, and payers will find sufficient value in telemedicine to make it a part of daily practice.

Wireless Networks

Installing the wires that form the office network presents a significant cost and several challenges. There are various grades of computer cable that must be matched to the computer system and to the distance of the devices from the server. Building codes require certain computer cable specifications. Even details such as avoiding electromagnetic interference from fluorescent lights and other electrical power sources must be considered. The new wireless network technology may eliminate many of these issues. Wireless networks connect devices to the computer system through radio links rather than through standard computer cables. Wireless connectivity is typically accomplished by installing one or more wireless access points onto the wired network. An access point is a radio that transmits and receives information to and from other wireless-enabled PCs, printers, or modems that contain small radio receiver-transmitters. The wireless network connection eliminates the need for stringing cable and provides the ability to move devices about the office.

Wireless networks have their own set of issues, including security and encryption of the transmitted messages, bandwidth, interference, reliability, effective distance, and unauthorized access.

The cost of wireless networks has fallen and the reliability and ease of installation have improved considerably, making the wireless local area network a reasonable alternative or addition to the conventional wired office network. Careful planning of the wireless network is necessary and consultation with an IT professional is advised.

Other Hardware Issues, Privacy, and Portability

There are several hardware initiatives that can enhance security and privacy of patient information in the medical office.

Screen savers with passwords should be placed on all PCs and terminals that can be accessed by patients and non-staff persons, such as cleaning people, building maintenance persons, and building security personnel. Screen savers are programs that cause the monitor image to be replaced by a blank screen or pattern after a certain period of nonuse. Requiring that a password be entered in order to recover the screen will help prevent inappropriate browsing of computer information. The time-out period for activation of the screensaver should be short, perhaps one to three minutes.

All applications that contain confidential information should be password protected. Passwords should be unique to each user and should not be shared. The health IT community has developed standards for password management. Each health care entity should develop and periodically review its own password and security policies.

A commonly overlooked risk for confidentiality is the inappropriate management of paper output from the computer. Reports that contain patient-specific information should be discarded properly by shredding or burning or by cutting the patient identifier from the documents. Paper output should not be left in areas where patients may be tempted to read about other patients.

Back-up media, such as computer tapes, floppy disks, and CDs, should be closely guarded. Any media that leaves the office and contains personally identifiable health information should have encrypted data files so that, if the disk or tape is lost, others cannot read confidential patient information. Many physicians are beginning to carry laptops from the office to home or to the hospital in order to have current patient information at their finger tips. These laptops can be lost or stolen. Confidential information in the files on these mobile computers should be protected by password and should be encrypted.

The medical office embarking on an EHR project should become familiar with HIPAA security and privacy standards. The HIPAA rules contain important guidelines that may be used to develop policies and operational procedures surrounding the EHR.

Protecting Computer Equipment and Data

A very important hardware consideration for the medical office is protecting computer equipment from electrical disasters. The quality of the electricity supplied by the outlets in the office is often quite variable. The voltage drifts up and down. There are occasional spikes of electrical current, as occurs when the power is turned on or off in the building or during electrical storms. All of these unexpected electrical events can damage delicate computer equipment unless the equipment is protected. To protect against unexpected surges of electrical power, all of the office computer equipment and peripherals should be protected with surge and spike protectors. To guard against power failure, an uninterruptible power source, called a UPS, should power the server. The UPS is a battery that can give the server a few minutes to shut itself down in an organized manner rather than crashing to a halt and damaging data or hardware when the power goes off. Higher priced UPSs with larger batteries can power the server for hours.

In addition to protecting hardware, software and data should be protected with regular backups. Decisions about the backup process include:

◆ What media to use: magnetic tape, CDs, DVDs, network attach storage on hard drives, off-site hard drive stored service.

◆ How often and when to do full backups: backups are usually performed during non-work hours because the backup process often degrades server performance.

◆ How often to do incremental backups: incremental backups back up only the data that has changed since the last full backup and saves backup disk storage space and backup time.

The backup process copies data from the computer's hard drive to removable media or off-site media, usually magnetic tape or CDs. PC workstations should be backed up as well as the server. Backups of irreplaceable billing data and medical records should be made daily. It helps to automate the process. Not only should one plan to prevent electrical events from corrupting data, one must also worry about physical disasters, such as fire, flood, and storms. Whole servers have been stolen from offices. While hardware can be replaced easily, replacing data is impossible without backups. Every office with an EHR or a computer practice management system should have a disaster recovery plan. Backup tapes should be removed each day from the office premises and stored in a secure environment. Another form of off-site backup is to send backup data over the internet to a commercial off-site storage facility. The medical office is obligated to follow HIPAA requirements when working with an off-site storage company.

Choreographing the Doctor-Patient-Computer Interaction

Successful implementation of a computer system in the doctor's office requires many skills. In addition to developing a business case for computerizing the medical office, one should analyze the flow of patients, personnel, and work through the office. The movement, spatial relationships, and timing of how people and computers interact in the office is similar to chore-ographing a dance. Where and when patients, personnel, and doctors walk, sit, stand, and talk are important factors to consider when choreographing the doctor-patient-computer interaction.

Consider who can view the information on the computer screen. On the one hand, sharing the screen information with a patient may be impor-tant when doing patient education in the privacy of the exam room. On the other hand, when scheduling a patient for a follow-up visit, the patient should not be able to see other patients' names and diagnoses on a com-puter schedule.

The amount of physical space taken up by computer equipment is an important consideration. The desk space required by a desktop or tower PC, a 15-inch CRT monitor, and a printer may consume all the available desk space at the nurse station. Because space is often limited, think about space-saving alternatives such as the new, smaller PCs. Consider placing PCs under the desk or on a sturdy bookshelf high off the desk. Think about sharing network printers in order to decrease computer clutter in the exam room. Flat panel monitors save a lot of desk space, generate less heat than CRTs, and are now quite affordable. Laptop, sub-notebook, and small net-work PCs may save space in your work environment.

When using a computer in the exam room, think carefully about the placement of the doctor, the patient, and the computer equipment. A trian-gle arrangement often works best with the patient, the computer, and the doctor at the corners of the triangle. This arrangement allows the doctor to sit directly facing the patient, maintain eye contact, and occasionally glance at the computer screen at the other corner of the triangle. Avoid placing computer equipment between the doctor and the patient. If the patient is encouraged to view information on the computer screen, such as an anatomic diagram or a problem list, the display must be large enough and positioned properly so that both doctor and patient can see the image. This will require the triangular relationship noted above among doctor, patient, and computer screen.

Be wary of extraneous noises. Computer noise can distract from the doctor-patient conversation. Choose a quiet keyboard. Avoid keyboards that produce irritating mechanical key clicks. Some keyboards are pro-grammed to generate key click sounds through the computer speaker. If possible, disable these computer-generated key clicks. Turn down the vol-ume of alarms from the computer.

Some physicians report successful use of speech recognition in the pres-ence of patients in the exam room. Potential benefits of using speech recognition in the exam room are:

◆ The patient enjoys hearing what the doctor is putting in the record.

◆ The patient is able to correct the doctor when necessary ("Doc, it was my right foot, not my left foot").

- The encounter documentation can often be completed by the time the patient leaves the exam room.

- Patients or caregivers can be given a copy of the note at the time they leave the exam room.

There must be an artful arrangement of patient flow, workflow, computer hardware, and geographic space in the medical office to implement a computer system successfully.

Where Do I Start?

Start by planning your EHR project well. Whether you are in a small medical office or a large health care enterprise, you should define the function of your EHR in detail before you consider the form of your hardware.

First consider the relationship of the EHR project to your business strategies and goals and key workflows in the context of an EHR. (This topic, although beyond the scope of this chapter, is covered in detail in Chapters 7 and 8).

After you have completed analysis of your business strategies and goals, you can begin to consider which EHR system satisfies your needs. After choosing your EHR and understanding the functional components that are important to your outcome targets, you can begin to define the hardware and physical environment of your EHR. Remember, form follows function.

Begin a detailed analysis of the hardware and physical environment requirements for your EHR project by making a list of each of the issues discussed in this chapter. Then analyze each hardware issue with respect to your key outcome measures and EHR functions. For example, if one of your deliverables is to succeed in a pay-for-performance program that values diabetes management, you may need a lab interface to automatically track hemoglobin A1c. You may need a method of scanning diabetic eye exam results into the EHR and tracking the results in a flow sheet. You may need reporting capabilities to discover which of your diabetic patients have not completed their eye exam this year.

Choices of basic computer hardware should be determined primarily by a careful analysis of the workflow and function of the persons using the computers in the office. The hardware configurations required by the front office receptionist or by the back office clerk are likely to be different from the physician who is using the computer in the exam room.

Your EHR vendor and IT consultant should be able to address many of these functional and hardware questions. Avoid the mistake of allowing your vendor or IT consultant to make all the decisions. The more you understand about the link between your medical practice's desired outcomes and the form of your EHR implementation, the more successful you will be in achieving your desired outcomes.

Summary

A successful computer system for the medical office requires thoughtful business planning, a clear understanding of office functions and workflow, and reasonable knowledge about computer hardware and software. The hardware and network configuration chosen for the office is always defined by office functions, workflow, and software requirements. Form (the hardware) follows function (workflow and software).

An understanding of fundamental computer concepts and how basic hardware works will help with planning the office system and will allow appropriate adoption of new technologies (Appendix B provides information on hardware technology resources). Different computer technologies have different strengths and weaknesses. Understanding these weaknesses can help avoid computer disasters like lost data. Understanding the strengths of new technologies will help the clinician provide better care. Like choreographing a dance, thoughtful attention to space (the placement of hardware, doctor, and patient), to timing (workflow process), and to roles (office personnel, clinicians, and patients) will enhance the doctor-patient-computer interaction.

3

Operating Systems and Programming Languages

Stephen E. Brossette, MD, PhD

Operating systems and programming languages are cornerstones of modern computing. Although they are appropriately hidden from most users, practitioners with a basic knowledge of each can better understand and appreciate computing systems and applications software. This chapter briefly describes the historical development of the operating system, highlights features of the modern operating system, and surveys popular modern operating systems. Good in-depth treatments of operating systems can be found elsewhere (1,2).

Operating Systems

Users of computers are more accurately users of operating systems and the programs that run on them. An operating system is itself a program that sits between the user (and application programs) and computer hardware. The job of the operating system is to insulate the complexities of the hardware from the user and other programs.

Operating Systems History

Early computers were entirely dedicated to running one program at a time, and each program was responsible for controlling the entire computer: input/output (I/O), the central processing unit (CPU), and memory. Even though different programs performed different tasks, they often contained significant amounts of redundant code that was used to control hardware subsystems like I/O devices. Separating this redundant code from the main programs led to the creation of device drivers, programs that control I/O devices and provide interfaces for other programs to communicate with them.

Device drivers freed application programmers (scientists) from writing and maintaining device-specific code. Modern operating systems contain thousands of device drivers that control everything from printers, video cards, keyboards, hard disks, and memory to network adapters and wireless devices.

Because early computers were also very expensive, minimizing the time they were not computing was critical. At first, computer operating schedules were maintained by hand. Scientists arrived (or not) at their scheduled times to load, run, and debug their programs. Since many scientists were not efficient computer operators, valuable computing resources were wasted. To minimize downtime, dedicated computer operators were hired. Scientists queued their programs with the operator, who was more efficient at loading and executing programs. Unfortunately, as a side-effect, many scientist-program interactions were eliminated.

Soon computer scientists created another program, the *resident monitor program* (RMP), to replace the operator. When one program finished, the RMP simply started the next one. If a program crashed, however, human intervention was often required and RMPs, like human operators, still limited scientist-program interactions. Together with device drivers, though, the RMP comprised the first computer operating system.

Multitasking

Even computers with RMPs were entirely dedicated to running one program at a time. A single running program, however, inefficiently utilizes the CPU and I/O devices. For example, in the time between the keystrokes or double mouse clicks, a modern CPU can perform millions of operations. Therefore, when a program needs data from an I/O device, even a hard disk, the CPU sits idle for relatively long periods of time waiting for the I/O device to return data. On the other hand, if a program keeps the CPU busy, the I/O devices idle. In either case, computers dedicated to one program at a time underutilized valuable computing resources.

To solve this problem, computer scientists created ways for computers to switch between programs so that when one program is waiting for I/O, another can use the CPU. This framework of multiple program management is called *multitasking*. Multitasking requires two important operating system features: interrupts and context switching.

An *interrupt* is a signal generated by an I/O device that tells the operating system when work from the device has been completed. For example, if a program needs data from the keyboard, it sends a request to the keyboard's device driver and then waits for that device to return data. When a key is pressed, the keyboard generates an interrupt to inform the operating system that a key has been pressed. The operating system recognizes the signal, retrieves the data, then continues running the main program.

Context switching allows the operating system to change running programs. Each program in a multitasking operating system can be in one of three states: running, blocked, or ready. When a program requests service from an I/O device, information about the current state of the program is saved, and the operating system marks the program as *blocked* (awaiting I/O). In the meantime, the operating system, through its *scheduler*, selects another program that is ready to use the CPU. When the *interrupt handler* (also part of the operating system) receives an interrupt for the blocked program, the operating system moves the blocked program to the ready state. Any program in the ready state can use the CPU when it becomes available.

Unless a program requests the service of an I/O device and enters the blocked state, it will not relinquish control of the CPU to allow another program to run. This behavior in which programs voluntarily relinquish the CPU is called *cooperative multitasking*. In reality though, programs are not so cooperative, and the performance of older PC operating systems that depended on cooperative multitasking was unpredictable.

Multiple Users and Preemptive Multitasking

To solve the problem of cooperative multitasking, programs have to be forced from one state to another at regular intervals. To do this the operating system uses a fixed rate (e.g., 60 per second) *timer interrupt* generated by hardware. At each interrupt, the scheduler saves the state of the running program and loads a ready program. Since the time between interrupts, the *time slice*, is very short compared to the speed of human-computer interactions, the computer can run many programs in a short period of time. To the user, this makes it seem as if the computer is running programs simultaneously. This scheme where the operating system interrupts a running program to start another is called *preemptive multitasking*. Preemptive multitasking is standard in all modern operating systems.

It should be noted that the scheduler is selective in picking the next program for execution. It does so based on how I/O intensive the program is, to keep the CPU and I/O devices busy, and how important the program is, to give important programs, or those owned by important users, higher priority. But now with multitasking and multiple users, the operating system has new problems to address.

Protection and Security

Safeguards against programs corrupting other programs are necessary in multitasking environments. Without them, any program can control any device or write to any location in memory, even if that memory contains another program or data for another program. But the operating system is also a program. So the CPU must distinguish between it and other programs and allow for two distinct modes of operation: user mode (other programs) and protected mode (the operating system). In *user mode*, CPU instructions responsible for memory management and direct control of I/O are disabled. Without direct access to these resources, programs must request these services from the operating system. When the CPU enters *protected mode* where privileged instructions can be executed, the operating system can satisfy these sensitive requests. Before giving control back to the other programs, though, the operating system switches the CPU back to user mode. In this way, the operating system is in sole control of the direct manipulation of vital resources. Larger computers have supported protected mode operation for some time. PCs offered protected mode operation with the introduction of the Intel 80386 microprocessor.

Files and File Systems

All computer data are stored and manipulated as bits (zeroes and ones). A *file* is nothing more than a set of bits. A *file system* is a structure for organizing files on one or more storage devices (e.g. memory, hard drives, external storage). Operating systems create and maintain file systems and provide functionality that programs use to create and delete files, locate them, and transfer data to and from them. The operating system controls the details of file manipulation. For example, if a program needs data stored in a particular file, it asks the operating system to open the file, locate the data, and copy it into memory. File systems also determine things like how many files can be stored on a disk partition and how files are secured by ownership and access privileges.

Multithreading

A *thread* is a single pathway of instruction execution through a program. Many programs have one thread. However, some programs can be separated into more than one thread. Such a program is *multithreaded* and usually consists of a primary thread that may, for example, handle user interaction, and one or more secondary threads that perform background tasks, such as rendering images on the screen.

In a multitasking operating system, each thread of a multithreaded program is handled separately so that the program can take advantage of multitasking. While one thread is running, others can be blocked or ready, thereby improving the performance of a single program. UNIX, Mac OS, and Windows (XP, 2003, Server, and Vista) support multithreaded programs.

Memory Management and Virtual Memory

Just as the operating system manages files stored on external media, it also manages programs and data stored in memory. A secure operating system prevents a program from accessing memory that it does not own by assigning each program its own address space and not allowing other programs to access it. The operating system also allocates memory for running programs, keeps track of data and programs scattered through memory, re-claims unused memory, and manages virtual memory.

Virtual memory is not really memory at all, but a file on disk. When a program requests memory but none is available, the operating system can use a piece of the hard disk as virtual memory. To do this, the operating system moves less frequently used pieces (pages) of memory to the virtual memory file so that the space cleared in memory can be used for the new request. When data in virtual memory are needed again, the operating system moves them back to physical memory by swapping them for other pages in memory at the time. The extra overhead required to swap pages in and out of memory makes accessing data in virtual memory slower than accessing data in physical memory but gives application programs the illusion that there is more physical memory than actually exists. For this reason, memory-intensive applications run relatively slowly when they are required to use virtual memory. In these cases, more physical memory (RAM) will improve performance substantially.

User Interfaces

Operating systems provide one or more user interfaces (UIs). Common UIs include text-based interfaces such as the DOS command line and the UNIX bash shell, or graphical user interfaces (GUIs) such as X-Windows for UNIX, the Macintosh OS UI, and the Microsoft Windows UI.

Multiprocessing

Multiprocessing is the operating systems's ability to support more than one CPU. This is different from multitasking. Multitasking refers to a single-processor using timer interrupts to change running programs. On a two-CPU computer, two programs can truly run simultaneously, one on each CPU. Newer CPUs often contain more than one CPU per chip. When two CPUs are present on a single chip, it is referred to as dual-core.

A number of schemes exist for dividing work between two or more processors, and some of the ways that operating systems do this are complicated. The most complex, powerful, and reliable of these is *symmetric multiprocessing* (SMP) in which all processors are connected to a common memory, share the same I/O devices, and are capable of performing the same tasks. UNIX, Mac OS X, and newer versions of Windows support SMP.

Network Services

Network services allow the computer to communicate with other computers in a network. Some computers run programs that act primarily to serve information to different programs on other computers. The serving programs are called *servers* and the receiving programs are called *clients*. This *client-server* paradigm is responsible for most of the data transferred on the Internet. (Client-server computing also describes two or more programs on a single multitasking machine that interact with each other in a client-server relationship.) By tradition, computers that run important server programs, like an HTML server for web pages, are themselves called *servers*, while computers that run client programs, like a web browser, are called *clients*.

The term "network operating system" is usually reserved for operating systems that only run on LAN servers. Network operating systems are not used on client machines. UNIX and Microsoft NT, for example, can run on servers, but are also used on client machines. Novell NetWare, on the other hand, is found only on servers.

A Survey of Popular Modern Operating Systems

UNIX

UNIX is the legendary multiuser, multitasking, network-capable operating system first developed at AT&T in the late 1960s and early 1970s, and later developed at the University of California at Berkeley. Originally created for computers in academic and government environments, UNIX can now be found on computers of all types, from supercomputers to PCs, and in all work environments from major corporations to the home.

UNIX has many robust features. It is secure and stable, multiuser, multitasking, and multiprocessing. It can act as a network server, and is available for virtually any hardware platform. Additionally, many distributions come with compilers and other useful software not found in other operating system distributions, and many vendors and independent organizations offer training and certification. Unix also supports file systems that can handle large hard disks and other external storage devices efficiently.

There are many versions of UNIX from many vendors. HP, IBM, and Apple are but a few companies that sell versions of UNIX. There is also a free Unix called Linux, originally developed by Linus Torvalds and a small army of programmers in an effort that has come to exemplify the Open Source movement.

In the past, Unix was considered an expert's operating system, which was not as user-friendly as operating systems with sophisticated GUIs and self-configuring installation programs. Apple has changed that and has placed UNIX at the core of Mac OS X.

MS-DOS

MS-DOS (or simply DOS) was, for all practical purposes, the original operating system of the personal computer. Developed by Microsoft for the first IBM PC, MS-DOS version 1.0 was released in 1981. Since then, it has gone through many versions, gaining features such as a hierarchical file system (v2.0), installable modular device drivers (v2.0), a background print spooler (v2.0), some networking capabilities (v3.0), the support of several communication ports (v3.3), the support of 1.44MB floppy disks (v3.3), the support of 2GB hard disks (v4.0), and improved memory management (nearly all versions). The last version of MS-DOS, unofficially known as version 7, is the foundation for Microsoft's Windows 95 and Windows 98 operating systems. While DOS has been eclipsed in many ways by more sophisticated operating systems, it maintains a strong presence in the PC world due to its popularity in the 1980s and the fact that many computers still run DOS and DOS-based applications.

DOS has served the personal computer well, but it has many limitations. It is 16-bit, single user, single-tasking (vs. multitasking), has poor memory management, and does not support virtual memory. Perhaps the most notorious shortcoming of DOS, however, is its inability to run in protected mode. As a result, DOS cannot stop application programs from directly writing to memory or controlling I/O devices. This has been used to the advantage of some programmers (especially game programmers) to get direct control of hardware to maximize program speed. Ultimately, however, this feature makes DOS unsafe and unstable.

The inability of DOS to run in protected mode also restricts DOS programs to 1 MB of addressable memory, only 640 KB of which are famously available to application programs. This 640 KB addressable memory ceiling is the remnant of the maximum addressable memory of the Intel 8088 and 8086, which were the 16-bit CPUs of the first IBM PCs.

Although Microsoft stopped developing MS-DOS in favor of its Windows line of operating systems, DOS programs are still supported by DOS emulators in Windows, Unix, and MacOS.

Microsoft Windows

Microsoft Windows dominated the PC operating systems market in the 1990s. The successor to MS-DOS, Microsoft Windows (or just Windows) evolved through many product generations including Windows 3.x (which includes Windows 3.0, 3.1, and 3.11), Windows 95, Windows 98, Windows NT, Windows 2000, Windows XP, Windows Server, and Windows Vista. In addition to giving the PC a Mac-like GUI, the Windows operating systems have provided a number of desirable operating system features unavailable in DOS. These include memory access beyond 640 KB (Windows 3.0), virtual memory (Windows 3.0), a 32-bit architecture (Windows 95), built-in networking (Windows 95), plug-and-play hardware support (Windows 95), true preemptive multitasking (Windows NT), improved security and stability (Windows NT), symmetric multiprocessing (Windows NT), and server capabilities (Windows NT Server). With the exception of Windows Server, all are single-user operating systems.

Windows 3.x, 95, and 98 all depend to some extent on DOS version 7. Otherwise, Windows 3.x is significantly different from Windows 95 and Windows 98. In addition to the new GUI style, the most notable difference between Windows 3.x and Windows 95/98 is that the latter have a 32-bit architecture whereas Windows 3.x has a 16-bit architecture. This means that with Windows 95/98, 32-bit application programs can use the ability of the Intel 80386 and newer CPUs to transfer information around the hardware 32 bits at a time. Windows 3.x has a 16-bit architecture designed to run on the Intel 80286 CPU.

Multitasking improved from Windows 3.x to Windows 95/98. Windows 95/98 can preemptively multitask 32-bit Windows programs, but must still cooperatively multitask 16-bit programs.

Windows 95/98 support the FAT32 file system, which allows more efficient data storage and supports larger hard disks than the FAT16 file system. The maximum hard disk size supported by FAT16 is 2 GB (32K/page x 216 pages). Anything bigger must be divided up (partitioned) into logical partitions, each no larger than 2 GB. FAT32, on the other hand, with 32-bit addressing, supports disks up to 2 terabytes on a single partition.

Windows 95 supports *plug-and-play*, a hardware standard that allows the operating system to determine the identification of plug-and-play I/O devices so that it can automatically install their device drivers. Windows 95 also provides built-in networking with TCP/IP support (the data transfer protocols of the Internet), as well as support for other network communication protocols.

Windows NT was the first in a new line of operating systems from Microsoft, and along with its successors Windows 2000, XP, Server, and Vista, contains many features that the DOS-based Windows systems do not. These include preemptive multitasking for 16 and 32-bit programs, multithreading, symmetric multiprocessing, support for the NTFS file system, and improved stability and security.

MacOS

The Apple Macintosh set the standard for user-friendly personal computing with a revolutionary graphical user interface and plug-and-play capabilities long before Microsoft offered these features in Windows. Since its release in the 1980s, the Macintosh has enjoyed a loyal following and continues to be the preferred computer of visual artists and desktop publishers. It also has a strong and growing following of scientists.

The Macintosh OS (MacOS), has also gone through many versions and, like Windows, has become more feature rich over time. Originally designed for the Motorola 68000 line of CPUs, the MacOS has never been confined to 640 KB of addressable memory. Until 1999, however, MacOS did not support advanced operating system features such as preemptive multitasking, memory protection, multiple users, or symmetric multiprocessing. It was also inferior to Windows 95/98 in memory protection and multitasking capabilities. Apple has addressed these deficiencies by combining the core of UNIX with traditional MacOS technologies to create the MacOS X operating system.

MacOS X combines the advanced operating system features of UNIX, including preemptive multitasking, server, and multiuser capabilities, with an advanced, easy to use MacOS GUI. MacOS X is also the first Mac operating system to run on Intel microprocessors. Combined with powerful Intel-based Mac computers, MacOS X is a very capable and elegant operating system.

Programming Languages

Programming languages, like operating systems, are a cornerstone of modern computing. Hundreds, if not thousands, of programming languages have been created, and entire texts are devoted to the subject. In this section, some programming language basics will be presented, and several popular modern programming languages will be surveyed.

Many programming languages were created for specific disciplines and applications. FORTRAN was designed for science and engineering, Lisp and Prolog for artificial intelligence, C for operating system development, COBOL for business, and BASIC to teach programming. Other languages were developed to embody new programming paradigms. Prominent among these are the object-oriented languages C++ and Java.

Machine and Assembly Languages

A computer program is a sequence of bits that direct the CPU to perform simple operations: add two numbers, store bits in memory, send bits to a to another device, etc. Unfortunately, bit-encoded instructions (machine language) are difficult to write and understand. They are also CPU-specific. A machine language program for a Dec Alpha will not run on an Intel x86, a PowerPC, or any other type of CPU. Therefore, machine language programs are not *portable*. Exceptions exist within families of microprocessors. For example, the Intel x86 microprocessors are backward compatible: each CPU supports the instruction set of its predecessors. Therefore, a machine language program that runs on the 80286 will run on the 80386 through the latest generation Intel chip. The reverse, however, is not true. Machine language programs that take advantage of features (and instructions) of newer microprocessors cannot run on older ones.

Assembly language is a low-level programming language that uses text to represent machine instructions and allows programmers to assign names to variables. Each assembly language instruction is translated by a program called the *assembler* into a single machine language instruction. Therefore, Assembly language allows for very precise control of hardware. Before

UNIX, which was written in C, many operating systems were written in assembly language. Today, sometimes pieces of operating systems and other types of embedded systems are written in assembly language, although C or C++ is usually the language of choice.

Compilers and Interpreters

Most programmers do not write programs in assembly language. Instead, they use high-level programming languages like C++ and Java.

There are three ways high-level programs are executed by computers. They can be compiled into machine language, interpreted by another program without compilation, or compiled into an intermediate language that gets interpreted by another program. C and C++ do the first, scripting languages (VBScript, JavaScript) the second, and Java and C# (and other Microsoft .NET supported languages including Visual Basic) the third. Each approach has advantages and disadvantages, and each programming language supports one or more approaches.

Programs that are compiled to machine language can be executed directly by the CPU. Compilation occurs by a program called a *compiler* that turns a program written in a high-level language into assembly language, which is then assembled into machine language. Since most programs depend on calls to the operating system for I/O, the machine language program is then *linked* by a program called the *linker* to operating system code to form an *executable*, which runs directly on the CPU.

Compiled programs (executables) are fast compared to interpreted programs, but compiled programs are CPU-specific. Therefore, when porting a program written in a compiled language from one computer type to another, the program must be recompiled and reassembled. Compiler principles and construction are interesting subjects and are necessary for the construction of new compiled programming languages. An excellent treatment of compiler principles can be found in Aho, Setthi, and Ullman (3).

Interpreted programs are translated on the fly by an *interpreter*, a program that acts as a go between for the source program and the CPU. The source program is not executable. While theoretically portable, interpreted programs are typically slower than their compiled counterparts, often making them inappropriate for computationally intensive tasks. For most applications though, interpreted programs are fast enough.

Between compiled and interpreted programs are hybrids that use both compilers and interpreters. The most popular programming languages that use this approach are Java and the languages supported by the Microsoft .NET development framework, including C#. A Java program is compiled by the Java compiler into Java *byte code*. Java bytecode is then interpreted by the Java interpreter, called the Java Virtual Machine (JVM). .NET has its own compilers and a JVM equivalent called the Common Language Runtime (CLR). Both the compilers and the interpreters (JVM and CLR) are machine-specific executables. Java byte code and .NET CLR code, however, are portable and can be run on any hardware/operating system platform that supports the Java Virtual Machine or CLR, respectively.

The hybrid approach to programming language implementation is a compromise between a purely compiled and a purely interpreted implementation. The intermediate representation of the source program produced by the compiler (e.g. Java byte code) is easier and faster to interpret than the original source language program, which makes for faster programs and simpler interpreters. Programs in languages with hybrid implementations, however, are still slower than their purely compiled counterparts like C++. For most programs, however, this is not significant.

Object-Oriented Programming

Object-oriented programming is supported by object-oriented programming languages like C++, Java, and C#. Object-oriented programming facilitates code reusability by supporting five fundamental concepts: objects, classes, inheritance, polymorphism, and dynamic binding. While a detailed discussion of each is beyond the scope of this text, all except dynamic binding will be briefly explained. Extensive treatments of all of these concepts can be found elsewhere (4-7).

An *object* is a variable that has, in addition to data, associated semantics and functionality. Each object has a state, described by its *member data*, and each can be selectively manipulated by its interface, which are its *member functions*. For example, an object is like a telephone. It is not necessary to know how a telephone works in order to use it. All that is required is a basic knowledge of the interface: microphone, speaker, and keypad. The internal workings are hidden.

A *class* is a blueprint for an object. It specifies the types of member data and the member functions. Classes can be related to each other by *inheritance*. This is useful when objects of one class are "kinds-of" objects of another class. For example, in a program that draws on the screen, a class *Shape* with member function draw() might have child classes *Circle*, *Rectangle*, and *Triangle*.

Each child class must support every function of the class from which it was derived, the *parent class*. This is accomplished in one of two ways. If the function implementation of the child class is no different from the parent's, then the parent's implementation can be used by default. If, however, special requirements exist for the child class implementation, or if the parent class does not provide an implementation for the function, then the child class can specify the function implementation itself. For example, since the method for drawing a circle differs from the method for drawing a triangle, both the *Circle* and *Triangle* classes provide their own implementations for the parent-class function draw().

Polymorphism allows objects of a child class to be used as objects of its parent class. Continuing the previous example, a function that moves a shape on the screen can be specified broadly to use a *Shape* object. Since shape has child classes *Circle*, *Rectangle*, and *Triangle*, polymorphism allows the same function to move a circle, rectangle, or triangle. This eliminates the need for different move() functions for each type of shape. If another kind of shape class is added in the future, e.g. *Ellipse*, then it too can use the same function. This is an extremely powerful idea that allows for old code to use objects of future classes.

Developer's Toolkits

Software developer's toolkits (SDKs) and integrated development environments (IDEs) are software packages that contain everything needed to build application programs. SDKs and IDEs contain a compiler or interpreter, a debugging tool, an editor, libraries of reusable source code, and a GUI builder that allows the programmer to easily add graphical elements such as buttons, display boxes, and drop-down lists. While SDKs and IDEs are not necessary to build software, they make the process much easier.

A Survey of Popular Programming Languages

C

C is a compiled programming language that was developed at Bell Labs for the construction of the UNIX operating system. Many of C's features were borrowed from ALGOL 68 including block structure, recursion, dynamic memory allocation, machine independence, conditional expressions, and for-loops.

C is a very popular programming language, and much of its success can be attributed to its free distribution with UNIX. C is not, however, a beginner's programming language, since it requires familiarity with pointers and dynamic memory management. Still, C is very flexible, powerful, and popular. It also forms part of the basis of C++. Additionally, C compilers are widely available, including the free GNU C/C++ compiler *gcc* distributed with UNIX and Linux.

C++

C++ is a compiled, object-oriented programming language developed at Bell Labs. C++ was not designed as an object-oriented programming language from the ground up. Instead, C was used as the foundation, and object-oriented programming features were added. As a result, C is a subset of C++, and C++ compilers and SDKs can be used to develop C programs.

To program in C++, it is helpful to have knowledge of C, but not necessary. For those that do, the temptation to write C programs instead of object-oriented C++ programs must be avoided. For long-time C programmers, this is sometimes difficult.

Like C, C++ requires knowledge of pointers and memory management, which are often confusing for beginning programmers, and error prone for even experienced ones. If learning object-oriented programming is a goal, Java or C# is a better choice. Since C++ is compiled and not interpreted, its programs are faster than equivalent ones in Java or C#.

Good resources are available for the C++ programmer. Excellent books for both the motivated beginner and more experienced programmer include *Thinking in C++* by Bruce Eckel (7). Advanced authoritative texts include *The C++ Programming Language* by Bjarne Stroustrup, the creator of C++ (5).

C++ compilers, SDKs, and IDEs are available for nearly all computing platforms including UNIX, Windows, and Mac OS.

Java

Java is an object-oriented programming language for creating platform-independent, Internet and intranet applications. Developed by Sun Microsystems in the early 1990s, Java is an interpreted language that resembles C++ but has added features such as operating system independent multithreading, a singly-rooted class hierarchy, and platform-independent GUI classes.

The success of Java has been remarkable, and this can be attributed to several factors. First, Java is a full-featured, object-oriented programming language. Second, it resembles C++, but it is simpler. And third, it was designed from the beginning with platform-independent, network computing in mind.

While Java is ultimately an interpreted language, Java source code is compiled into an intermediate language called *byte code*. Byte code is run by the Java interpreter, known as the Java Virtual Machine, which is included in popular web browsers and operating system distributions. The Java Virtual Machine is also available as a *plug-in* for browsers that do not have one built in, and as a standalone executable for UNIX, Windows, and MacOS.

A Java program that runs in a web page is called an *applet*. When a Java-capable browser requests a web page that has an associated *applet*, the server sends the applet to the browser as byte code. The browser then starts the Java Virtual Machine and runs the applet, which appears on the web page. Therefore, a Java applet can run on any hardware/operating system platform so long as a Java-capable web browser is available for that platform. This browser-facilitated portability makes Java programs accessible across the Internet and allows program maintenance and distribution from a single location. When a new version of a Java program is released, it can be stored on one server and all users have access to it across the network. This paradigm of software development and distribution is very attractive for organizations that have many users of an application program. Instead of installing a copy of the software on each user's machine, the program can be made available as a Java applet stored on one intranet server.

Java also supports platform-independent database access through JDBC (Java Database Connectivity), a programming interface that allows Java programs to access data in relational databases such as Oracle, SQL Server, and Sybase. JDBC functionality is provided through the JDBC class library.

Java is an interpreted language. Therefore, programs in Java are slower than their C++ counterparts. If faster execution speed is needed, however, Java compilers that generate fast machine language executables are available. Unfortunately, the resultant executable programs, like C and C++ executables, are machine-specific and are not portable.

Java compilers, browser plug-ins, stand-alone interpreters, class libraries, online books, and documentation are all available free of charge from Sun Microsystems at www.java.sun.com. The Java Developer Kit (JDK), available at the same site, contains the latest compiler, interpreter, debugger, and class libraries all in one package. Excellent books include *Thinking in Java* (6,7) and an ongoing series published by Sun Microsystems Press (www.sun.com/books).

.NET

.NET is Microsoft's Java-like programming paradigm. Like Java, .NET uses an intermediate compiled language and an interpreter; however, in .NET the interpreter is called the Common Language Runtime. Unlike Java, .NET supports the compilation of several high-level programming languages including C# and Visual Basic. C# is an object-oriented programming language that resembles C++, and just like Java, hides pointers and memory management. Visual Basic (VB) is a popular programming language that is a descendent of BASIC (Beginner's All-purpose Symbolic Instruction Code). The latest versions of Visual Basic have also incorporated object-oriented programming features. C# and VB, like Java, are relatively easy to learn, and contain few of the complexities of C-like languages that confuse some beginning programmers. Unlike Java, .NET compilers and interpreters are currently only available for Windows-based computers. Java compilers and interpreters are available for nearly all OS and hardware platforms.

MUMPS

MUMPS (also known as M) is an interpreted, general-purpose programming language developed at the Massachusetts General Hospital Laboratory of Computer Science in the 1960s. MUMPS was designed for medical records processing, and supports some unique and sophisticated data handling features such as persistent variables, multi-dimensional associative arrays, and advanced string handling capabilities. MUMPS maintains a loyal following in the medical community.

Although MUMPS has its own database, it is not a relational database management system (RDBMS) like Oracle, Sybase, or Microsoft SQL Server. MUMPS does, however, support RDBMS access through embedded SQL and ODBC, like other popular programming languages. MUMPS databases, which are really persistent associative arrays, are highly-portable because they are composed of and indexed by a single data type: character strings. Therefore, a MUMPS database can be shared between MUMPS programs on radically different hardware/operating system platforms.

Versions of MUMPS are available for many popular operating systems including Windows, UNIX, and MacOS. A guide many MUMPS resources can be found at www.mcenter.com/mtrc/.

Web Scripting Languages

Web scripting languages such as JavaScript, VBScript, and Tcl/Tk are supported by web browsers and browser plug-ins. While they are not programming languages, per se, they are convenient and useful for creating interactive user interfaces on web pages. Although the same could be accomplished with Java, scripting languages are simpler, easier to learn, and easier to implement for certain routine web programming problems.

Summary

Knowledge of operating systems and programming languages is not required to understand, purchase, or use an EHR. A basic understanding of each, however, will provide valuable insights to the motivated practitioner and a better understanding and appreciation of computing.

References

1. Silberschatz A, Galvin P, Gagne G. Operating System Concepts, 7th ed. Reading, MA: Addison-Wesley Publishing;2005.
2. Mosberger D, Eranian S. ia-64 Linux Kernel: Design and Implementation, Upper Saddle River, NJ: Prentice Hall PTR;2002.
3. Aho AV, Sethi R, Ullman JD. Compilers: Principles, Techniques, and Tools. Reading, MA: Addison-Wesley Publishing;1986.
4. Cline MP, Lomow GA. C11 FAQs, 2nd ed. Reading, MA: Addison-Wesley Publishing;1998.
5. Stroustrup B. The C11 Programming Language, 3rd ed. Reading, MA: Addison-Wesley Publishing;1997.
6. Eckel B. Thinking in Java, 4th ed. Upper Saddle River, NJ: Prentice Hall PTR;2006.
7. Eckel B. Thinking in C11, 2nd ed. Upper Saddle River, NJ: Prentice Hall PTR;2001.

4

Databases, Warehouses, and Data Repositories

Ashwin B. Philar, MSEE, Jerome H. Carter, MD

D ata and information have become an integral component of human civilization. Over thousands of years of existence, through observation and measurements, humans have gathered data, which forms the basis of information.

With the rapid advancements in the fields of computing and technology over the past few decades, it is becoming easier to gather and store large amounts of data from disparate sources with relative ease. Whether it is businesses trying to maximize profits, astronomers looking for life on other planets, or clinical researchers searching for gene mutations, everyone has become dependent on data-driven electronic systems. Data-driven systems have become indispensable tools for the normal operation and advancement of society. Although data collection has become easier, organizing and storing data in a manner that supports effective processing and delivery is an on-going challenge.

Large database systems such as data repositories and data warehouses are technologies and tools designed to meet the need for information systems that are optimized for patient care and clinical research knowledge requirements.

Evolution of the Database

Herman Hollerith, an American statistician, who completed his PhD at Columbia University in 1890, developed the first "database" application using punched cards. This system was successfully used by the U.S. Census Bureau for the census of 1890, which was completed in 2.5 years compared to the 1880 census, which took almost 7 years to complete (1).

New inventions and discoveries in the field of computing led to advancements in the field of database technology in the 1950s. The earliest known use of the term "data base" was in June 1963, when the System Development Corporation sponsored a symposium under the title *Development and Management of a Computer-Centered Data Base*. **Database** as a single word became common in Europe in the early 1970s, and by the end of the decade it was being used in major American newspapers (2).

A *database model* can be described as a structure for organizing and managing data. Over the past five decades, numerous database models such as hierarchical, network, relational, and object-oriented have been invented. We will study these different database models in the coming sections.

Database Systems

Fundamental Concepts

Data: "Data" is plural for the Latin word *Datum*, which means a single piece of information. In the context of information technology, this word is now acceptably used as either singular or plural.

Field: If we wanted to discuss the properties of a book, a natural place to begin might be properties such as the title, publisher, number of pages, and reviewer rating. Each of these properties is referred to as a "field" or an "attribute" in the world of databases.

Record: A record is a collection of fields. Every record of the same type has identical fields.

Database: In its simplest form, a database is a collection of records. In relational database models, databases consist of a collection of one or more tables where each table is a collection of records of the same type.

Models

Flat File Database

A flat file database is the most basic form of database and is conceptually similar to the punched card system developed by Herman Hollerith. It consists of a single file (e.g., collection of data) that contains many records: the fields of each record may be of fixed width, where the fixed width could be achieved by padding data with spaces, or the fields of the record may vary in size, in which case they may be separated by a field separator such as a comma. A flat file database containing patient information where the fields are of fixed width is shown Figure 4-1, and one where fields are delimited using a comma is shown in Figure 4-2.

Flat file databases provide the minimum functionality for organizing, managing, and analyzing data and are generally used for simple information needs such as mailing lists. Flat file databases are often used for simple data transfers between systems.

00001	John	Doe
00002	Mike	Gates
00003	Bill	Buffet
00004	Joey	Geller

Figure 4-1   Flat file data layout, fixed width.

Hierarchical Database

The next step in database evolution was the hierarchal database model, developed in the late 1950s. It allowed data to be organized in a hierarchical fashion in the form of a tree. This model permitted a single parent record to have many child records.

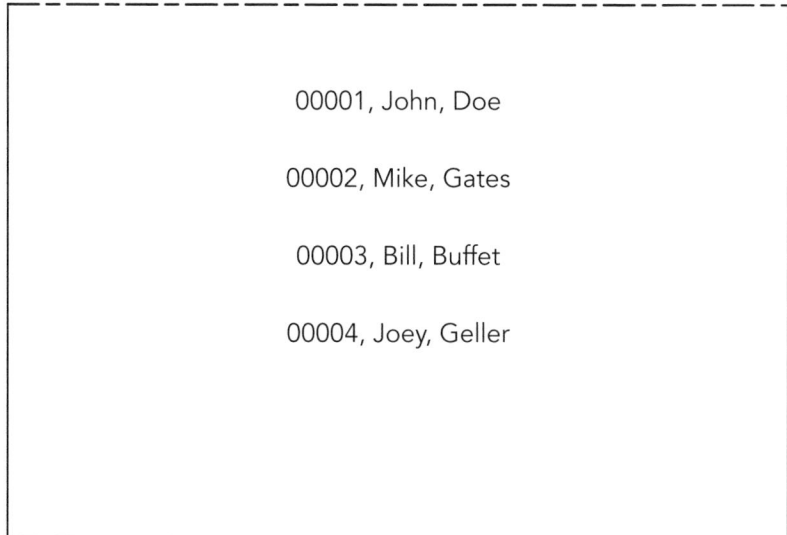

00001, John, Doe

00002, Mike, Gates

00003, Bill, Buffet

00004, Joey, Geller

Figure 4-2   Flat-file comma delimited.

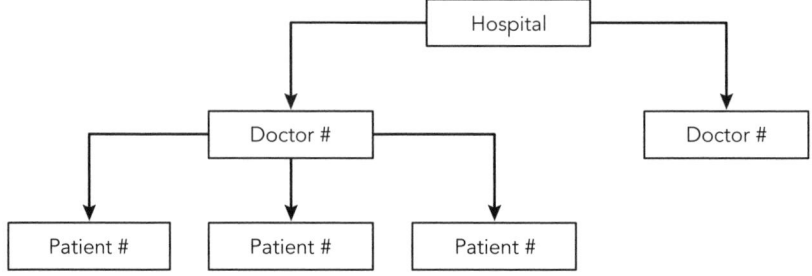

Figure 4-3 Hierarchical database structure.

Figure 4-3 shows how data about doctors, patients, and medications are organized using a hierarchical data model. A hospital (parent) has many doctors (children), and each doctor (parent) can attend to many patients (children).

Although this model facilitates a one-to-many relationship between records (i.e., a parent record can have many child records), it does not allow a child to have more that one parent; thus, if a patient were to see more than one doctor this data model would be incapable of depicting this relationship.

Network Database

Charles Bachman, a prominent computer scientist, invented the network database model, which was later developed into a standard specification published in 1969 by the Conference on Data Systems Languages (CODASYL) Consortium.

The network model proposed a structure for organizing data that could easily represent and clearly describe real world entities (people, places, and things) and the relationships between them.

This model overcame the limitations of the hierarchical model: not only could a parent have many children but the child itself could have multiple parents. For example, the fact that a patient (child) can have multiple doctors (parent) or that a doctor (child) can work at many hospitals (parent) can be easily stored in a network database as shown in Figure 4-4.

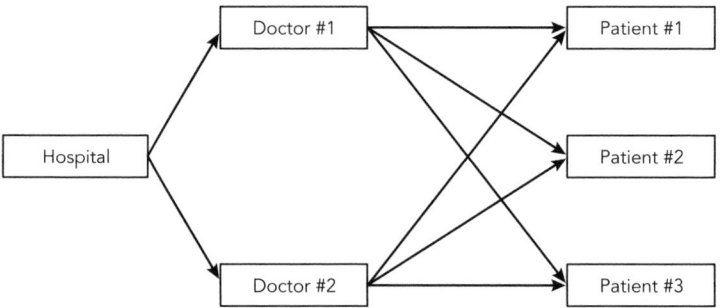

Figure 4-4 Network model database structure.

Although the network model was successful in overcoming the challenges of the hierarchical model, it did not become a popular model for storing data because of resistance on the part of the database vendors to change a profitable product and because of the advent of the more capable and powerful relational model.

Relational Database

E.F. Codd, a British computer scientist, created the relational model for organizing data and introduced it in an academic paper in June 1970 (3).

Hierarchical and network database models presented major challenges to users in terms of data retrieval. In both models accessing data required a deep knowledge of the structure of the database. Retrieving data from a database with thousands of parent and child records required understanding all the links between them well enough to write a computer program that would correctly identify and access each record. This proved to be a very time consuming and problematic task for all but the simplest databases. The relational model sought to make it possible to accurately retrieve data without the user having to know the exact manner in which the data were ordered, indexed or connected (3).

The goal of the relational data model was to describe data in a more natural form without additional structural changes for storing it in a computer system (3). The relational model aimed to separate the concepts of data access from the actual relationships that existed between the entities (3). In the relational model, E.F. Codd eliminated these dependencies, thereby addressing a major weakness of the hierarchical and network models.

A relational database is made up of relations, also called tables. These relations are made up of attributes, also called columns or fields, and the domain (number, text, date), which defines the values that the attributes are allowed to take. Relations (tables) may represent an entity (person, place, or thing) or the result of an interaction (event or transaction) between two or more entities. For example, assume that Patient and Formulary represent two entities. Medication History would then be a relation (table) representing the interaction between them (Figure 4-5). The main advantage of a relational database design is that neither the order of the fields in a record nor the order of the records within a table is important when storing or retrieving data. The most important concept in this database model is not the table itself but the ease with which relationships may be defined between tables (relations/entities).

Keys

As a rule every record in a relational database must be uniquely identifiable. This is accomplished through the use of a *Primary Key*. The primary key is formed using one field, or a combination of fields in a record. Medical record numbers and social security numbers are examples of fields that

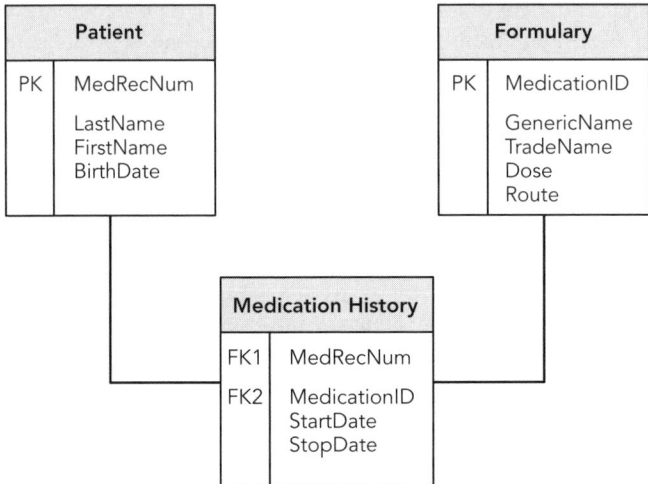

Figure 4-5   Foreign keys from patient and formulary tables to medication history table.

could be used in a demographics table as primary keys because no two people should have the same number. When two tables are used to create a relationship, each provides a copy of its primary key to a third table that represents the relationship. The primary keys that are now located in the newly created table are referred to as *Foreign Keys*. This is illustrated in Figure 4-5 where the Patient table uses the Medical Record Number as the primary key and the Formulary table uses Medication ID. Both tables participate in the relation "Medication History", which has MedRecNum and MedicationID as foreign keys.

The challenge in designing a relational database system is in organizing the data in tables so there is minimal or preferably no redundant information in the database (the same data should not exist in multiple tables) and so relationships between tables represent correct and important concepts in the real world, a process referred to as *data modeling*.

The process of eliminating redundancy in a database is referred to as *normalization*. There are multiple levels to which a database can be normalized; these levels are called *normal forms*. E.F. Codd proposed the three main normal forms, namely, the *first normal form, second normal form,* and the *third normal form,* and as of today, there are eight different normal forms (4,5). *De-normalization* is the exact opposite process of normalization, where it sometimes becomes necessary to de-normalize a database to improve efficiency by reducing joins (connections made between tables to answer a query).

Data stored in a database, however organized and clean as it might be, is useless until it can be extracted and combined to form useful information. Structured English Query Language (SEQUEL; commonly referred to

Name	DOB	Medication1	Medication2
Doe, John	1/1/1960	Acetaminophen	Cough syrup
Gates, Warren	1/1/1975	Cimetidine	Ibuprofen
Doe, John	1/1/1960	Acetaminophen	Aspirin
Gates, Warren	1/1/1975	Mouthwash	Saline

Figure 4-6 Non-normalized relational table.

as "SQL") has been standardized as the language for manipulating data stored in a relational database (6). SQL is the language used for all database-related operations, whether it is adding new rows, deleting existing rows, modifying existing rows, creating tables, deleting tables, joining tables, etc.

Figure 4-6 shows a medication history table that has not been normalized. It contains a table that has the patient data and the patient's medication data stored in a single table. Notice that patient "Warren Gates" appears twice (redundancy).

Figure 4-7 shows the same database in third normal form where there are three separate tables (Patients, Formulary, Medication History). The first table contains only the patient data, the second table contains only the formulary data, and the third table relates the patient data with the medication data (Medication History).

Patient ID	First Name	Last Name	DOB
1	John	Doe	1/1/1960
2	Warren	Gates	1/1/1975

Patient

Medication ID	Name	Route
1	Acetaminophen	PO
2	Cimetidine	PO
3	Acetaminophen	PO
4	Mouthwash	PO
5	Cough Syrup	PO

Formulary

Patient ID	MedicationID	StartDate	StopDate
1	1	05/01/2006	
1	5	03/01/2007	
2	2	10/21/2005	05/01/2006

Medication History

Figure 4-7 Third normal form relational tables derived from Figure 4-6.

Object-Oriented Databases

The object-oriented paradigm for building computer programs was widely adopted in the 1990s. Here, computer programs are designed using objects (collections of data and programs), which aim to model real world objects in terms of their properties and behavior (7).

The fundamental concepts of object-oriented systems are classes and inheritance. A *class* is an abstract representation of a real world entity that includes the characteristics as well as the behavior of the entity. An *object* is a particular instance or example of a class. Classes have *methods,* which are functions that object of the class can perform.

Class: Patient

Properties: Name

   Address

   Phone

   Medical Record Number

Methods: Take Medication

   Make Appointment

For example, we can create a class called *Patient* having characteristics (properties) such as first name, last name, medical record number etc. and can perform functions (methods) such as "take medication". Any patient could then be represented by a patient object in a computer program, where the characteristics of the patient would be set based upon the actual patient.

Object: Patient

   123 Elm

   555-555-5555

   123456

Methods: Take Medication

   Make Appointment

Object-oriented databases excel at managing data that are not easily represented as rows and columns such as maps. Objects allow modeling of complex hierarchies, aggregates, and other data associations that are very difficult to do efficiently in relational databases. Even so, relational databases still dominate the data management landscape.

Data Dictionary

During the process of creating a data model, entities, relationships between the various identities, types of data associated with the entities, and descriptions of the entities are identified. This collection of information is very useful as a reference when building applications that interact with the database and is referred to as a *data dictionary*. The data dictionary concept has been expanded in many health care environments to encompass more than one database. Clinical data dictionaries are enterprise-level data stores that contain information about key data elements across different databases and applications (8). Clinical terminologies are but one example of the type of data that may be found in a clinical data dictionary.

Database Management Systems

A database management system (DMBS) is a software system that is used for managing a database. A DBMS includes a modeling language, data structures, a database query language, and a transactional mechanism (9). Oracle, DB2, Postgres, MySQL, and SQL Server are examples of DMBSs.

A DBMS provides mechanisms for creating a database, managing the storage of database files on physical storage media, and managing the security of the database in terms of controlling who can access the database and what operations a user may perform on the database. It also provides a query (SQL) language that can be used to perform various operations such as inserting, updating, deleting, and retrieving data. The DBMS also provides features that ensure the integrity of the data stored in a database in situations where many people are performing operations on the same data at the same time.

Database Technology in Healthcare

In its report, *To Err Is Human: Building a Safer Health System*, the Institute of Medicine estimates that 44,000 to 98,000 Americans die in hospitals each year as a result of medical errors that could have been prevented (10). Health care providers are under increased pressure to enhance clinical productivity, reduce medical errors, improve quality of care, improve quality of life, and reduce the cost of care. As a result there is an increasing emphasis on using information technology for error reduction and quality improvement. Access to timely and accurate patient information and medical knowledge that is harmonious with clinical workflow is critical to providing quality care.

Sophisticated medical research that collects thousands of data values across a range of clinical variables also relies on DBMSs to meet its data management requirements. Clinical research databases, electronic health records (EHRs), clinical data repositories, and data warehouses have become foundational components of advanced clinical information systems that are appearing in major hospitals and health centers nationwide.

Evolution

In the 1960s as computer technology started developing, many hospitals began using computerized systems for automating payroll and patient accounting functions. The focus was on building a hospital information system as a way to manage hospital administrative information and little attention was given to development of clinical information systems to support patient care (11).

As computer technology evolved during the 1970s, computers became widely available and affordable, which encouraged small physician practices, clinics, and hospitals to embrace information systems. Some clinical systems were developed for laboratory systems, radiology departments, and pharmacies (11). In the 1970s, two separate approaches for building the hospital information system began to develop. One proposed the development of a single computer that would host multiple clinical applications, and the other supported the idea of hosting individual special applications on smaller computers. The common idea between the two approaches was to use a central database for storing patient information.

With the development of microchips, personal computers, and networking technology in the 1980s, computer technology and applications became affordable to individuals. The use of personal computers for practice management in a physician's office became very common during the 1980s.

The healthcare information systems scene changed dramatically during the 1990s. The emphasis was on building clinical information systems for managing patient care, improving the quality of medical research, and building decision support systems for helping clinicians in the management of diseases. Advancements in the fields of telecommunications, networking, and the Internet contributed to the development of distributed clinical information systems and made collaboration on multiple levels over geographically disparate locations a reality.

Clinical Database Applications

EHRs are the highest profile clinical database application. The architecture of EHR applications depends largely on where they are deployed. Generally they can be divided into two groups: ambulatory systems and hospital-based or enterprise systems.

EHR systems intended for use in outpatient settings are usually composed of two major components: the underlying database and the user interface. With few exceptions, the database component is based on the relational model and consists of tables organized around common medical record concepts. Typical table groups would be laboratory, diagnoses, medications, demographics, referrals, etc., with each group consisting of sub-tables that represent key relationships (medication list, allergies, problem list, etc.) (Figure 4-8). Even simple EHRs may have 100 or more tables.

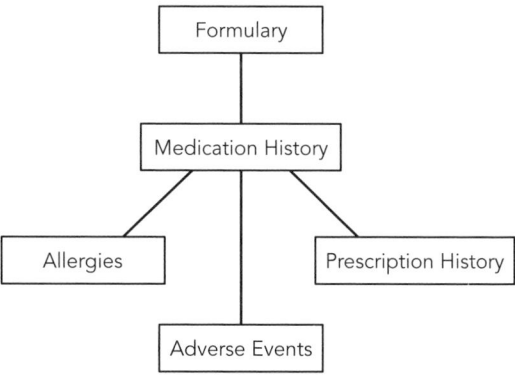

Figure 4-8 Medications table sub-group.

Outpatient EHRs are stand-alone systems and have relatively simple external interfaces (e.g., EKG, clinical laboratory downloads, practice management system). This permits the design of the database component to remain uncomplicated.

Inpatient EHRs are much more complex in design and have at their core clinical data repositories (CDR) Figure 4-9. A CDR is a:

> real-time database that consolidates data from a variety of clinical sources to present a unified view of a single patient. It is optimized to allow clinicians to retrieve data for a single patient rather than to identify a population of patients with common characteristics or to facilitate the management of a specific clinical department. Typical data types that are often found within a CDR include: clinical laboratory test results, patient demographics, pharmacy information, radiology reports and images, pathology reports, hospital admission/discharge/transfer dates, ICD-9 codes, discharge summaries, and progress notes". (12)

CDRs grew out of the need to integrate data from departmental systems (e.g., pharmacy, laboratory, radiology, etc.) into a central data store that would make it easier to access patient information. Due to its role as an integrator of patient data from disparate systems, CDR designs must address a number of issues in areas such as clinical concepts, terminology, and patient identifiers.

Clinical Concepts

Data amassed from multiple systems may have very different ways of representing the same information. For example, some lab systems may report using CPT Codes, while others use Logical Observation Identifiers Names and Codes (LOINC). More subtle discrepancies are possible: some systems may capture patient first and last name as one data field, while others may use a separate field for each name. Keeping track of the meaning, origin,

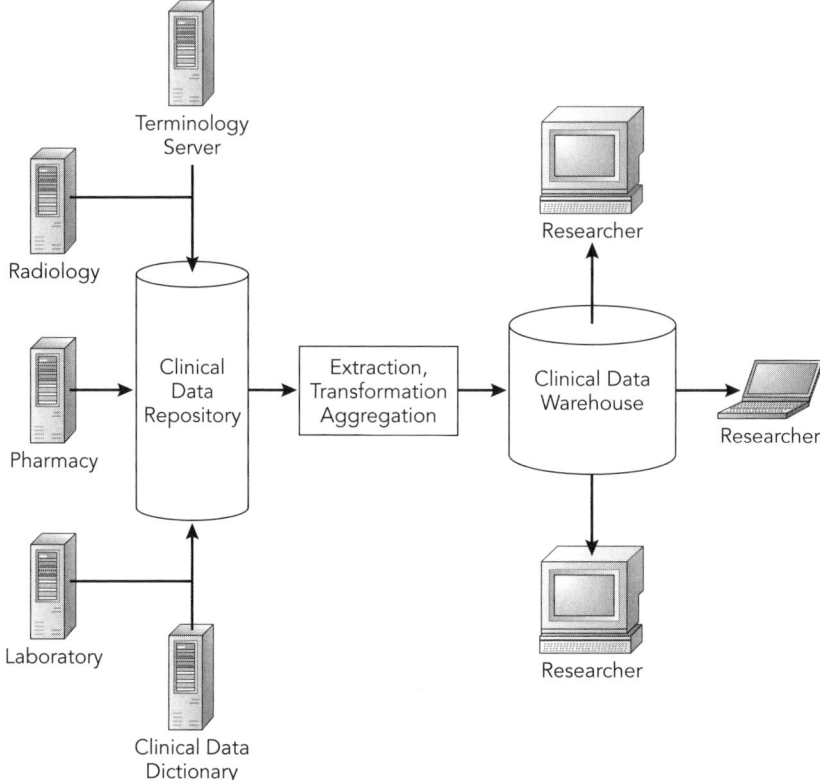

Figure 4-9   Clinical data repository and data warehouse.

and characteristics of all data elements is the job of the clinical data dictionary (CDD). CDDs are specialized databases that manage information about the data (meta-data) in the CDR. The best known example of a CDD is the Medical Entities Dictionary of Columbia–Presbyterian and New York–Cornell Medical Centers. The MED currently contains over 100,000 concepts and adds approximately 6,000 new concepts each year (13).

Vocabulary and Terminology

Standard codes and classifications such as ICD and CPT have been around for a while and are widely used. However, as more clinical information is obtained from doctors, nurses, and other care providers a more expressive vocabulary is required to capture the data contained in patient documentation. Terminology servers, computer systems dedicated to managing terms used in clinical descriptions, are becoming more common as attempts to capture granular data for outcomes analyses increases (14,15). SNOMED-CT, a clinical terminology consisting of over 300,000 terms, has been adopted by the federal government as the official terminology for EHRs (16). Managing terms sets is more difficult than might be expected due to the laxity permitted in human languages (17). Here is a simple example to explain the problem. Consider a term such as "resting blood pressure". In reading this, a specific set of concepts comes to mind. However, they are not likely to be the same for everyone. Does "resting" mean sitting, lying down, or simply standing still for a while? Each of these positions could affect the blood pressure reading. Yet, each does conform to some idea of resting. Lack of a standardized language is a major barrier to seemless data sharing between different computer systems and institutions. Even with the availability of SNOMED it continues to be an ongoing challenge (18,19).

Patient Identifiers

The ability to uniquely identify every patient is essential to safe high-quality care, making duplicate patient identifiers a particularly dangerous problem. Patients in large health systems may seek care at many different sites and, regardless of the degree of patient movement throughout the system, proper identification must be ensured. Additionally, organizations may have many different sets of demographics information and may use different sets of attributes to uniquely identify each patient in the database. In order to be able to store this patient data from multiple online databases, there is a need to create a master patient index (a software system that uses special algorithms to assign and cross-check patient identifiers). This master patient index will assign a global unique identifier to all the patient records while maintaining their original database identifiers.

Clinical Data Warehouses

As organizations evolve and grow, so do the databases that they use to store patient-related data. Often data is stored in databases of different computer systems (pharmacy, radiology, laboratory), and in the course of time they become islands of information. As the amount of data in these systems grows, the level of effort and time required to prepare data for analysis becomes more difficult. However, if data are collected, cleaned (a process of ensuring that data is complete and free of errors), aggregated, and stored in a manner that makes analysis easier, questions concerning important issues such as cost, quality, and safety become much easier to answer. This is the essence of a clinical data warehouse.

The term "data warehouse" was coined by William Inmon in 1990 and is defined as a "subject-oriented, integrated, time-variant and non-volatile collection of data in support of management's decision making process" (20). Stated less technically, a data warehouse is a collection of data extracted from a variety of sources within an organization that is set aside specifically for the purpose of asking questions to support decision making.

Clinical Data Warehouse vs. Clinical Data Repository

Clinical data repositories consist of data received from a number of systems and integrated to provide patient information to clinicians as they are in the process of providing care (i.e., real-time). The clinical data repository is where a provider goes to find the latest laboratory result, current medication list, and other information required to deliver care. Clinical data repositories are designed to deliver data for only one patient at a time.

Clinical data warehouses, on the other hand, are not intended for use during the process of care. Rather, they are used to answer population-level questions. Data are moved to the clinical data warehouse on a scheduled basis (weekly, monthly, quarterly), depending on the question the clinical data warehouse was designed to answer. Patient data in clinical data warehouses are population-based and often have most identifier information removed, making it difficult or impossible to identify a specific patient. Providers would access data in a clinical data warehouse only when they have questions that apply to a group of patients. For example, if you wanted to know Ms. Jones' most recent blood glucose level, you would use the clinical data repository. If you wanted to know the average blood glucose level for every patient admitted for the last year, you would go to the clinical data warehouse.

Evolution

In the mid-1970s, rapid advancements in the field of storage technologies led to the development of Direct Access Storage Devices (DASD). This technology was far superior compared to the magnetic tape technology that was prevalent at that time. The only way to access the data stored on magnetic tapes was to start at the beginning of the tape and continue until the desired data were located, whereas data stored on a DASD could be directly accessed. This drastically reduced the time for locating a record to the order of a few milliseconds. The availability of storage devices that supported rapid searching of large data sets encouraged the development of very powerful and capable database systems. During the mid 1970s, high-performance transaction systems that provided fast access to data became very popular and were adopted by large businesses and became known as Online Transaction Processing Systems (OLTP). OLTP systems were used for key business applications such as airline reservation systems, banking systems, and retail purchasing (Table 4-1).

With advances in the field of computer technology and computer programming languages in the 1980s, it became obvious that computerized database systems could be used for more than just routine data entry. Soon, the idea that transaction data could be analyzed and used as an aid to decision making caught on, and online analytic processing (OLAP) and data warehouses were born. These new technologies contributed to the devel-

Table 4-1

UNDERSTANDING DATA WAREHOUSES: OLTP vs OLAP

Online Transaction Processing (OLTP)	A "transaction" occurs when data is either written to or read from a database. Databases were used to design applications that did thousands of transactions per second such as bankteller systems, airline reservations, and computerized cash registers. These came to be known as Online Transaction Processing Systems.
Online Analytic Processing (OLAP)	Databases with large collections of transaction data contain information potentially useful for decision making. The process of using these large databases for analysis/decision-making is referred to as "Online Analytic Processing".

opment of Management Information Systems, which are now commonly known as Decision Support Systems and were used to produce sophisticated reports that drove management decisions.

After a while it became clear that a single database was incapable of supporting both the routine operations of the organization and the analytic processing required for decision making. This led to the development of a process whereby data would be extracted from an online transaction database to an offline analysis database where it could be reviewed without slowing the performance of transaction databases. However, the extraction process was rarely well thought out. In many companies that made use of OLAP, "spider webs" were created. Spider webs arise when data extracts are taken predominantly from other extracts instead of the original OLTP system. Eventually the origin and credibility of the data are called into question. This haphazard process of data extractions came to be known as the "naturally evolving architecture" (20).

The naturally evolving architecture was, of course, plagued with numerous problems such as a lack of data credibility (too many data sets of questionable origin and content) and loss of productivity (managing multiple extracts from different departments), resulting in the inability to readily transform data into information.

The architected environment was a reaction to the lack of a standardized way of creating data stores for analysis. In the architected environment, there are four levels of data: the operational level (day-to-day data from business applications), the atomic or data warehouse level (granular data for analysis), the departmental (data owned by an organizational unit) or data mart level, and the individual level (data used by someone answering a question, ad-hoc) (20). An orderly process is used whereby data is extracted from multiple databases, cleaned, transformed, and loaded into a data warehouse for analysis. Data is periodically refreshed so that decisions can be made based on the most recent data, and older data is purged and archived on a regular basis (21). Figure 4-9 shows a generic information systems layout for a hospital or integrated delivery system consisting of operational systems (laboratory, pharmacy, radiology), CDR, and data warehouse.

Building a Data Warehouse

Modeling for a data warehouse is different from modeling for transaction processing databases. Whereas OLTP systems are designed with the goal of optimizing reading and writing speed through the process of normalization, OLAP systems are read-only in regular use and are usually denormalized so that they are optimized to answer questions. The standard data modeling technique used when building data warehouses is dimensional modeling using the star schema (Figure 4-10).

Dimensional Modeling

Star schemas generally include two types of tables: facts and dimensions. Fact tables contain the measurements, metrics, or facts of the business process and correspond to the *how much* or *how many* aspects of a ques-

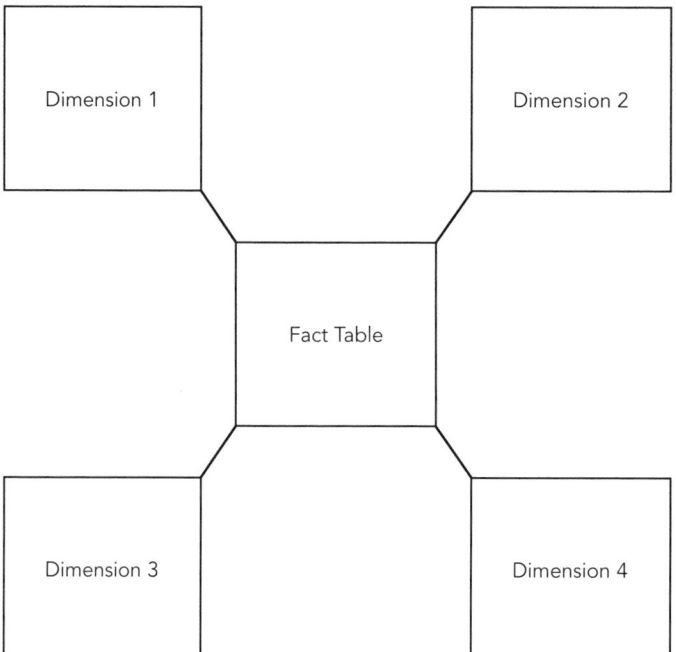

Figure 4-10 Generic start schema.

tion. Fact tables consist of foreign keys plus the information of interest to the data warehouse user (Figure 4-10). The dimension tables are companions to the fact tables. They provide summarized, "reference" information that helps to fully explain the facts to which they are linked (22). By using this model it is possible to step through the fact table one record at a time and easily view all data related to that record. This model makes querying simpler. This is best understood through a simple case study.

STUDY CASE

Integrated Delivery Systems, Inc., a health network consisting of a hospital and five outpatient sites, wishes to review antibiotic use due to concerns about over-prescribing for upper respiratory infections (URIs) (sinusitis, pharyngitis, common cold, laryngitis). The hospital is paperless and has a clinical data repository that contains radiology, laboratory, pharmacy, Admission-Discharge-Transfer (ADT), computerized physician order entry (CPOE), and clinical documentation data. All outpatient sites use the same EHR system, which is run from a central location using an application service provider model. They decide to build a data warehouse to answer the following series of questions:

1. How often are antibiotics prescribed for URIs?

2. What percentage of those patients have negative cultures?

3. How often are cultures taken for a diagnosis of sinusitis?

4. Are patients who present to the emergency department more likely to have a URI that requires an antibiotic than those who present to their primary care providers?

5. What are the annual costs of URI diagnoses in terms of antibiotics, lab costs, and number of emergency department and primary care visits?

Data warehouse designers use a star schema to model the important facts and dimensions. Since there is an interest in relating antibiotics to URI diagnoses, which occur mainly in an outpatient setting, the decision is made to use Patient Visits as the "fact" table and Antibiotic, Patient, Visit Location, Provider, Diagnosis, and Test Result as dimensions. Figure 4-11 shows the final schema.

Data Warehousing Issues

Problems such as patient identifiers, clinical concepts, and terminology are issues for all clinical databases. Even so, data warehouses present additional data and technology related concerns (21,22).

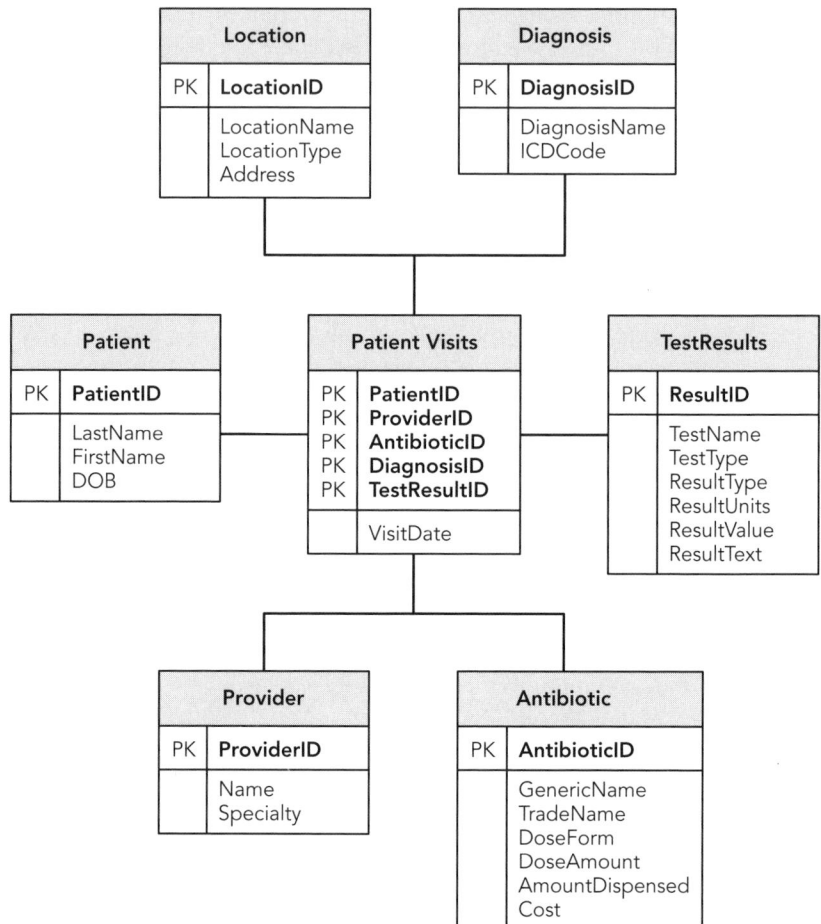

Figure 4-11   Star schema for data warehouse case study.

Technology Integration

A major challenge in creating a data warehouse is the integration of technologies. Billing systems, accounting and other legacy systems may reside on minicomputers and use older database models. Exporting data from these systems can be quite problematic due to obsolete data formats, poor communications capability of older computers systems, and outmoded programming languages and tools.

Data Loading

The data warehouse has to be loaded with data from archival systems, and current operational databases. The main challenge is determining what has changed in operational and archival systems since the last refresh to the data warehouse which may included new data types as well as new data (20).

Data Temporal Properties

Temporal relationships are extremely important in healthcare. The time between an intervention such as drug dosing and a change in patient status (e.g., skin rash) is a major factor in medical reasoning. Typical retail and banking data, for which data warehouses were originally created, are much simpler and the time dependencies for data elements are less important. When data is moved from operational systems to data warehouses, many of these temporal relationships are lost or are too difficult to model (23).

Data Accuracy

Missing or incorrect data is always a problem. Data validation and integrity checking must occur at the operational level. Once data is removed from operational systems and arrives at the data warehouse, it is too late to capture missing values or to catch and correct errors without a significant amount of extra time and effort. This makes data warehouses very sensitive to deficiencies in front-end systems (24,25).

Variety of Data Types

There are many types of medical data (numeric, images, text, sound, and combinations of the four), making it difficult to create a data structure that contains all the pertinent data about a patient. This can be seen in the example of a complete blood count. Some data are numeric (white blood cell count), while others are text based (peripheral smear report). In situations in which it is important to know not only cell counts but also to have descriptions of the data, creating an efficient structure to allow for OLAP is challenging.

Data Granularity

Since there are no standards for recording medical data, the issue of having data of the required granularity for analysis is a problem. Common clinical concepts are often captured differently, leading to difficulties when combing data for analysis. For example, patient medication data may be recorded in the form of 1) a medication list (drug with start and stop dates); 2) a prescription history (each time the drug was prescribed); 3) a dispensing history (each time the patient obtained the medication); or 4) an administration history (each time the patient was given the medication) (25,26).

Regulatory Issues

Data collected for internal quality improvement efforts does not require any additional approvals on the part of the patient. However, if data sets are used for formal research studies, often patient approval is required. This will create a problem unless approval was obtained at the time of data collection. Obviously, attempting to determine which patients provided approval for any particular use of the data is a difficult problem to sort out at the level of the data warehouse, making this a major issue for those building data warehouses (25).

Technical Skills

A data warehouse is more than just a big database. Building a clinical data warehouse will require the input of database administrators, programmers, administrators, clinical researchers, and statisticians in order to ensure that the data and the structure of the warehouse are capable of answering the questions being posed. Because data warehousing is fairly new in most clinical environments, many organizations do not have all required skills on hand.

Future Trends

Database servers and database management systems are becoming more and more powerful and sophisticated with improvements in technology. The latest version of Microsoft's SQL Server database empowers database developers to write database objects such as stored procedures using mainstream high-level programming languages. It has also added the capability of making database functionality available over the internet as web services.

Extended Markup Language (XML) and related technologies are becoming standards when it comes to data interchange between various systems. XML is an open standard that is driven by the users and simplifies the processes of storage, extraction, transformation, delivery, and sharing of data across heterogeneous database systems.

Open source is a relatively new concept in the information technology industry whereby the software code of sophisticated software products is managed by a community instead of a particular organization. The popularity of open source database products is rapidly growing in the industry, and these systems are becoming powerful and capable of meeting data storage and management needs of larger organizations.

Summary

In this chapter, we have seen how database technology has evolved during the past five decades and how clinical databases are helping to shape the future of health care. Clinical data repositories and data warehouses are enabling health care organizations to use data to guide clinical and administrative decision-making in a manner that is impossible using paper-based record systems.

Given the advances of the past 10 years, it is reasonable to be guardedly optimistic about the future. New analytical tool sand database models will play a major role in transforming health care into a more consistently reproducible activity. They may provide a means of capturing in analyzable form the many variables that allow us to understand what is safe, effective, and appropriate.

References

1. http://en.wikipedia.org/wiki/Flat_file_database, 01/14/2007.
2. http://en.wikipedia.org/wiki/Database, 01/21/2007.
3. Codd EF. A relational model of data for large shared data banks. Communications of the ACM. 1970;13:6.
4. Kent W. A simple guide to five normal forms in relational database theory. Communications of the ACM. 1983;26:1205.
5. http://en.wikipedia.org/wiki/Database_normalization, 01/21/2007.
6. King K, Jamsa K, eds. SQL Tips and Techniques. 2002. ISBN:1931841454.
7. Kim W. Introduction to Object-Oriented Databases. The MIT Press; 1990. ISBN 0-262-11124-1.
8. AHIMA e-HIM Work Group on EHR Data Content. Guidelines for developing a data dictionary. Journal AHIMA. 2006;77:64A-D.
9. http://en.wikipedia.org/wiki/Database_management_system, 1/22/2007
10. Corrigan JM, Donaldson MS, Kohn LT, et al for the Committee on Quality of Health Care in America. To Err is Human: Building a Safer Health System. Washington, D.C.: National Academy Press; 2000.
11. Austin CJ, Boxerman SB. Information Systems for Healthcare Management, 6th ed. Health Administration Press. Foundation of the American College of Healthcare Executives; 2003. ISBN:1567932029
12. Sittig DF, Pappas J , Rubalcaba P. Building and using a clinical data repository, http://www.informatics-review.com/thoughts/cdr.html. Accessed May 25, 2007.
13. Cimino JJ. From data to knowledge through concept-oriented terminologies: experience with the Medical Entities Dictionary. J Am Med Inform Assoc. 2000;7:288-97.
14. Rosenbloom ST, Miller RA, Johnson KB, et al. Interface terminologies: facilitating direct entry of clinical data into electronic health record systems. J Am Med Inform Assoc. 2006;13:277-88. Epub 2006 Feb 24. Review.
15. Chute CG, Elkin PL, Sherertz DD, Tuttle MS. Desiderata for a clinical terminology server. Proc AMIA Symp. 1999;42-6.
16. Chalmers RJG. Health care terminology for the electronic era. Mayo Clin Proc. 2006;81:619-24.
17. Chute CG. Standards move to center stage. MD Computing. 1999;29-32.
18. Chiang MF, Hwang JC, Yu AC, et al. Reliability of SNOMED-CT coding by three physicians using two terminology browsers. AMIA Annu Symp Proc. 2006;131-5.
19. Andrews JE, Richesson RL, Krischer J. Variation of SNOMED CT coding of clinical research concepts among coding experts. J Am Med Inform Assoc. 2007.
20. Inmon WH. Building the Data Warehouse, 4th ed. 2005. ISBN: 0764599445.
21. Chaudhuri S, Dayal U. An overview of data warehousing and OLAP technology. ACM SIGMOD Record. 1997;26:65-74.
22. Pavliashvili B. Dimensional databases: building a data warehouse, http://www.phptr.com/articles/article.asp?p=336255&rl=1. Accessed 5/25/2007.

23. Pedersen TB, Jensen CS. Research issues in clinical data warehousing. Scientific and Statistical Database Management, 1998. Proceedings. Tenth International Conference. 1-3 Jul 1998;:43-52.

24. Stein HD, Nadkarni P, Erdos J, Miller PL. Exploring the degree of concordance of coded and textual data in answering clinical queries from a clinical data repository. J Am Med Inform Assoc. 2000;7:42-54.

25. Wisniewski MF, Kieszkowski P, Zagorski BM, Trick WE, et al. Development of a clinical data warehouse for hospital infection control. J Am Med Inform Assoc. 2003;10:454-62.

26. Gray GW. Challenges of building clinical data analysis solutions. J Crit Care. 2004;19:264-70.

5

Internet and Intranet Technologies

Daniel R. Masys, MD

During the past decade, the Internet is one of two technologies (the other being cell phones) that have altered the nature of human existence on a global scale. With over a billion users worldwide (1), the Internet holds both promise and peril for electronic medical records. This chapter will give the reader an overview of how the Internet works, its technical vocabulary, and the strengths and weaknesses it brings to medical applications. Special variations on Internet technology, called Intranets and Virtual Private Networks, will be described, along with current and evolving standards for communicating both data and computer programs over the Internet.

History of the Internet

Much of the power and usefulness of computers derives from their ability to share and retrieve information as needed via data networks. The term "internet" is a short form of "internetwork," and was originally used to describe any network that connected two or more computer networks to each other. Internetworks and today's Internet have their historical roots in the 1960s, when computers were expensive and "few and far between". The problem of creating communications to and among computers that did not suffer from single points of potential failure was the subject of a series of seminal theoretical papers by researchers at the Massachusetts Institute of Technology and the RAND Corporation in 1961 and 1962 (2). These treatises proposed the idea of "packet-switching" networks, built on the idea of an electronic envelope or packet containing a destination address, a return address, and up to a few hundred bytes of data. These packets would be passed via what might be thought of as a "bucket brigade" of specialized computers called routers, whose job would be to read the address information on the packet and send it to the next router on the route to its final destination. Multiple routes would be available to each router, so that if a single line failed the router would simply re-route the packet via a different route.

In 1968, the Advanced Research Projects Agency (ARPA) of the U.S. Defense Department initiated a project to build a network using these design principles. This new network, called the ARPANET, became a reality with the connection of computers at four research sites: UCLA, the Stanford Research Institute, UC Santa Barbara, and the University of Utah. In 1971 there were fifteen "nodes", i.e., participating computers on the ARPANET; by 1972 there were thirty-seven. By the second year of operation, however, an interesting phenomena emerged. ARPANET's users developed tools to turn the computer-sharing network into a dedicated, high-speed, federally subsidized electronic post-office. The main traffic on ARPANET was not long-distance computing. Instead, it was news and personal messages. Researchers were using ARPANET to collaborate on projects, trade notes on work, and engage in informal "conversations". This unexpected and personal focus of network usage was a harbinger of events that would occur on a much larger scale two decades later.

The technical building blocks of the Internet as we know it today evolved quickly. In 1974, the creation of a set of rules for movement of packets throughout the network called the "Transmission Control Program/Internet Protocol" (TCP/IP) were developed and published as an open standard that replaced the original ARPANET technology in 1983, and flourishes today as the basis for communications among billions of computers worldwide.

The specifications for network functions essential to today's Internet were developed in the 1980s and 1990s. These included the "Domain Name Service" (DNS), a form of "white pages" directory service that translates human-readable computer names (e.g., google.com) into the computer-readable string of numbers representing the unique address, called the IP address, of each computer reachable by the network. A set of rules, called "protocols" in engineering terms, were also created for newsgroups (named "nntp" for Network News Transport Protocol), for posting messages on electronic community bulletin boards. The standard for error-free transfer of computer files, called "ftp" for File Transfer Protocol, was developed and formed the basis of the "click to download" functionality now ubiquitously available.

The turning point that propelled the Internet into homes and businesses occurred in 1991, with the development of the HyperText Transport Protocol (http) that underpins the functionality of the World-Wide Web. The idea of Hypertext is based on linkages between related information sources, where those related sources may be additional "pages" (downloadable files, each representing a "page" of information) located anywhere on the network: on the same computer or on another network-connected computer tens of thousands of miles away. The World-Wide Web is based on the notion of "server" computers that make information available on request, and "client" computers the make requests, receive the information, and display it.

A simple set of rules for describing the content of pages called the HyperText Markup Language (HTML) was developed with the concept of a "hyperlink", which is a word, a phrase, or a picture that is associated with the address on the Internet of another, related page. The user of a World-Wide Web browser program generally sees the hyperlinked text or image highlighted in a way that, when he or she clicks on the link, the browser program makes a request of the server whose name is "hidden" behind the link.

This remarkably powerful set of ideas was embodied first in a World-Wide Web viewing program called "Mosaic", developed at the University of Illinois and now available on virtually every Internet-connected computer in the form of browsing programs such as and Microsoft Internet Explorer, Safari, and Firefox. The ease and low cost of both publication and viewing via the World-Wide Web have made it the foundation of electronic commerce (i.e., online shopping) and fueled an explosive growth in both server and client computers. As of this writing, the Internet is used by over 230 million people in the U.S. and Canada, and worldwide the milestone of 1 billion estimated users was reached in 2006. Still, this represents less than 20% of the world's current population, and the "Internet revolution" is still in its early phases with respect to the full impact it will have on the human condition globally.

The decade of the 90s saw the emergence of thousands of local "Internet Service Providers" (ISPs) offering a variety of ways for individuals and organizations to connect their computers to the Internet. Connections based on dial-up phone lines were supplemented by a growing array of technologies capable of communications speeds in the millions-of-bits-per-second range. The pace of change and innovation continues to accelerate, and the near-term future promises a veritable alphabet soup of communications alternatives from phone, cable, and wireless communications companies, all holding the promise of higher communications speeds and lower costs.

How the Internet Works

Since the Internet may be thought of as a "telephone system for computers", enabling them to "talk" to one another in the way that we use the telephone system for voice communications, it is useful to compare the Internet to the phone system to highlight its strengths and weaknesses.

The design of the phone network has its roots in the original model developed by Alexander Graham Bell. Two or more phone devices that convert audible sound into electrical signals are connected by a "circuit", a set of wires connecting them. In early phone systems, these connections were physical wires connected via physical switches that could make an electrical pathway between any two phones for the duration of a single phone call. Now, switching is done electronically but the notion of a dedicated circuit, a channel used solely by the communicating parties for the duration of the call, persists as a design feature of the phone network. This "circuit-switched" model guarantees a certain amount of bandwidth, which is the term used for the transmission capacity and speed of a particular connection between two devices (in this case, telephones) connected to the network. In the circuit-switched phone network, one either gets a full allotment of bandwidth, or none, resulting, for example, in the familiar "I'm sorry, all circuits are busy" message on Mother's Day, the heaviest calling day of the year. If a circuit is lost, all communication ceases. A complex, centralized control scheme is required to maintain the proper operation of local and long distance phone circuits.

In contrast, the Internet was designed to have no central authority and to be tolerant of disruptions of parts of the network. The principles of this "fault-tolerant" network are simple. The network is assumed to be unreliable at all times. All of the specialized router computers that serve as the hands in the bucket brigade that pass packets are equal in status to all other routers, and each has its own authority to originate, receive, and forward messages. The messages themselves are divided into packets, and each packet is separately addressed. Each packet begins at some specified source computer, and ends at some other specified destination computer, but each packet can potentially wind its way through the network on an individual basis.

The particular route that a packet takes is unimportant; only final results count. Each packet is tossed like a hot potato from router to router, more or less in the direction of its destination, until it ends up in the proper place. In the Internet, the TCP (which started as the Transmission Control Program and is now the Transmission Control Protocol) converts messages into streams of packets at the source, then reassembles them back into messages at the destination. The IP, or "Internet Protocol", handles the addressing, seeing to it that packets are routed across multiple router computers and even across multiple networks with multiple standards for exchange of information, worldwide.

By design, Internet networks can be loosely characterized as either access networks or backbone networks. Access networks are those to which users connect directly, and often serve a limited geographic region. These include dial-up networks that serve consumers who access the Internet using the public telephone network, and a variety of emerging network technologies described below. Backbone networks typically have wide geographic scope and are used to interconnect the access networks as well as large corporate customers. One important consequence of this architecture is that a packet moving through the Internet will normally traverse networks owned and operated by many different providers enroute to its eventual destination. This has implications for two aspects of the network especially important for healthcare, which are quality of service (QoS) and security, described below.

The Internet Backbone

Within the U.S., the Internet backbone is currently operated by a small number of independent companies. The major backbone providers interconnect with each other at numerous points, some of which are "private" (typically a connection between only two providers), others of which are public. The public interconnection points are used not only by backbone providers but also by local providers to gain access to the backbone. Backbone networks carry highly aggregated traffic, representing the combined traffic flows of millions of customers connected to access networks. Backbone networks connect to access networks and to each other at Points of Presence, or PoPs. PoPs are locations where service providers house switching hardware and transmission equipment. PoPs are interconnected by long distance transmission lines. They are also the places where providers make connections to each other and to their customers.

A useful metric of backbone bandwidth is the capacity of a single inter-PoP trunk, a link from one PoP to another. Providers typically have PoPs in major urban areas; a large provider might have thirty or more PoPs in the U.S. Within the backbone networks, today's trunk speeds are typically on the order of ten to forty billion bits per second (Gbps). Providers upgrade link capacity constantly, either replacing slower links with faster ones or installing new links. The key driver for backbone providers is to enlarge capacity to keep up with demand, in order to avoid congestion in their networks. Over the years, traffic measurements on the Internet persistently indicate that such efforts are not always successful, i.e., that some of the backbone links are at or near capacity. This has important implications for some types of healthcare applications.

The Last Mile: Dial-Up Connections, DSL, and Cable Modem Service

"Last Mile" is the term used to describe the access link to end-users, especially residential users. In the US as of this writing, a majority of residential users (approximately 60%) still connect to the Internet using a dial-up connection, i.e., they use a modem connected to a conventional telephone line to connect to an ISP (3). These consumer-oriented ISPs then aggregate traffic from large numbers of residential customers and provide connectivity to the rest of the Internet by interconnecting with other ISPs.

The fastest modem connections are generally capable of providing 56,000 bits per second, or about 5600 characters per second (56 kbps) connections. Many residential users still connect at 28.8 kbps or less. Other options for connecting at higher speed, including both wired and wireless networks, are becoming more prevalent. Limitations on bandwidth have important implications for some types of healthcare applications. While having a bottleneck in the access link will always prevent one from achieving high end-to-end throughput, the converse is not necessarily true. Even with a high-speed access link, congestion at other points in the network may limit the throughput to a small fraction of the access speed. The issue of obtaining ensured end-to-end bandwidth is one of the essential components of QoS.

Businesses have a range of options for connecting to the Internet, depending on their ability to pay. At the low end, they have the same options as residential users. At the high end, many businesses connect over dedicated lines (i.e., not dial-up) at speeds ranging between 1.5 million bits per second, called "T-1" in communications parlance, and 622 million bits per second, called Optical Communications standard 12 or OC-12, since it uses and requires fiber optic lines. Prices charged for these services vary by geographic region and depend to some extent on market forces within local regions. Prices for dedicated lines are generally high enough to preclude use by residential customers (hundreds to thousands of dollars per month).

In between these two extremes, Frame Relay and Digital Subscriber Loop (DSL) are popular methods of connection. Frame Relay connections are typically sold at speeds from 56 kbps to 1.5 Mbps. Unlike a dedicated line, the bandwidth on a frame relay connection may be shared with other customers. Thus, for example, a business with a T-1 (1.5 Mbps) Frame Relay circuit might only be able to send 100 kbps at a certain time. DSL is a family of digital telecommunications protocols designed to allow high speed data communication over the existing copper telephone lines between end-users and telephone companies. Typical maximum data transfer rates for DSL are generally 384 kbps for downloads and 128 kbps for uploads.

A competing technology to DSL is cable modem service provided by cable TV companies, which uses the coaxial cable distribution system designed for television to deliver broadband connectivity to homes and businesses. Like DSL, cable modem service involves asymmetric speeds that are optimized for rapid downloading of information (1 to 5 megabits/ second) rather than uploading from the client computer (generally limited to 384 kilobits/second). Unlike DSL, the actual amount of bandwidth available on a cable modem connection is a function of how many other subscribers are sharing a "local loop" that may have up to fifty household connections attached to it. Much has been made in advertising wars between DSL and cable providers about which service is theoretically superior; actual experience has shown that both DSL and cable are cost-effective and useful ways to obtain a persistent high-bandwidth connection to the Internet if the service provider has well trained staff and support services.

Limitations of the Current Internet

As noted above, the Internet is a "best effort" network that provides no guarantees with respect to several key communications parameters. The most important of these from a healthcare perspective are assured QoS and security.

Quality of Service Issues

QoS refers to the ability of a network to provide several levels of performance assurance. Performance is characterized by metrics that include the following.

◆ Bandwidth: the throughput that is actually obtained between two points in the network (which may be dramatically less than the link speeds in the path between those points due to resource sharing and contention).

◆ Packet loss rate: the percentage of packets transmitted that are dropped inside the network.

◆ Latency or delay: the time taken to get a packet from one point in the network to another.

◆ Jitter: the variation in delay over time.

Note that these metrics are not independent of each other. For example, a high packet loss rate is likely to lead to low throughput. Note also that QoS is distinct from reliability. Reliability refers to the likelihood that a service remains available at all times. A network may be highly reliable in the sense that it is always possible to obtain connectivity to a given destination, but the same network may lack any assurance of performance and thus QoS as defined above.

A few numbers will help to illustrate the nature of best effort service. For example, while round trip times (or latency) from east to west coast across the Internet are frequently in the range of 100 milliseconds (1/10 of one second) or less, latencies in the range of a second can occur during periods of high network traffic. Although this amount of delay is not significant for asynchronous applications such as e-mail, it may make interactive applications such as videoconferencing unusable. There is nothing that a customer of an ISP can do today to ensure that this type of latency will not be encountered. This variation in latency might even be observed in the lifetime of a single connection, making it hard for a user or application to adapt to the prevailing latency. Similarly, packet loss rates range from fractions of a percent to tens of percent, which results in degradation of quality or the need to re-transmit packets. Re-transmission, in turn, results in increased latency. In addition, many applications reduce their sending rates in response to lost packets as they attempt to reduce congestion. As a result, packet loss directly affects the time taken to complete a transaction such as an image transfer over the network. While some links are chronically congested (e.g., between the U.S. and Europe), some links display high loss rates only sporadically. There are no mechanisms deployed in the Internet today to address this issue, but it is high on the list of issues to be addressed soon, as discussed below.

QoS is important for any application that involves interactive audio or video motion. Of the two, audio is the more sensitive to delays and disruptions. For example, in transmitting normal speech, a pause of 50 milliseconds is noticeable to the speaker and listener but does not disrupt communications. Difficulty understanding speech increases as pauses or periods of silence lengthen, until at 300 milliseconds of pause, speech becomes largely unintelligible to the listener. Thus the necessary quality of signal provided by the circuit-switched phone network is simply unavailable in the current packet-switched Internet. Voice-over-IP "Internet telephone" programs are growing in popularity, but they depend on an availability of bandwidth which may or may not be present in the network at any particular moment, and thus are not as reliable as standard telephone voice service, which is based on guaranteed minimum availability of a full "voice channel" equivalent (about 56 kbits/second) of bandwidth.

Because the Internet lacks QoS guarantees, a variety of adaptations have been developed for time-sensitive information such as audio and video. So-called "streaming media" players are based on the sending of a continuous series of packets containing audio and/or video data by a server computer. The client computer program receives and stores ("buffers") several seconds worth of data before beginning to play or show it, and continues to play the audio or video at a precise and regular pace while accumulating additional data, often irregularly, in the background due to the unpredictability of packet delivery from the Internet.

Security

Security is a fundamentally important aspect of healthcare data communications, and the Internet presents special challenges and vulnerabilities in this regard. First, it is important to understand the basic functions that are needed to make an information system of any type secure. These include:

1. Identification of the persons and computers that will be involved in the acquisition, storage, and communication of information within the system. Identification is a process that computer security professionals refer to as "out of band". An example of such a process would be a human being that compares an identifying document such as a passport with your personage to establish for

the system that you are authorized to have access in some way. As a general rule, the network cannot be used to identify parts of the network.

2. Authentication is the function that ensures that the user or system, at the time of each use of the system, is who or what it represents itself to be. In contrast to identification, which occurs once or generally at relatively long intervals (e.g., renewing of a driver"s license), authentication in a secure system occurs every time a person or machine makes its presence known to the system, such as during a system login.

3. Access control is the set of functions that ensures that people, computer systems, and processes, once authenticated, can use only those resources (e.g., files, directories, database records, computers, networks) that they are authorized to use and only for the purposes for which they are authorized.

4. Confidentiality is provided by functions that ensure that sensitive and/or private information is protected from unauthorized disclosure. While access control mechanisms define what one is authorized to see, and thus what the system should do, confidentiality mechanisms provide assurance that the system is not doing what it should not do.

5. Integrity is maintained by functions that ensure that data, computer programs, and system resources are as they are supposed to be and that they cannot be modified by unauthorized people, software, or computer equipment.

6. Attribution (also called non-repudiation), which are functions that ensure that information and actions that occur in the system are reliably traceable to the users and/or computers involved.

These six functions are required of any information or communications system that is designed to be secure, ranging from tin cans on a string to computer networks. In contrast, the current Internet was designed to support open communications and collaboration among mutually trusting entities. Thus issues relating to authenticating the identity of the attached computers and users and protecting the contents of IP packets simply was not an issue that the IP protocol needed to address. The Internet as it exists today has a number of vulnerabilities:

♦ The Internet provides no positive means of identifying systems. No reliable means exists to positively bind IP addresses to specific computers. Indeed, there is an Internet standard for a Dynamic Host Configuration Protocol (DHCP) that has capitalized on this "vulnerability" by enabling IP addresses to be assigned in real-time. Using this approach, ISPs generally maintain a pool of assignable IP addresses. As users dial-in to initiate a session, an IP address is temporarily assigned to that user's account; after the session is complete, the IP address is made available to the next caller as needed.

◆ The Internet provides no positive means of identifying users. In fact, the Internet does not recognize the concept of the individual user.

◆ The Internet provides no protection for confidential information. Information is loaded into the IP packets and passed from router to router ("node to node" in computer network parlance) in the clear. A "sniffer" program on any node through which the data passes can see the contents as it passes through, even packets containing sensitive information such as user passwords or medical test results.

◆ Vulnerabilities in attached systems can be exploited to further reduce the presumed security of the Internet. For example, "spyware" and "Trojan horse" programs, which provide some useful and visible service to users while performing actions in the background that are neither desired nor known to the user, such as transmitting information to malicious host computers on the Internet (4).

Measures for Achieving Internet Security

Encryption

The technology that makes it possible to authenticate users, protect the confidentiality and integrity of information, and ensure attribution or non-repudiation over a network is encryption, the age-old practice of scrambling a message to make its contents difficult to interpret. Two forms of encryption are in common use in the Internet: conventional or symmetric and public-key or asymmetric.

Symmetric encryption, also called private-key encryption, is based on the principle that the code or "key" used to scramble a message (formally called a ciphertext) is the same key used to unscramble it; in one form or another private key encryption has been used since the time of the Romans. Popular symmetric encryption algorithms include the Data Encryption Standard (DES) (5), which uses a 56-bit encryption key, and its successor, the International Data Encryption Algorithm (IDEA), which uses a 128-bit or higher key (6). The problem with private key encryption is that the parties must agree upon the key to be used before the encrypted communication is exchanged. If the key can be intercepted in the same way that an encrypted message can be intercepted, then little or no advantage of secrecy is gained by using encryption.

Asymmetric or public key encryption is based on a two-part key. What one part of the key pair encodes and only the other part of the key pair can decode; even the original key will not decode the message. This asymmetry has very useful properties. If one key of the key pair is kept private and the other, "public" key is made available to others, then a message successfully decoded by the public key must have been encoded by the private key. This effect makes public key cryptography well suited to creating digital signatures, establishing user authentication, and exchanging private (symmetrical) session keys in a way that does not permit eavesdropping. The RSA algorithm (7) was one of the first public-key encryption algorithms to be widely adopted. Named for its developers, Ron Rivest, Adi Shamir, and Leonard Adleman, RSA relies on the difficulty of factoring large numbers for its security.

In general, conventional private key encryption is used for protecting the confidentiality and integrity of large amounts of data, while public key encryption, which imposes a greater processing burden and, depending upon key length, may be a thousand or more times slower to decrypt, is often used for user authentication purposes and for exchanging private keys. The difficulty of attempting to decipher an encrypted message without use of the key, as might be attempted by an attacker, is proportional to the length of the key relative to the message; the longer the encryption key the more possible combinations that must be tried to unscramble the message simply by guessing all possible solutions. A 128-bit encryption key generates a ciphertext that has 300,000,000,000,000,000,000,000,000 (a three followed by 26 zeroes) times as many possible key combinations as there are for 40-bit encryption, and the standards for so-called "strong encryption" evolve to ever-longer key lengths as the computing power available at low cost increases.

Secure HTTP

The Hypertext Transport Protocol (HTTP) that underpins the functioning of the World Wide Web lacks protections for confidential data. The Secure HTTP protocol (SHTTP) was developed for secure and private exchange of information such as credit card numbers and has become an essential tool for web-based communication of health data. SHTTP is an application-level protocol (meaning that it is a set of procedures executed by the server program and the client browser program, not by the network) that provides encryption of messages transmitted in both directions between client and server, and for encapsulation of the message in a "wrapper" specifying the encryption method used, thus ensuring confidentiality. Any of a number of encryption mechanisms can be used; the particular mechanism is negotiated between client and server at the time the connection is made. An encrypted message may also incorporate a message digest, which guarantees the integrity of the data in the message, and a digital signature, which guarantees the authenticity of the sender. SHTTP is designed to be backward compatible with HTTP, so browsers that do not implement SHTTP can still access data on SHTTP servers.

Secure Sockets Layer

SSL is a secure communication protocol implemented as a layer between the transport layer (usually TCP) and applications that send and receive messages. It provides for message encryption and certification of public key authenticity, data integrity, and server authentication; client authentication is optional. It can provide these services to any application protocol, such as HTTP, telnet, or even SHTTP. When SHTTP and SSL are used together, SHTTP encrypts data at the application layer and passes it to SSL, which encrypts it a second time. As with SHTTP, SSL performs security services independently from the operating system and the network.

Public Key Infrastructure

As described above, an essential component of Internet security is based on public key cryptography, the two-part encryption scheme where one part of the key is held privately and one is made public. This technology has given rise to a growing industry that provides Certificate Authority (CA) services. These companies verify that a server computer's public key is valid and combines it with their own public key to create a unique digital certificate. A digital certificate is simply an electronic "statement" signed by an independent and trusted third party in a format that is standardized so that its contents can be decoded by client programs such as web browsers. CA services are built on a combination of out-of-band identification (e.g., calling individuals associated with the organization to verify the authenticity of the request for a public key certificate) and technology that "wraps" the public key of a given server with the CA's own cryptographic key. The most common digital certificates on the Internet follow a standard named X.509 (8). In healthcare, state medical boards are responsible for certifying and licensing practitioners within their jurisdiction; thus, it can reasonably be expected that in the future such regulatory agencies will perform the functions of a medical CA for practitioners and institutions. The technical and documentary relationships for certifying the authenticity of the public keys of server (and potentially also client) computers on the Internet is referred to collectively as a public key iInfrastructure.

Encryption of Health Data on the Internet

In 1999, the Health Care Financing Administration (HCFA) issued an Internet Security Policy that requires encryption of all person-identifiable health data communicated to HCFA (9). The policy specified a minimum level of encryption as "triple DES", which means encrypting a message with the DES 56-bit key, and then encrypting the resulting message twice more. A single 128-bit encryption is equally acceptable, which is important for web-based clinical systems because commonly used domestic webserver programs (such as Microsoft Internet Information Server, which is available as a no-added-cost option for Windows servers) are capable of and easily configured to be compliant with the HCFA 128-bit standard.

In contrast to web-based communication of health data, the use of Internet electronic mail is currently problematic. The use of electronic messaging for clinical care highlights an important set of risks. Standard ("smtp", simple mail transport protocol) e-mail is currently passed in cleartext format over the Internet, which makes the "snooping" of message contents trivially easy to do using a variety of network management and hacker tools. Although encryption utilities such as PGP and standards for privacy-enhanced e-mail exist, they are, as of this writing, not widely installed or used. The Pew Internet and American Life project, which monitors trends in use of the Internet in America, notes that approximately 75% of the adult U.S. population has access to the Internet; of those, 91% have sent or received e-mail; and more than half use e-mail daily (10). This exuberant acceptance of e-mail has not been reflected in growth of e-mail communications between physicians and patients, however. A 2005 survey of all physicians in the State of Florida reported that only 16% had communicated with patients using e-mail, and only 3% used it regularly for this purpose (11).

Given that common e-mail does not protect confidentiality but may still contribute significantly to improved patient care, the American Medical Informatics Association Internet Working Group published in 1998 a set of guidelines for e-mail communications between patients and providers that emphasize the establishment of orderly procedures for the handling of provider-patient e-mail (12). A partial list of the recommendations of that white paper are summarized in Table 5-1; these recommendations provide

Table 5-1

GUIDELINES FOR E-MAIL USE WITH PATIENTS

- Establish a turnaround time for e-mail responses to patient inquiries; do not use e-mail for urgent matters.
- Inform patients about privacy issues: who sees e-mail in the practitioners' office, and that e-mail becomes part of the medical record.
- Establish types of transaction (e.g., prescription refills, appointment scheduling) that are appropriate for e-mail, and the limits on message content in terms of sensitivity (e.g., HIV test results).
- Instruct Patients to put category of transaction in e-mail subject line (e.g., "Med refill").
- Acknowledge receipt of all messages and request that patients do also.
- Print all messages, replies, and confirmation of receipt and place in paper chart.
- Request Patients to put name and MRN in body of message.
- Use encryption as soon as it is feasible and practical.
- Do not use unencrypted wireless communications for Patient-identifiable information.

a reference point for some of the challenges and difficulties associated with electronic healthcare communications.

While representing a pragmatic approach to the management of clinical messages that are now flowing in increasing numbers between patients and providers, the guidelines advise practices that heighten the risk of breeches of confidentiality (e.g., putting patient name and MRN in the body of the message). They also serve to highlight the lack of currently available security mechanisms and the lack of tools to integrate electronic messages easily into the increasingly electronic medical record.

Intranets

The networking technologies developed for the open Internet can also be applied to a private network. The term Intranet is given for a local area network that is configured to use the networking protocols (TCP/IP) and services (World-Wide Web, smtp E-mail, ftp file transfer protocol, etc.) of the larger Internet. An Intranet can either be isolated unto itself, or connected so that information can also be transmitted to and received from the Internet (Figure 5-1). In the case where an Intranet is connected to the Internet, it inherits the security challenges and difficulties (such as the risk of unauthorized access by malicious users) of the larger network. As a result, most Intranets are designed to have only a single point of contact with the Internet, through which all incoming and outgoing communications streams must pass. At this point, a specialized communications filtering computer called a firewall is installed. As their name implies, firewalls are designed to protect an internal network from external threats. A variety of rules regarding the types of incoming and outgoing message traffic allowed, and the machine identities (IP addresses) of authorized internal and external computers, can be implemented via software programs. Rules can relate both to types of services (e.g., no incoming file transfers allowed except from specific "trusted" sources) and to the contents of the IP packets (e.g., no e-mail attachments allowed that are executable programs). Firewalls can also inspect the communications stream for patterns that indicate malicious programs such as computer viruses. Currently, the majority of large corporations and a growing number of healthcare enterprises have some form of corporate Intranet.

Extranets and Virtual Private Networks

The popularity of Intranets gave rise to the idea of extending the same forms private communications found within an Intranet to selected sites (such as branch offices, affiliated clinics, or business partners), using the open Internet to pass data communications traffic between two or more geographically distant Intranets. The general idea of this has been called an Extranet but this term does not imply a specific set of technologies (Figure 5-2). In some cases

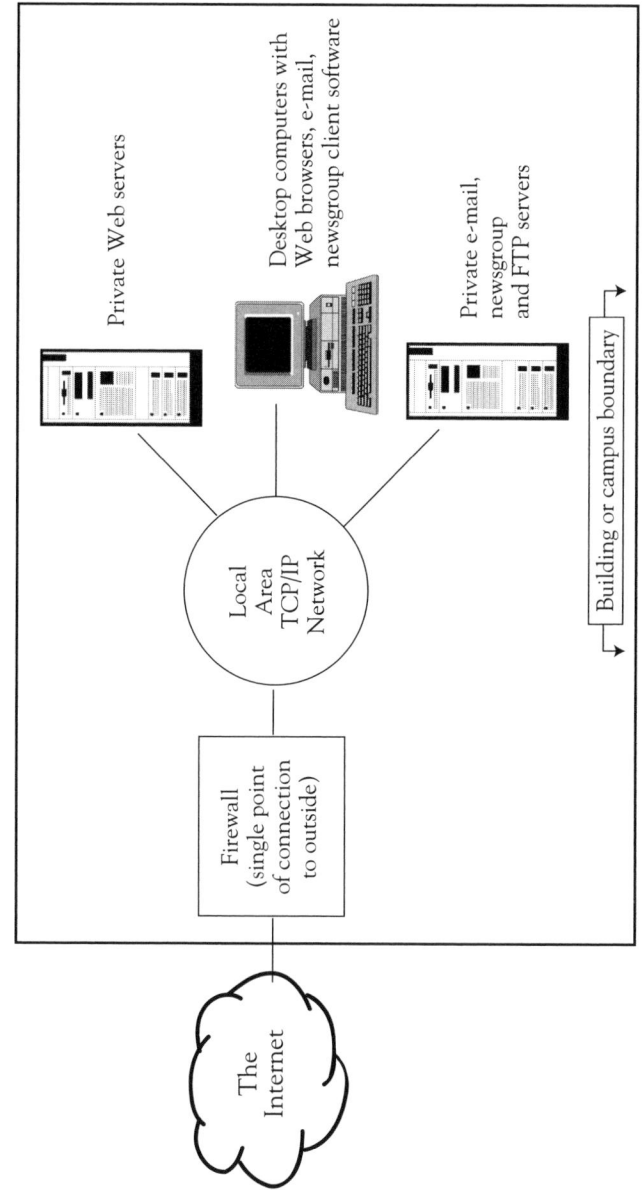

Figure 5-1 Intranet architecture.

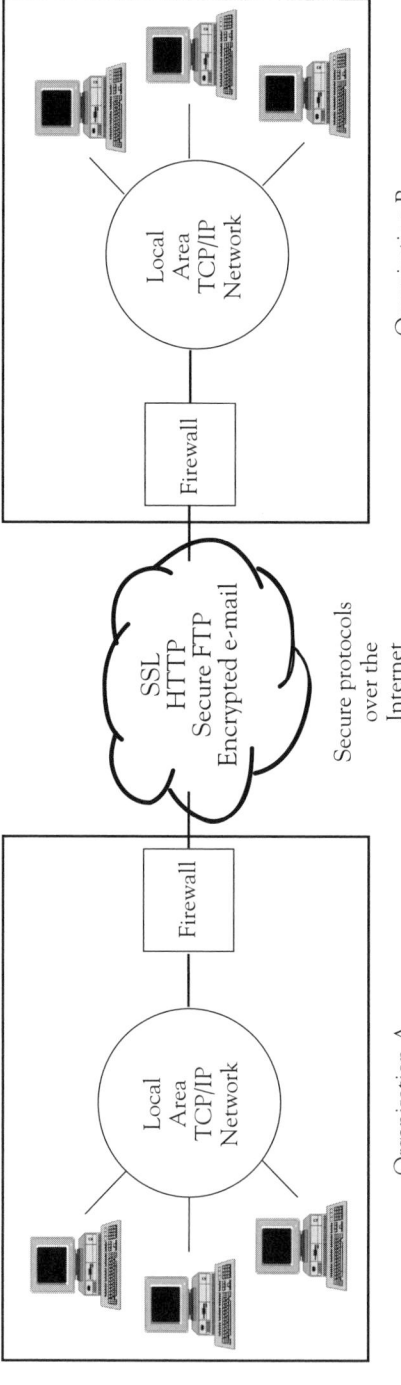

Figure 5-2 Extranet architecture.

what is called an Extranet is simply the use of open Internet protocols, such as secure HTTP and Secure Sockets Layer among organizations known to one another.

In contrast, a Virtual Private Network (VPN) has a specific technical definition. Like an Extranet, it involves passing communications between Intranets using the open Internet. However, a VPN is based on specially configured routers that are programmed with a private encryption key and the IP addresses of the other routers comprising the VPN. The router computers perform "link level encryption" of packets and may adopt a private and nonstandard messaging protocol known as a "tunneling protocol", so-called because it effectively creates a tunnel for communications that can only be interpreted correctly by the routers of the VPN. VPNs provide strong security and predictable paths (unlike the open Internet where packets are passed in a generally unpredictable series of hops) but have the disadvantage that the specialized routers must be pre-configured with the security keys and destination information of the other members of the network.

Extending the Web via Markup Languages

The World-Wide Web began as a publication metaphor, based on servers providing electronic data representing individual pages with content encoded in the Hypertext Markup Language (HTML). HTML is a formatting language based on the Standard Generalized Markup Language (SGML) developed by the publishing industry to specify page layout and text appearance. SGML and HTML use simple text tags of the form:

<TAG>This is text affected by the instruction in the tag</TAG>

The tags themselves are not displayed, but provide instructions to a web browser on how to treat the information contained between the tags, so that an HTML construction such as:

This is <B>Bold</B> text and this is <I>*italic*</I>.

will be displayed as:

This is **Bold** text and this is *italic*.

HTML is a limited and "improper" subset of SGML. This means that an SGML document can be translated to HTML, but information is lost in the translation so that an HTML document cannot be translated back to SGML, which has additional requirements for specifying a formal document type description (DTD) and structure.

The power and utility of specifying document structure and content via embedded tags has given rise to an evolving set of standards called Extensible Markup Language (XML). XML is a flexible way to create common information formats and share both the format and the data on the World

Wide Web, intranets, and elsewhere. There is intense activity currently underway to develop XML specifications for elements of healthcare records (15,16). Using XML as a standard for representing documentation of clinical encounters, laboratory results, dictated operative reports, etc., facilitates both the consistent formatting of this information by web browsers and the ability to analyze content via computer programs that look for and extract specific tagged elements.

XML is "extensible" because, unlike HTML, the markup symbols are unlimited and self-defining. Thus, XML tagging of a initial history and physical could include healthcare-relevant tags such as <CHIEF COMPLAINT>....</CHIEF COMPLAINT> as well as the formatting information carried by standard HTML tags.

Extending the Web with Downloadable Computer Programs

In addition to these evolving standards for describing viewable "document" or "page" content on the Web, there is no barrier to a server sending executable computer programs to a client upon request. The idea of transmitting on-demand programs to a client computer has given rise to a variety of programming languages developed specifically for use via computer networks, the most widely deployed of which are Java and Javascript (see "Survey of Popular Programming Languages" in Chapter 3).

Java

Java is a programming language developed by Sun Microsystems specifically to expand the interactive possibilities of the Web. Java can be used to create complete applications that may run on a single computer or be distributed among servers and clients in a network. It can also be used to build small application modules called "applets" that are downloaded to a client computer as part of a Web page (for example, an interactive Body Surface Area calculator displayed within a page providing guidance on drug dosage).

JavaScript

Although it has a similar sounding name, JavaScript is a more limited "scripting language" with a much different syntax. JavaScript can be embedded within an HTML page. Originally called "LiveScript", JavaScript was developed by Netscape, and soon modified and renamed in order to tap into the Java craze sweeping the Internet. As with Java, most major browsers provide support for interpreting its scripts. It is used primarily for animating and enhancing navigation on web pages; the now-familiar Web motif of buttons which "glow" when the mouse cursor is passed over them is most commonly implemented by JavaScript scripting within the web page.

CORBA

Providing access to and control over network-accessible programs is the goal of another set of emerging standards called CORBA. CORBA is an acronym for Common Object Request Broker Architecture. It is an architecture and specification for creating, distributing, and managing distributed program objects in a network. It allows programs at different locations and developed by different vendors to communicate in a network through an "interface broker", which is a set of software functions that examine requests coming from programs running on client computers, and determine how and where to route those requests to the appropriate server. CORBA was developed by a consortium of vendors through the Object Management Group (OMG), which currently includes over 500 member companies. Industry-specific committees and working groups are developing standards for CORBA, including a CORBA MED group focused on the functionality unique to healthcare computing (14).

A notable hold-out from CORBA is Microsoft, which has its own distributed object architecture, the Distributed Component Object Model (DCOM). However, CORBA and Microsoft have agreed on a gateway approach so that a client object developed with the Component Object Model will be able to communicate with a CORBA server (and vice versa).

WEB 2.0: Anyone Can Be a Publisher

The first generation of websites were based on the idea of technically proficient publishers (mostly organizations) providing public information via a set of "Internet storefronts." This motif fundamentally was based on the economics of web publication: the technology was new and somewhat arcane, required a set of compuer programming skills to work well, and was therefore expensive. Web 2.0 refers to the second generation of web technologies, which feature new ways of sending and receiving information, "e-commerce" applications such as online shopping carts and credit card approvals for business, and an emphasis on providing tools for nontechnical users to publish their own material to a potentially global audience. There is no single definition of what is and is not included among Web 2.0 services, and it has become in some ways a label for anything related to the Web that is new and contemporary. A new vocabulary of web-based services has entered the popular lexicon. Some of the more widely known and adopted Web 2.0 innovations are described here.

Blogs

Blogs are the shorthand form of the term "web log" that generally feature personal commentary about a topic or event, more or less in the spirit of a published and continuously updated diary, to which the readers can also submit comments. A distinctive feature of blogs is that they show contributed text (and sometimes uploaded pictures, links, and other multimedia content) in reverse chronological order, so that the latest happenings and conversations are at the most prominent position on the site, and readers can follow the trail of earlier contributions (usually called "threads" when a blog has multiple topics under discussion at the same time) by reading down the web page.

Wikis

Wikis are similar to blogs in their ability to accept input from users and immediately publish it as a web page. The word Wiki is derived from the Hawaiian word for "quick." Unlike blogs, wikis are designed to be group authoring tools where all users are able to contribute to the content of a shared document, often a single web page, thus pooling the accumulated group understanding of a particular topic. It is therefore not surprising that the most famous Wiki is the Wikipedia (www.wikipedia.org), which is a multilingual global encyclopedia constructed essentially entirely by volunteer authors who wish to publish something they know about almost any topic that can be found in a traditional published encyclopedia (as well as many that are not, since Wikipedia pages appear within days of the usage of a new technical term or popular slang).

One potential concern about public wiki sites is that they are open to misleading, opinionated or malicious entries. As a result, most wikis do have an administrator who serves as editor-in-chief to permit or withdraw submitted content. In spite of fears that wikis would become the bully pulpits of a few highly opinionated and perhaps malevolent authors, the community ethic of shared information that is validated by other volunteer contributors works remarkably well in most instances. Wiki software that is free can be used in Intranet settings to provide a private group editing environment within an organization that functions as an internal community bulletin board.

RSS

Most web technologies are passive in the sense that a user must choose to visit a website using their web browser in order to see if the content has changed. A complementary "push technology" that sends new content from the website to a user whenever new information is added is based on an internet protocol called RSS, which stands for "Really Simple Syndication."

Most major commercial websites and a growing number of "private individuals" sites provide RSS feed capability. To take advantage of it, users install an RSS reader software program on their local machine, which receives the new content from the multiple sites that they have designated as wishing to follow, and in essence builds a dynamic table of contents representing new information available from all sites since the last time the user viewed the site. An interesting intersection of consumer electronics exists when RSS feeds are used for "podcasts", which are online audio and video content that can be automatically downloaded into the ubiquitous Apple iPod and other forms of personal multimedia storage devices.

Mash-Ups

As the amount of information available on the web expands to virtually every sphere of human endeavor, the value added by dynamically combining the content of two or more websites grows. A "mash-up" is a website that merges the content from other sites in response to a specific query. For example, a real estate website may merge data showing the sales prices of properties with data from a geographic mapping site to display a map of recent sales with hyperlinks that show financial data and images of the homes involved. It can be easily predicted that analogous services for patients will spring up, showing a variety of publicly available health data such as provider report cards mashed-up with maps, provider's credentials and services, and other information that may bear on a patient's decision to choose a particular provider or healthcare organization.

Harnessing Community Intelligence

The world of Web 2.0 recognizes that there is a new class of information sometimes called "herd intelligence", which represents the aggregation of thousands or millions of individual decisions and actions taken by web developers or users. The most prominent example of this is the Google page-rank algorithm. Many general-purpose Internet search engines existed before Google, but its unique contribution has been to present websites in a ranked order determined largely by how many other websites point to the website being indexed. This approach harnesses the intelligence of many individual decisions made by web creators to create links to other valuable sites. Similarly, websites devoted to "social bookmarking" gather and count the URLs submitted by users who have found those sites particularly interesting or useful. The evolution of these types of user-to-user sharing of information is in its early stages, and the full power of a global village whose citizens can communicate freely and nearly instantly, without respect to geopolitical boundaries, has yet to be realized.

Internet-Accessible Medical Records

The description of the various Internet-related technologies described above serves as a preamble to the use of the Internet for communicating person-specific clinical data. Vendors of electronic medical records systems have been under increasing pressure from purchasers to create Web-based information access methods to complement their existing products. The Healthcare Financing Administrations implementation in 1999 of a set of security standards for transmission of person-identifiable health data established an acceptable set of technical measures for satisfactory information security, opening the floodgates for a vast array of new commercial products. Currently, it would be exceptional if vendors did not have a web interface to their EHR product either available or in development. As with most new technologies that eventually achieve widespread acceptance, the first applications tend to be evolutionary and incremental modifications to existing systems. Later, revolutionary applications appear that support a redefinition of roles, responsibilities, and workflow. The Internet is currently being used to support the former but will almost certainly change the very nature of electronic medical records as the latter emerge. Examples of both are provided below.

Web Interfaces to EHR Systems

Currently, the most common approach to making EHR data from existing systems available via the Internet is to create an accessory "wrapper" system that accepts queries from client computers via HTML forms and translates those queries into a syntax compatible with the existing (often mainframe-based) clinical data repository (CDR). The CDR responds as it would to a request originating from any workstation in the existing system architecture and sends back data to the web server machine. The server then re-encodes that data as a dynamic-generated HTML page and sends it to the requesting web client. If the client is located outside of the organization's local area network, the web client-server communications are encrypted and travel though the firewall computer to the open Internet (Figure 5-3).

The strength of such a model is that it does not require a fundamental redesign of the CDR, since the incoming transactions appear to the existing system to be "just another workstation" sending and receiving data. The disadvantage is that designs of this type have several additional layers of information processing and reformatting and are consequently relatively inefficient and difficult to scale up.

New Internet-Based EHR Designs

Though most Web interfaces to EHRs are "grafted on" to the existing architecture using the design described above or a variant of it, the emerging technologies and growing ubiquity of the Internet will enable a new genre of EHR designs that include:

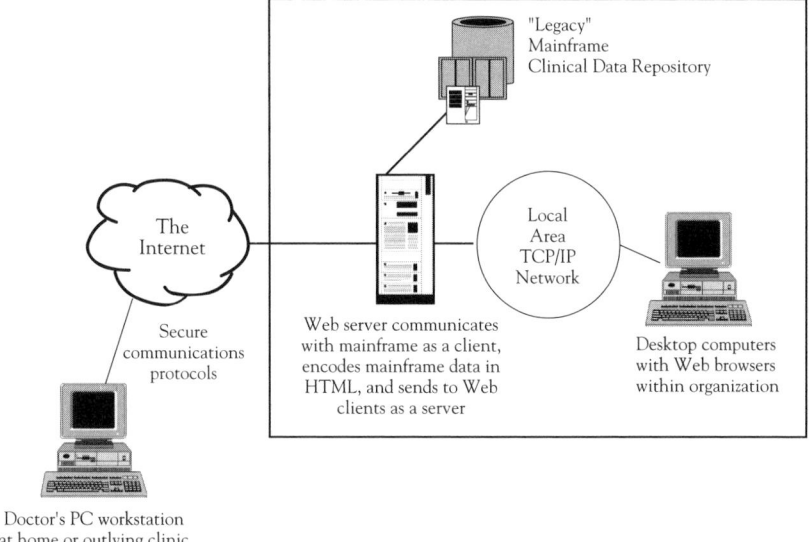

Figure 5-3   Web "wrapper" architecture.

♦ Java-encoded EHR client programs that connect directly via the Internet to an organization's CDR database without the need for an intermediary web server, thereby improving data access efficiencies, while giving an organization control over the user interface and the security aspects of the data communication. Since the Java code is downloaded each time a user session is initiated, this design has the additional benefit that all client workstations are guaranteed to be running the most up-to-date version of the client program.

♦ Clinical data repositories that are in reality just a logical view of data that is physically located on many different servers located at geographically-distant sites. The Internet will provide, via "middleware" services such as CORBA, an environment where requesting client computers do not need to know or be concerned about the location of servers. Though health care organizations have historically viewed their computer systems as a necessary local resource, computer networks loosen the requirement for physical facilities and enable strategies such as outsourcing to medical "data warehouses" located hundreds or thousands of miles from the hospital or clinic. The most provocative (and perhaps inevitable) model would locate the electronic records of care delivered in a network-accessible "neutral repository" database, encrypted with a private key unique to each patient, and with access controlled by the patient. On entry into a healthcare plan or system, the patient would grant access privileges to their providers via a public key infrastructure as described in the encryption section above.

The Future of Data Networks in Healthcare

The importance of the Internet and Internet-associated technologies for EHRs will continue to grow for the foreseeable future, driven by dual forces of innovation and societal change. It can be reasonably predicted that four key areas of data networking that have an impact on healthcare will see substantial change and improvement over the next several years. They are bandwidth, QoS, security, and ubiquity.

Bandwidth

The first and most obvious difference between the current Internet and the networks that will evolve from it in the future is a dramatic increase in transport speeds. Currently, speeds of OC-12 (625 Mbits/sec) to OC-48 (2.5 Gbits/sec) are being deployed in research settings and are expected to become commercially available in some metropolitan areas within the next several years. From a healthcare perspective, requirements for bandwidth of this magnitude tend to derive from the aggregate traffic of dozens to thousands of data streams, rather than from individual applications that have stringent requirements for extremely high bandwidth. One might assume that many data-intensive clinical transactions require very high-bandwidth communications. However, empirical telemedicine studies conducted over the past decade by and large have concluded that a relative minority of clinical applications, such as cardiac cineangiography, require application bandwidth in the range of 768 kb/sec (e.g., 6 bonded ISDN channels). Most interactive video telemedicine, such as telepsychiatry and routine general medical follow-up, can be effectively delivered with bandwidth as low as 128 kb/sec. (17-20). More importantly, very high bandwidth alone will not be sufficient for interactive telemedicine unless it is also accompanied by guarantees of QoS.

Quality of Service

As noted previously, although best-effort service is the only option available via the Internet today, a range of different services will be available within the next several years. The two main approaches to offering Internet QoS are typically referred to as "integrated services" (int-serv) and "differentiated services" (diff-serv). Both int-serv and diff-serv improve upon the current best-effort service model.

As the name implies, in diff-serv the intention is to deliver a differentiated set of qualities of service beyond best effort. As a simple example, a clinic might purchase "Premium service" from an Internet Service Provider at a certain transmission rate, say 128kbps. Such an agreement would mean that the organization could send up to 128kbps of packets into the network and expect them to receive "better" service than a best-effort packet would receive. Exactly how much better would be determined by the provider. An important limitation of differentiated service is that it goes only as far as the boundary of a single ISP's network.

The term integrated services (int-serv) is used to refer to an overall architecture for providing QoS in IP networks such as the Internet. An important component of the architecture is the signaling protocol Resource ReSerVation Protocol (RSVP), and the int-serv model is sometimes referred to as the RSVP model. Unlike diff-serv, int-serv attempts to provide quantifiable end-to-end guarantees to applications such as "this video conference from host A to host B will receive 128 kbps throughput and 100 ms end-to-end latency". It also includes a signaling mechanism (RSVP) to provide "on-demand" guarantees, which appears to be ideal for many healthcare applications.

The major concern that has prevented widespread deployment of int-serv and RSVP is scalability. As currently defined, every connection (e.g., a single video call) needs its own reservation, and each reservation requires information about the connection to be stored at every router along the path that will carry the application data. The prospect of having per-application state in backbone routers is not attractive to ISPs, for whom scaling is a major concern. In addition, an ISP would need to have mechanisms to control which users were able to make reservations, and to bill for such reservations. In spite of these problems, an int-serv model remains attractive. It provides a service model that more closely resembles that of the telephone network than diff-serv does. Service is requested as needed. If resources are available to provide the requested service, then the service will be provided; if not, a negative acknowledgement (equivalent to a busy signal) is returned. For this reason, int-serv is already being used in "Voice over IP" networks that are small enough to avoid the scaling issues mentioned above.

Security

IPSec refers to a security architecture and set of standards developed by the Internet Engineering Task Force. The standards provide for a variety of services such as encryption and authentication of IP packets. One of the main areas of deployment of these technologies to date has been to support Virtual Private Networks (VPNs) across the Internet. A number of products are now available to enable the establishment of an "encrypted tunnel" across the Internet. Such a tunnel is created between a pair of IPSec gateways, which might be located at two geographically separated locations of a single healthcare organization. Each gateway encrypts the data sent from one site to the other and sends the encrypted data as the payload of a standard IP datagram to the other gateway. The receiving gateway then decrypts the data before passing it on to the final recipient at the second site. Because the data are encrypted using a key that is known only to the two gateways, it cannot be "snooped" as it crosses the Internet. Furthermore, the receiving gateway can authenticate the data as having come from the sending site and not some other source in the Internet. Thus an IPSec tunnel provides a viable way to build a VPN. Like other approaches to VPNs, it requires a priori knowledge of where connectivity will be required, as the gateways must be configured with appropriate keys and routing information to create the tunnel.

Ubiquity

The importance of understanding and taking advantage of Internet technologies comes as much from their projected future growth as it does their current functionality. Global computer data networks will become ubiquitous to a degree that equals or surpasses voice telephone service (and in fact will likely become the default carriers of both voice and data as networking technologies converge). Surveys of Internet users in the U.S. are showing that user demographics are "regressing to the mean" so that access to the Internet, once the province solely of the affluent and well educated, will be the norm in most or all segments of society.

A major trend that will help propel the Internet into homes and offices is the appearance of "smart" appliances and machines that communicate over IP data networks. The marketplace has begun to see the appearance of devices such as "Internet refrigerators" that record food items as they are removed from the refrigerator in a shopping list database that is automatically transmitted to an online grocery as needed. The tongue-in-cheek vision of "toaster net" that is a current joke among Internet afficianados will have an analogous impact in the medical office, where the vision of "sphygmomanometer net" will become a reality in an increasingly paperless healthcare environment.

One prominent computer company has for over a decade had a slogan that states "the Network is the Computer" (18). The impact of the Internet, though already substantial in healthcare, is at an early stage along a path that may lead eventually to a similar assertion: the Network is the Healthcare Organization. Internet-based EHRs will be an important component of that future.

References

1. Internet world statistics, http://www.internetworldstats.com/stats.htm accessed 26 December 2006.
2. For a complete technical history of the Internet, the Internet itself is, not surprisingly, a rich source of information. Readers interested in pursuing this may wish to navigate the Internet subject area of catalog sites such as http://www.yahoo.com or the Electronic Commerce Resource Center site at http://www.becrc.org/nethistory.htm.
3. Pew Charitable Trust Home Broadband Adoption Project 2006, at http://www.pewtrusts.org/pdf/PIP_Broadband_0506.pdf accessed 26 December 26, 2006.

 4. Masys DR, Baker DB. Patient-centered access to secure systems online (PCASSO): a secure approach to clinical data access via the world-wide web. J Am Med Informatics Assoc. 1997;4(Suppl):340-3.

 5. Federal Information Processing Standard Publication 46-2. Data Encryption Standard (DES), available from the National Institute of Standards and Technology at http://www.itl.nist.gov/fipspubs/fip46-2.htm.

 6. http://csrc.nist.gov/encryption/aes/aes_home.htm.

 7. http://www.rsa.com.

 8. For more information on public keyiInfrastructure and digital certificates, see the National Institutes of Standards and Technology PKI site at http://csrc.nist.gov/pki/.

 9. HCFA Internet Security Policy, available online at http://www.hcfa.gov/security/isec-plcy.htm.

10. http://www.pewinternet.org/index.asp. Accessed December 31, 2006.

11. Brooks RG, Menachemi N. Physicians' use of email with patients: factors influencing electronic communication and adherence to best practices. J Med Internet Res. 2006;8:e2; http://www.jmir.org/2006/1/e2/.

12. Kane B, Sands DZ. Guidelines for the clinical use of electronic mail with patients. The AMIA Internet Working Group, Task Force on Guidelines for the Use of Clinic-Patient Electronic Mail. J Am Med Inform Assoc. 1998;5:104-11.

13. For a comprehensive overview of Java, consult the Sun Microsystems Java page at http://java.sun.com.

14. The Object Management Group provides introductory tutorials and additional technical information on CORBA, including activities of the CORBA MED group, at http://www.omg.org/.

15. Kahn CE Jr, de la Cruz NB. Extensible markup language (XML) in health care: integration of structured reporting and decision support. In Chute C, ed.. Proc AMIA Symp. 1998;725-9.

16. Dolin RH, Rishe W, Biron PV, et al. SGML and XML as interchange formats for HL7 messages. In Chute C, ed. Proc AMIA Fall Symp. 1998;720-4.

17. Anogianakis G, Maglavera S, Pomportsis A, et al. Medical emergency aid through telematics: design, implementation guidelines and analysis of user requirements for the MERMAID project. Int J Med Inf. 1998;52:93-103.

18. Stewart BK, Carter SJ, Cook JN, et al. Application of the advanced communications technology satellite to teleradiology and real-time compressed ultrasound video telemedicine. J Digit Imaging. 1999;12:68-76.

19. Stoloff PH, Garcia FE, Thomason JE, Shia DS. A cost-effectiveness analysis of shipboard telemedicine. Telemed J. 1998;4:293-304.

20. Phillips CM, Murphy R, Burke WA, et al. Dermatology teleconsultations to Central Prison: experience at East Carolina University. Telemed J. 1996;2:139-43.

21. Sun Microsystems, Inc. http://www.sun.com.

6

Informatics Standards

Naveen Maram, MD, MSHI, MPH

S tandards play a pivotal and yet often indiscernible role in our lives. Every facet of our day-to-day activities is supported by innumerable standards. In everything from power sockets to automobiles, we interact with standards at various levels. Without standardization, chaos ensues. Yet in a data-intensive discipline like healthcare, the push for wide adaptation of well-defined informatics standards is surprisingly recent. For years, key stakeholders in healthcare saw no compelling business case for standardization, especially for clinical data, because the focus was on billing and financial systems. The challenge is fundamental to healthcare where providers are trained to use the expressive power of spoken and written language to describe their impression of a patient's state. Natural languages, while working perfectly for analog systems like humans, do not translate well to information systems, which are not as well equipped to resolve ambiguities that appear in documenting problems, findings, and outcomes (1). Standards offer the possibility of capturing clinical data in an analyzable form suitable to support the needs of researchers, educators, and providers.

In its very first position paper in 1994 (2), the American Medical Informatics Association (AMIA) identified that "lack of standards" (e.g., identifiers, message exchange, and structured medical data) was one of the biggest stumbling blocks in the adoption of information systems in healthcare. This chapter introduces the reader to some of the main standards development organizations, along with key standards that facilitate the capture and storage of clinical data and allow the exchange of data across organizational boundaries.

Standards Development Organizations and Facilitators

International Organization for Standardization

The International Organization for Standardization (ISO) (3) is a nongovernmental umbrella organization for developing standards across various industries with a global reach. National standards institutes of more than 150 countries are members of the ISO network. Standards developed by ISO have been incorporated in several areas. Some of the popular standards include the compact disk image file (commonly referred to as ISO, in actuality it is an ISO 9660 file type) and ISO 9000 (quality management). To date ISO has developed 16,000 standards covering almost every aspect of our lives. Though voluntary, due to its global reach any standard that achieves ISO approval in essence becomes an international de facto within that area.

Within ISO, the process of standards development is driven by technical committees that draw upon experts from across the globe in their respective domains. Technical Committee 215 (TC 215) focuses on health informatics and the issues surrounding it. To date, TC 215 has released 37 standards within this domain, covering areas such as medical devices, individual identifiers, and interoperability. ISO/TS 17117:2000 is a standard that reviews controlled health terminology and their structures.

Department of Health and Human Services

While the Department of Health and Human Services (HHS) itself is not directly involved in standards development, any standard that receives its backing becomes official, at least within the United States, and hence it is being included in this discussion. In 2004, an executive order established the Office of the National Coordinator (ONCHIT: Office of the National Coordinator for Health Information Technology) to assist the Secretary of HHS in achieving the objective of providing access to an interoperable electronic medical record for most Americans by 2014.

Following the recommendation of the ONC, the HHS Secretary created AHIC (Table 6-1), consisting of public and private sector leaders to accelerate adoption of interoperable electronic health IT.

The Department of HHS, through the office of ONC, awarded contracts to:

◆ Identify interoperability standards
   1. This led to the Health Information Technology Standards Panel (HITSP) (4)
◆ Define a process to certify health information technology products
   1. This led to the establishment of CCHIT
◆ Develop prototypes for National Health Information Network
   1. Awarded to consortia led by Accenture, IBM, CSC, and Northrop Grumman

Table 6-1

ENTITIES COMPRISING THE AHIC

American Health Information Community (AHIC)
The Certification Commission for Health Information Technology (CCHIT)
Health Information Technology Standards Panel (HITSP)
Health Information Security and Privacy Collaboration (HISPC)
National Health Information Network Architecture Projects (NHIN)

2. The Standards Harmonization Collaborative (a consortium of eighteen independent entities led by ANSI) won the contract and established the Health Information Technology Standards Panel (HITSP) with a mission "…to serve as a cooperative partnership between public and private sectors for the purpose of achieving a widely acceptable and useful set of standards specifically to enable and support widespread interoperability among healthcare software applications in the US".

The Panel has representatives from a broad group of stakeholders. Currently over 200 organizations participate in HITSP activities. HITSP's usage of the term "standard" refers to more than just standards in a generic sense to include:

◆ Specifications
◆ Implementation Guides
◆ Code Sets
◆ Terminologies
◆ Integration Profiles

In August 2006 HITSP approved three sets of "Interoperability Specifications" that were recommended by AHIC to the Secretary of HHS. Following the Secretary's acceptance of these interoperability standards, the federal government committed to use these standards in future health IT solutions.

American National Standards Institute

Founded in 1918, the American National Standards Institute (ANSI) (6) may well be regarded as the guardian of the voluntary standards system in the US. Initially christened American Engineering Standards Committee, reflecting its engineering roots, ANSI adopted its current name in 1969 in line with its expanding role and influence in shaping the standards debate within the US and globally. Along with 25 other member nations, it was the founding member of the International Organization for Standardization (ISO). ANSI is the US voting member on ISO and the International Electrotechnical Commission (IEC).

ANSI provides the forum for dialog and information exchange between public and private sector stakeholders to develop consensus standards. Currently there are over 11,500 American National Standards covering a range of subjects such as Consumer Products (e.g., bicycle helmets, baby cribs), Financial Industry, Healthcare Industry, Homeland Security, and Defense Industry

While ANSI itself doesn't develop any standards, using openness, balance, consensus, and due process as measures, it can accredit standards developing organizations (SDOs) to develop the standards in their respective areas of expertise. Since ANSI is the representative on ISO, once a standard has been approved by an ANSI-accredited SDO, ANSI can work with ISO to get it approved as an ISO standard either in part or completely. Examples of organizations in US healthcare industry that are ANSI-accredited include HITSP, HL7, and SNOMED.

American Society for Testing and Materials

The American Society for Testing and Materials (ASTM) is probably one of the largest standards development organizations (7) in the world, with over 30,000 active members across 100 countries. Founded in 1898 in Philadelphia, it initially was tasked with improving the standards of the steel used in railroad construction. From there, it expanded its mission to develop standards that enhance the reliability of materials, systems, products, and services. In 2001, it renamed itself ASTM International to reflect its global reach.

ASTM Technical Committee E31 on Healthcare Informatics was established in 1970 to develop standards addressing the architecture, content, security, functionality, and communication of information used within the healthcare domain.

American Dental Association

The American Dental Association (ADA) was established in 1859 to advance the public's oral health, with a mission to provide leadership through advocacy and research initiatives. ADA is an ANSI-accredited SDO. The ADA Standards Committee on Dental Informatics (ADA SCDI) (8) and Standards Committee on Dental Products (ADA SCDP) are the consensus bodies for standards development. ADA represents the US in the TAG (Technical Advisory Group) for ISO/TC 106. The US TAG is composed of seven sub-TAGs covering areas such as orthodontic and restorative materials, dental instruments, dental equipment, oral hygiene products, dental terminology, and dental implants. The ANSI/ADA Specification No 33-2003 focuses on Dental Terminology.

American Medical Association

The American Medical Association (AMA) (9) is a professional organization established in 1847 with a mission "to promote the art and science of medicine". It also has been involved in the development and maintenance of Current Procedural Terminology (CPT) codes used throughout the US for billing and reimbursement.

American Medical Informatics Association

The American Medical Informatics Association (AMIA) (10) is a non-profit informatics professional body that is focused on advancing the field through grants, advocacy, and partnerships with industry. Due to its academic role, it helps shape the debate regarding standards and provides guidance on gaps that may require additional research.

Healthcare Information and Management Systems Society

The Healthcare Information and Management Systems Society (HIMSS) is a non-profit healthcare information technology industry organization focusing on providing leadership in usage of information technology within healthcare. Founded in 1961, it has more than 20,000 individual members and more than 300 corporate members (11). Due to its commercial heritage, it serves to bridge the gap between theory and practice, helping to focus discussion as standards move to real-world systems.

Terminology Standards

Two categories of standards will be discussed: terminology standards that support capture and storage of patient information and data interchange standards that support sharing of data between information systems (Table 6-2).

International Classification of Diseases-9 Clinical Modification

International Classification of Diseases (ICD) (12) is probably one of the most popular terminologies and also represents the earliest attempt to structure clinical content for administrative purposes. The origin of the ICD system is in the UK, where the Bills of Mortality were used as a way to warn the general public of plague epidemics. John Graunt and William Farr of the General Registrar Office of England and Wales did early pioneering work in developing a working statistical classification of morbidity and mortality reporting. Their work was synthesized by Bertillon at the 1893 gathering of the International Statistical Institute in Chicago. The Bertillon

Table 6-2

TERMINOLOGY STANDARDS

Standard	Domain
Terminology	
CPT	Procedures, Laboratory
SNOMED	Clinical findings
ICD	Diagnosis
LOINC	Procedures, Laboratory
RXNORM	Medications
HUGN	Genome
DRG	Diagnosis
NANDA	Nursing
Data Interchange	
HL7	Message exchange
DICOM	Image exchange
NCPDP	Pharmacy
XML	Data exchange

Classification of Causes of Death, as it was initially known, was adopted by the American Public Health Association in 1898. This classification was revised every ten years and in 1948 its sixth revision was adopted under the stewardship of the World Health Organization (WHO).

In 1975, work on the ninth revision of ICD began with the intention of updating just the content in line with the new knowledge. Due to the enormous interest in ICD from insurance carriers, and national governments, the classification itself had to be modified with special coding provisions to accommodate various needs. ICD-9 has about 7000 categories organized in a hierarchical manner. Users in the United States felt that the ICD-9 codes must be more precise to better support statistical reporting. Hence, a clinical modification (CM) with the intent of capturing the patient's clinical state in greater detail was adopted (ICD-9-CM) in the US for reporting purposes, expanding the content to about 12,000 categories. Although WHO published ICD-10 in 1993, ICD-9-CM codes remain prevalent within the US for reporting purposes.

ICD codes consist of at least three digits (e.g., 410 acute myocardial infarction), indicating the main concept with a decimal followed by fourth and fifth digits to denote variants or sub-types of the main concept (e.g., 410.1 of the anterior wall, 410.7 subendocardial infarction). If knowledge is assumed to be static, this classification holds well, but when new knowledge arises, codes are revised. Hence, it is hard to ascertain if a particular code has carried the same meaning over time through multiple revisions.

Although clinical modification allows capturing patient state in greater detail, ICD-9-CM is primarily intended for billing and administrative purposes. Some of the features of ICD-9 that negatively affect the value of data for analysis are the *Not Otherwise Specified* (NOS) and *Not Elsewhere Classified* (NEC) categories. These categories provide coding flexibility at the expense of data quality.

Systematized Nomenclature of Medicine

Systematized nomenclature of medicine SNOMED (13) is a terminology that originated as systematized nomenclature of pathology (SNOP) in the early 60s under the guidance of the College of American Pathologists (CAP). In the late 70s, the content of SNOP was expanded to encompass most of the domains in medicine and changed itself into SNOMED.

SNOMED has been one of the earliest to forge relationships with other content developers, and its evolution over time reflects this heritage. In 1979, SNOMED II was released with approximately 45,000 terms. SNOMED International (SNOMED III) was released in 1993 with over 130,000 terms. Working primarily with Kaiser Permanente, in 1999 SNOMED Reference Terminology (SNOMED RT) was released. Partnering with the National Health Service (NHS) of the UK, it was decided to combine SNOMED RT with Read Codes to create SNOMED CT (Clinical Terms). In 2000, CAP was accredited by ANSI as a standards developing organization. SNOMED CT currently has over 350,000 concepts and over 1,000,000 descriptions. Unlike ICD-9 codes, where the code implicitly denotes a hierarchy, SNOMED codes are randomly generated unique IDs. Such an approach allows easy addition of content as new knowledge becomes available.

SNOMED core content includes text files such as the concepts, descriptions, relationships, ICD-9 mappings, and history tables. The concepts table contains terms with unique meanings. The descriptions table contains various descriptions for the concepts to support synonyms. Finally, the relationships table defines the relationships between various concepts to define their meaning. In terms of content coverage, although SNOMED is quite comprehensive relative to other terminologies, it still has problems in certain areas. For instance, SNOMED has "phimosis" as a synonym for both Congenital and Acquired variants. This can be a source of confusion, especially during data conversion. Assessments such as Cough, Claudication, Headache or Neurological assessments are some of the other areas where content coverage may be unclear. Another issue is that of post-coordination. Post-coordination refers to the practice of combining concepts to create new concepts. For instance, Thrombosis of the superior vena cava can be a single SNOMED CT Concept (Concept ID: 281596000) or can be post-coordinated from two concepts: Thrombosis (Concept ID: 264579008) and Superior Vena Cava (Concept ID: 48345005). Post-coordination extends the coverage of terminology by allowing composition of new concepts from existing concepts. However, it is an extremely challenging effort to define the rules or the grammar that ensures that only meaningful concepts can be derived and, more importantly, prevent nonsensical combinations (e.g.,

Female (Concept ID: 248152002) Prostate (Concept ID: 181422007]). Post-coordination can lead to inadvertent creation of synonyms of existing concepts. Subsequently, the tasks of data retrieval and data analysis become extremely difficult, if not impossible. In April 2007, CAP officially transferred the ownership of SNOMED to an international entity, International Health Terminology Standards Development Organisation (IHTSDO). HHS has adopted SNOMED CT as the official clinical terminology for EHRs.

Logical Observations, Identifiers, Names and Codes

Developed under the stewardship of Clement McDonald of the Regenstrief Institute in Indiana and Stanley Huff of Intermountain Healthcare in Utah, the Logical Observations, Identifiers, Names and Codes (LOINC) (14) database is available as a free download from the Regenstrief website. Though it was introduced as Laboratory Observations, Identifiers, Names and Codes in 1994, its scope was expanded to include other clinical observations and hence renamed as LOINC in 1996. Along with the database, a navigational tool called RELMA (Regenstrief LOINC Mapping Assistant) is also provided to assist in searching and mapping local codes to LOINC codes. Currently LOINC includes over 45,000 terms covering lab and clinical subject areas. LOINC can be used in messaging standards such as DICOM, and HL7 for encoding observations. LOINC also is available in a variety of other languages such as Spanish, Swiss French, and German.

A LOINC code can be anywhere from three to seven characters, including the check digit as the last character (although for future expansion it is recommended to allow up to ten characters). A fully specified name for an observation has multiple parts: the actual name of component or analyte being measured; its property (e.g., MCNC:- Mass concentration; SCNC:-substance concentration; NFR:- numeric fraction); timing (e.g., PT:- point in time); sample type (e.g. BLD: -blood; URN:- urine;); method (e.g., QN:-quantitative; QL:-qualitative); and method (e.g., IB:- immune blot). An example of a LOINC observation is illustrated in Figure 6-1.

Since detailed structured information is included in the fully specified name, lab or clinical observations information from various entities can be semantically linked using LOINC to achieve interoperability.

LOINC #	Short Common Name	Component	Property	Time	System	Scale	Method
41995-2	Hgb A1c Bld-mCnc	HEMOGLOBIN A1C	MCNC	PT	BLD	QN	

Figure 6-1 A sample LOINC Concept (Hemoglobin) structure.

RxNorm

In 2001, as part of their effort to improve patient safety, the National Library of Medicine (NLM) began exploring ways of codifying information pertaining to drugs in the UMLS metathesaurus. Existing information systems use different terminologies to convey the same information regarding drugs. To accomplish interoperability between these semantically similar but syntactically different systems, NLM built the RxNorm (15) project around the HL7 model of order while content was primarily derived from other popular drug dictionaries such as First Databank, MediSpan, MediSource, SNOMED, VA's National Drug File, and FDA National Drug Code Directory, resulting in the RxNorm database. NLM also provides RxNav, a free browser to navigate through the RxNorm database.

The Semantic Normal Form (SNF) is the key construct of the RxNorm. The SNF has the generic names of the active ingredients, units, dose forms and strength in standard units constrained by rules and relationships. The SNF itself may be used in the context of a Drug Component (SCDC) or Clinical Formulation (SCD). The drug component's general structure is shown below with an example drug.

- CUI | ShortName | ActiveIngredient | PreciseIngredient | Basis | Strength | Units | Notes
  1. CUI: Concept Unique Identifier (from UMLS)
  2. Active Ingredient: the drug in its complete form, e.g., salt form like penicillin potassium
  3. Precise Ingredient: actual drug, e.g., penicillin

The clinical formulation allows combination of drug components to be dispensed and has the following general structure

- CUI | MetaID | ShortName | Component1/Component2... | OrderableDose Form | Notes

Human Gene Nomenclature

The HUGO Genome Nomenclature Committee (HGNC) (16) is a joint venture between the National Human Genome Research Institute of the US, the UK Medical Research Council, and the Wellcome Trust (UK). In the past decade, interest and activity in the area of genomic research has grown exponentially. The HGNC operates very closely with the Human Genome Organization (HUGO) to fulfill its responsibilities. HGNC is charged with assigning a name and a symbol to each of the genes identified by the Human Genome Project. Currently, over 24,000 symbols/names have been approved for use in information systems. The US Department of HHS, Veteran's Administration, and Department of Defense have approved HUGN for exchanging genetic information in translational and other research activities in the federal health system. Figure 6-2 shows a sample gene encoding for the aconitase enzyme.

Approved Gene Symbol	Approved Gene Name	Location	Sequence Accession IDs	Previous Symbols	Aliases
ACO1	Aconitase 1, Soluble	9p21.1	M58510 NM_002197	IREB1	IRP1, IREBP

Figure 6-2   Example of the nomenclature schema for a gene encoding for aconitase.

Diagnosis-Related Groups

Diagnosis-related groups (DRGs) began in the early 1980s, when Medicare (17) was on the brink of bankruptcy. Developed by researchers from Yale, the DRG prospective payment system interestingly enough was intended to be more of a quality assessment and improvement tool rather than a cost containment tool (18). ICD-9 CM codes were aggregated into categories that grouped similar procedures or diseases. More than 10,000 ICD-9 codes are grouped into approximately 526 DRG codes (Figure 6-3). As part of calculating the DRGs, while factors such as length of stay are included in the formula, the geographical boundary factor, which determines the Wage Index and thereby the reimbursement for labor costs, has been a huge challenge to manage socially and politically for Medicare. As part of its effort to overhaul the DRG codes, the 526 DRG codes are being expanded to 861 severity-adjusted categories to reflect the practice patterns more accurately.

As an example, ICD-9 code 482.9 for "bacterial pneumonia, unspecified" may be grouped under more than one DRG depending on the secondary diagnosis or related complications. For instance, it can be grouped under 79 or 80 (see Figure 6-3). CMS updates DRGs on an annual basis to support Medicare's prospective payment system.

DRG Code	Definition
135	Cardiac Congenital & Valvular Disorders Age >17
	With Complications, Comorbidities
136	Cardiac Congenital & Valvular Disorders Age >17
	Without Complications, Comorbidities
137	Cardiac Congenital & Valvular Disorders Age 0–17
79	Respiratory Infections & Inflammations Age >17
	With Complications, Comorbidities
80	Respiratory Infections & Inflammations Age >17
	Without Complications, Comorbidities

Figure 6-3   Sample DRG codes with their definitions.

Diagnostic and Statistical Manual of Mental Disorders

The Diagnostic and Statistical Manual of Mental Disorders (DSM) (19) is published by the American Psychiatric Association and is used extensively by psychiatrists in the United States and increasingly around the world. It has gone through four major versions since the first edition was published in 1952. The way psychiatric disorders are coded in the DSM is different from that in other classification systems in that a set of criteria is included along with the name of the disorder (Figure 6-4). Crosswalks have always been provided between the DSM and the corresponding ICD-9 equivalent. For instance, DSM-IV is mapped to both ICD-9 CM and ICD-10.

Unified Medical Language System

In 1986, NLM started work on the Unified Medical Language System (UMLS) as an attempt to address one of the fundamental barriers to applying computers in medicine: *the lack of standard language in medicine* (20). UMLS is a group of knowledge sources created in machine-readable format. The *Metathesaurus* is at the center of UMLS and is a collection of various terminologies that are, in the terms from source vocabularies, clustered into concepts with a Concept Unique Identifier (CUI). The 2007 AA UMLS release has more than 1.3 million concepts and over 6.4 million concept names from more than 100 source vocabularies. The *Semantic Network* (SN) describes over 54 hierarchical ('is a' relationship) and non-hierarchical (related to) relationships between the concepts. The SN groups terms into more than 135 subject categories like clinical drug or virus or disease/syndrome. Collectively, the semantic types and relationships set the groundwork for a semantic network of biomedical information.

Symptoms	Diagnosis	DSM Code
Sleep problems	Major Depressive Disorder (MDD), Single Episode. (To meet the diagnosis of MDD, patient must have 4 symptoms and depressed mood or anhedonia for at least 2 weeks.)	295.2x
Interest deficit		
Guilt, worthlessness, hopelessness		
Energy deficit		
Concentration deficit		
Appetite disorder		
(either increased or decreased)		
Psychomotor retardation or agitation		
Suicidality		
Fatigue		

Figure 6-4   DSM Code structure for Major Depressive Disorder (MDD).

```
26010  Drainage of finger abscess; simple
26011  Drainage of finger abscess; complicated (eg, felon)
26020  Drainage of tendon sheath; digit and/or palm, each
26025  Drainage of palmar bursa; single, bursa
```

Figure 6-5 Sample CPT Codes describing various types of abscess drainage.

The UMLS (21) is a unique resource that brings together all controlled medical terminologies currently in use within the US. This enables system developers and researchers to explore the relationships between terminology systems using sophisticated navigation and knowledge management tools. Published annually, NLM continually updates the syntax and semantics of UMLS content. UMLS is available in a free downloadable form, or a DVD of the content can be requested or accessed via the Internet from NLM.

Current Procedural Terminology

In 1966, the American Medical Association created current procedural terminology (CPT) codes (22) to document the procedures in medical records and also to help with insurance claims processing. While the first version covered surgical procedures, the next version was expanded to document diagnostic and medical procedures. The actual CPT codes consist of five-digit numbers. Some sample CPT codes are listed in Figure 6-5.

Nursing Terminologies

Within the informatics world, nursing groups are actively engaged in developing adequate standardized terminologies to reflect their clinical activities. While terminologies such as NANDA-I (North American Nursing Diagnosis Association-International) (23) and the Omaha system (24) have taken the early lead, further effort is required to deliver a comprehensive nursing terminology solution.

Data Interchange Standards

Health Level Seven (HL7)

Health Level Seven (25) is a messaging standard for exchanging information between various information systems within or across enterprise(s). HL7 is an ANSI-accredited SDO in the healthcare realm. HL7 membership is made entirely of volunteers who organize into technical committees (TC) and special interest groups (SIGs) to develop appropriate standards in their respective areas. It is a consensus-driven process, where any proposal is discussed between members of the TC or the SIGs and any negative comments have to be reconciled before allowing it to be put on the HL7 ballot as a standard. HL7 primarily focuses on developing standards in the clinical and administrative areas. Though it was founded in 1987 as an ad hoc standards development entity, in 1994 it became an ANSI-accredited standards developer.

HL7 messages are event driven, i.e., message flow is generated in response to some real-world event like an admission or a discharge or an order. Such an event triggers a message to be created in a sending system and sent to some receiving system(s) that needs to "know" of this event. Each of these messages is a collection of segments. A segment is composed of data elements whose order in the message and whether mandatory or optional, is defined by the corresponding version of the standard. As of the present, approximately six versions of the HL7 standard have been released. The latest version, HL7 version 2.5, was approved as an ANSI standard in 2003. HL7 standards V2.x are some of the most popular and well-implemented HL7 standards across the US and are gaining traction across the globe.

A sample lab order HL7 message is illustrated in Figure 6-6. Each HL7 message is made of a series of segments that are in turn made of elements separated by delimiters such as |, ~, \, and &. An MSH segment is required of all HL7 messages and stands for Message Header. It contains information such as field separators, sending and receiving applications/facility, and date and time stamp of the message. The next segment is the PID segment, which uniquely identifies the patient and includes the name, gender, address, contact information and IDs such as SSN or license information. The

---

MSH|^~\&|OADD|652|DADD||20070212124511||ORU^R01|20070430035413|T|2.2||||

PID||6916004||547621160^^^^UN|Doe^John||19561231|M||||||26387456

PV1||O|UCS^^^OP||||877^Smith^William^ZI^||||||OP|||||||||200701220000| 200701240000|||||||||

ORC|RE||A844542|||||||||33209^Doe^Jane^||||^|

OBR||T1606063:A844542|A844542|BMP^BASIC METABOLIC PANEL | 200701230848| ||||||20070123084900|^|33209^Doe^Jane^|T1606063||C|F| BMP^BMP^^^^^R|||||||||

OBX|1|NM|NA^Sodium^O|1.1|145|mmol/L|137–146||||

OBX|2|NM|K^Potassium^O|1.1|2.1|mmol/L|3.5–5.0|L^LL|||

ZLB|9|F|CE||FAFAM^If patient is African American, multiply estimated GFR by 1.21.^L^O|||||||

Figure 6-6   Sample HL7 version 2.x message (the segments have been altered for brevity).

next segment, PV1 segment, identifies information unique for a given visit such as the provider information, location, patient financial information, and location information such as outpatient, inpatient, or emergency.

The ORC (Common Order segment) segment contains the ID of the order and the provider who is ordering it. For instance, in the sample HL7 message above, the PID segment shows that this is a message generated for a patient named John Doe, his date of birth, gender, and his account number. Likewise, the PV1 segment (Patient Visit segment) shows the location of the patient (O for outpatient in the message above), the attending physician (William Z Smith) and the date and time stamps. The ORC segment (Common Order segment) is used to pass on any order data such as lab or radiology orders. For instance, in the message above, A844542 is an order by a provider whose ID is 33209 with a name Jane Doe. The OBR (Observation Request) segment contains further details of the ordering information such as the name of the tests being ordered, the provider information, and date and time. In the example above, for instance, Basic Metabolic Panel has been ordered for this patient by provider Jane Doe. The OBX (observation result) segment contains the results of the order such as labs. It is a segment that can be repeated. In the example above, the OBX segment has been repeated twice to illustrate the results of Sodium and Potassium as part of the Basic Metabolic Panel. And finally the Z-segment (ZLB segment) is also illustrated in the sample HL7 message. In a nutshell, the Z-segment is a custom segment that can be used in any HL7 message. Many of the multiple | | seen in Figure 6-6 are optional elements of the HL7 messages.

HL7 originally set out to address the problem of "interface explosion". Given the disparate proprietary legacy systems that comprise a typical HIS, as the number of systems that need to interface with each other increased linearly, the number of interfaces needed to facilitate information exchange between them increased exponentially. To address this, the HL7 standard focused on the message structure and the content while leaving its implementation to the vendors. To ensure the widest possible acceptance, HL7 messages contain both required and optional components. Since the implementation specifications were left to the vendor discretion, some vendors left the optional components of the message as part of their message while others dropped them completely from their message. In addition, the same information may be represented differently in different vendor implementation (e.g., Timestamp). Also, both the sender and receiving application should support the same version of the standard to ensure information exchange. As an acknowledgement of the inability to standardize all aspects of health information exchange across the enterprise, HL7 V2.x standards have the Z-segment. As this segment is defined locally, systems that do not understand it simply disregard it.

Recognizing the inherent limitations of the previous approach in developing messaging standards, HL7 started work in the late 90s on developing HL7 V3.0. HL7 uses a more formal model-driven object-oriented approach in defining and developing Version 3.0 specifications for messaging and non-messaging standards. At the heart of Version 3.0 is the Reference Information Model (RIM). The RIM consists of a set of core object classes including the *Act, Act Relationship, Participation, Role, Role Relationship*, and the *Entity* classes. The Act class is defined as a *discernible action of interest in healthcare domain,* e.g., Procedure, Order. Entity class is defined as *a physical thing or an organization/group of physical things capable of participating in Acts,* e.g. Person, Organization. Role defines how Entities take part in Acts. Act Relationship creates an association between two acts. Participation defines an association between an Act and Role e.g. subject, author, provider. Finally, the Role Relationship defines the association between two roles. If HL7 is understood as a language, RIM defines the grammar of the messages. HL7 version 3 is slowly gaining acceptance as vendors learn to adjust to its radically different approach compared to version 2.x.

Accredited Standards Committee X12

The Accredited Standards Committee X12 (ASC X12) (26) is an ANSI-accredited entity working in the electronic data interchange (EDI) domain. X12 draws its members from diverse industries such as transportation, insurance, finance, government, real estate, software, and law enforcement. ASC X12 messages are also similar to HL7 messages in that named segments are wrapped as transaction sets. The X12N sub-committee is involved in developing EDI standards relating to insurance. HIPAA requires HHS to adopt X12N standards for healthcare administrative and financial transactions (Table 6-3). Development and maintenance of the ASC X12 transaction sets are reconciled with the UN/EDIFACT messages, which are developed for international use.

Digital Imaging and Communications in Medicine

The Digital Imaging and Communications in Medicine (DICOM) standard (27) has been developed to facilitate exchanging and sharing of medical imaging content. DICOM is the fruit of cooperation primarily between imaging

Table 6-3

X12N STANDARDS FOR HEALTHCARE ADMINISTRATIVE AND FINANCIAL TRANSACTIONS

♦ Eligibility (WG 1: 270, 271. ICHEBI, ICHEBR)
♦ Healthcare Claim Attachments (WG2: Health Care Claim, Professional 837P; Health Care Claim, Institutional 837I; Health Care Claim, Dental 837D)
♦ Claim Status (WG5: Healthcare Claim Status Request 276/ Healthcare Claim Status Notification 277; WG9 Patient Information 275)
♦ Referral Certification and Authorization (WG10: Health Care Services Review 278)
♦ Claims, Encounters, and Coordination of Benefits (WG4: Enrollments 834)

device manufacturers (represented by NEMA: National Electrical Manufacturers Association) and the user community (represented by ACR: American College of Radiology). DICOM defines the hardware interfaces, connectivity protocols, media formats, and storage and retrieval information in great detail. DICOM is unique compared to other standards in that it requires a conformance statement from a manufacturer claiming compliance with the DICOM standard. While this does not completely resolve the issues of incompatibility between devices claiming compliance with a particular standard (e.g., HL7 compliant) it helps users understand how a manufacturers device implements the standard. While the initial two versions of the standard focused on point-to-point communication, the need for sharing information across multiple networks was compelling enough to warrant a redesign of the standard. DICOM 3.0 is built atop the TCP/IP stack (Figure 6-7) and follows the same layered architecture of the ISO Networking Model to accommodate any future connectivity enhancements.

Version 3.0 is object-oriented and has a key feature Service-Object Pairs (SOP). SOP can be understood as the mechanism through which DICOM ensures uniformity in implementation of the standard. SOP defines the nature of the transaction, the data being transferred, and how to deal with various actions. As part of the transfer process, during the handshake process, the receiving device has to acknowledge that it understands the information that the sending device is transferring. If it does not understand, it can

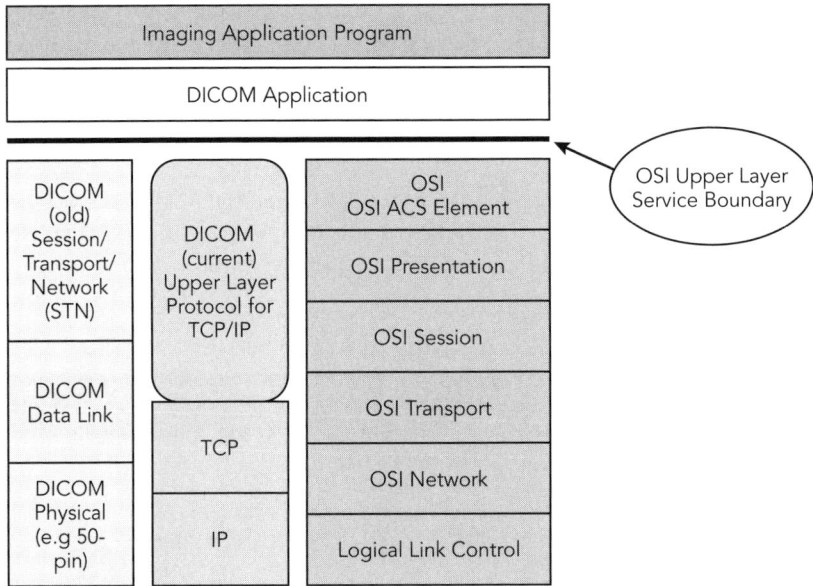

Figure 6-7 DICOM Communication Protocol Stacks – Any of the three architectures are supported for DICOM exchanges.

let the sending device know what it can support. A typical DICOM file consists of a header part, which contains information such as patient demographics, type of study, and the actual image data. A sample DICOM header is explored in more detail in Figure 6-8 for illustrative purposes.

By design, the information in the header is organized into groups followed by the elements that belong to that particular group. For instance, the group 0010 refers to information pertaining to the patient and has about seven elements such as name, ID, birth date, sex, age, weight, and additional patient history. Likewise, the group 0008 contains information about the study such as the modality (element: 0060 CT image) and the manufacturer of the device (element: 0070 GE Medical). Length describes the length of the value being stored for that particular data element (e.g. 0008 0008: image type has a length of 22 reflecting the value "ORIGINAL\PRIMARY\AXIAL"). Description provides a description of the particular field. VR refers to Value Representation, which describes the data type for that field (e.g., 0010 0030 shows DA for date value). VM, Value Multiplicity, defines the number of values for a particular field. Value Column contains the actual value being stored for a given field.

Grp	Elmt	Length	Description	VR	VM	Value
0008	0000	4	group_length_0008	UL	1	0x0000025e606
0008	0005	10	specific_character_set	CS	1-n	"ISO_IR 100"
0008	0008	22	image_type	CS	1-n	"ORIGINAL\PRIMARY\AXIAL"
0008	0012	8	instance_creation_date	DA	1	"20060110"
0008	0013	6	instance_creation_time	TM	1	"104123"
0008	0016	26	sop_class_uid	UI	1	"1.2.840.10008.5.1.4.1.1.2"
0008	0018	54	sop_instance_uid	UI	1	
"1.2.840.113619.2.55.1.1762938041.2227.1136911540.75.2"						
0008	0020	8	study_date	DA	1	"20060110"
0008	0060	2	modality	CS	1	"CT"
0008	0070	18	manufacturer	LO	1	"GE Medical"
0008	0080	16	institution_name	LO	1	"SLCER"
0008	0090	6	referring_physician_name	PN	1	"FRAME"
0008	1060	4	name_of_physicians_reading_study	PN	1-n	"UIA"
0008	1070	2	operator_name	PN	1-n	"RR"
0008	1090	12	manufacturer_model_name	LO	1	"Discovery ST"
0010	0010	14	patient_name	PN	1	"XTEST, LEGAL"
0010	0020	6	patient_id	LO	1	"111111"
0010	0030	8	patient_birth_date	DA	1	"19440609"
0010	0040	2	patient_sex	CS	1	"M"
0010	1010	4	patient_age	AS	1	"072Y"
0010	1030	4	patient_weight	DS	1	"84.0"
0010	21b0	26	additional_patient_history	LT	1	"OP,PRIOR PET/CT,LYMPHOMA

Figure 6-8 Sample DICOM Header (Partially represented).

National Council for Prescription Drug Programs

The National Council for Prescription Drug Programs (NCPDP) (28) is an ANSI-accredited standards development organization with a mission to create and promote standards in data transfer within the pharmacy sector of healthcare industry. HHS has adopted the NCPDP Telecommunication Standard and Batch Standard for part of pharmacy claims HIPAA transactions and code sets. The NCPDP standard is used for submitting retail pharmacy claims and verifying eligibility. Similar to DICOM, the NCPDP standard defines data types, supported transport protocols, data dictionary defining the possible values, the actual data that traverses the network and other relevant requirements.

eXtensible Markup Language

Extensible Markup Language (XML) (29) is a language that can be used to create other languages. XML derives its structure from Standard Generalized Markup Language (SGML), a language that has been around for a few decades. XML is extensible in that the tags used in an XML document can be defined by the end-user according to their industry or application. It is also platform-independent (i.e., XML is not locked into a particular operating system or hardware interface).

To understand the power of XML, it is necessary to understand another markup language, the Hypertext Markup Language (HTML). As the name implies, this language was intended to help in linking multiple documents through hyperlinks. This revolutionized the Internet and developed into what we know as the World Wide Web (WWW). HTML focused more on the presentation of the data. HTML also was caught in the cross-fire of browser wars. While Netscape-supported browsers tried to stick closely to the Internet Engineering Task Force (IETF) guidelines for HTML, Microsoft, with the lion's share of the browser market, injected its own proprietary tags to gain business advantage. This caused issues in rendering documents that may conform to the IETF standard and yet not be rendered properly by all browsers. As the number of web pages and web sites grew exponentially, the importance of semantic interoperability gained momentum. But HTML was of little help in addressing this growing and important concern. Sample HTML code that describes various types of diagnoses is illustrated in Figure 6-9.

Although other HTML tags can be used, for illustrative purposes, the tags have been oversimplified. Rendering the above code in a web browser would produce a web page with a single line that reads "Shoulder Pain Myocardial Infarction Myocardial Infarction Hypertension Acute Coronary Syndrome" (see Figure 6-9b). If someone were to view this file, it makes no sense whatsoever. At best, a web designer can beautify the above code by adding some formatting tags such as <b>, which bolds certain aspects of

```
<html>
<h1><Diagnosis></h1>
        <Preliminary>Shoulder Pain</Preliminary>
        <Discharge>Myocardial Infarction</Discharge>
        <Primary>Myocardial Infarction</Primary>
        <Secondary>Hypertension</Secondary>
        <Final>Acute Coronary Syndrome</Final>
</Diagnosis>
</html>
```

Shoulder Pain
Myocardial Infarction
Myocardial Infarction
Hypertension
Acute Coronary Syndrome

A   **B**

Figure 6-9   Sample HTML code of web page describing various types of diagnoses.

the data or <h1>, which makes something a header. But from a semantic perspective, it is hard to derive any meaning. With semantic interoperability, the stated goal of many standard developing organizations, the short comings of HTML become more acute.

The same code when defined in XML and viewed in a web browser (Figure 6-10 b) displays the hierarchy and clearly shows the nested nature of the data with quite self-explanatory tags. The kind of hierarchy present in XML allows searches and retrieval of data that are more advanced than anything possible with the HTML type of markup languages. In addition, different devices can ask for specific parts of the data to suit their needs. For instance, imagine the use case of an outbreak of some infectious disease. The local county health department might be interested in the preliminary

```
<?xml version="1.0" encoding="UTF-8"?>
<Diagnosis>
        <Preliminary>Shoulder Pain</Preliminary>
        <Discharge>Myocardial Infarction</Discharge>
        <Primary>Myocardial Infarction</Primary>
        <Secondary>Hypertension</Secondary>
        <Final>Acute Coronary Syndrome</Final>
</Diagnosis>
```

A

```
<?xml version="1.0" encoding="UTF-8" ?>
- <Diagnosis>
    <Preliminary>Shoulder Pain</Preliminary>
    <Discharge>Myocardial Infarction</Discharge>
    <Primary>Myocardial Infarction</Primary>
    <Secondary>Hypertension</Secondary>
    <Final>Acute Coronary Syndrome</Final>
  </Diagnosis>
```

B

Figure 6-10   Sample XML code of describing various types of diagnoses.

diagnosis rather than final diagnosis. In such a situation, queries can be tailored to deliver only the preliminary diagnosis. On the other hand, Medicare or other payers might be interested only in the final diagnosis for reimbursement purposes.

XML focuses more on describing the data rather than on the presentation of the data. The data and formatting information can reside separately. Due to this ability, the same data can be delivered via multiple channels such as the web, pagers, and print medium without taxing the resources too much. Advanced decision-support rules are possible due to the semantic understanding of the data. This also highlights the process of machine understanding. Though in its infancy, different information systems can comprehend the meaning inherent in the data and act on that understanding to help in the care delivery process. Hence, XML is considered to be the lingua franca of web 2.0. XML has also been used to create other languages such as WML (Wireless Markup Language: used to create Wireless Application Protocol), XSL (Extensible Stylesheet Language: specifies the presentation details of an XML document), and SOAP (Simple Object Access Protocol). SOAP deserves special mention as it empowers every connected device to share its information with other devices as needed through remote procedure calls (RPC). Through SOAP, distributed computing finally becomes a reality in healthcare, where instead of a single repository of patient data, multiple sites store various episodes of care provided, which can be pooled to generate a single view of it upon appropriate authentication. This type of model is being actively explored to support the Nationwide Health Information Network (NHIN) framework.

Finally, XML is the language used in HL7's RIM, and Clinical Document Architecture (CDA). XML also is central to ASTM's Continuity-of-Care-Record (CCR) and in the research arena through the Clinical Data Interchange Standards Consortium's (CDISC) Operational Data Model (ODM). These examples are intended to highlight the growing significance of XML in exchanging messages between devices in healthcare to transform pieces of data into meaningful information.

Electronic Health Records Functional and Content Standards

The HL7 EHR System Functional Model and Legal Record standards are welcome additions to the pantheon of informatics standards. The EHR Functional Model is used to create "profiles" that detail the requirements for EHR functionality within a specific care setting. These profiles are then used to create criteria used to certify EHR products (CCHIT). The Legal Record profile identifies a subset of requirements necessary to ensure data quality and integrity regardless of data usage or care setting. This work provides a global view of electronic heath records that can be shared by all stakeholders. Unfortunately, it does not at this time address issues related to data content (30).

Future Trends

Many of the expected benefits of electronic health records assume the ability to capture data that can be shared whether for real-time decision support or for secondary analysis to guide health policy. Standardization of concepts, terms, formats and content are required to address concerns of quality and safety. Increasingly, there is recognition that there is a clear business case for information standards use. Although not many studies have rigorously quantified the benefits of interoperability, a recent study (31) concluded that a fully standardized health information exchange and interoperability between providers and third parties could yield a net value of $77.8 billion per year. As experts lay out the case for standardization by quantifying the financial benefits, there is a growing belief that the clinical and public health benefits of standardization may far outweigh the financial benefits. For instance, preventive medicine and chronic disease management have traditionally been a tough sell. But standardization is expected to provide enhanced decision-support, and also better continuity of care to strengthen the therapeutic alliance between the patient and the provider thereby enhancing long-term care management.

While there may be a strong business case for standardization, provider organizations have been slow to embrace them. Several key issues may be at play here. First, demonstrating a return on investment (ROI) in implementing and utilizing standards is not an easy task. Due to the fragmented nature of the healthcare delivery system, the workflow may not reveal all the processes of care, and hence not lend itself to easy enumeration of the returns. Second, there are significant upfront costs in implementing standards without any guarantee of any tangible benefit. Third, the benefits of standards may not be spread out evenly. For instance, prescription modules provide a significant and obvious benefit by cutting down on the time and effort needed for prescription renewal. However, developing and defining a method to quantify, in monetary terms, for instance the value of a decision-support application's "Infobutton" (intended to provide more information about a diagnosis or a medication) is an extremely challenging task. Lastly, while providers bear the cost in implementing interoperable systems, in quite a few cases the savings are picked up by the insurers and the patients (e.g. reduced administrative overhead). As the healthcare emphasis changes from a focus on acute interventions to tracking cradle-to-grave outcome(s), the data elements, and the storage models needed to support it require rethinking.

While information sharing at the network level has dramatically improved, inability to map from one information system to another precludes meaningful data sharing. The proposed NHIN and the RHIOs (Regional Health Information Organization) are predicated upon organizational and provider ability to share their data in an unparalleled manner. Additionally, the general public has become more computer literate and Internet savvy where instant access to accurate and timely information is the norm rather than the exception. With most of the other service industries such as the food and beverage industry, finance industry, and travel industry delivering value-added services by embracing standards (e.g. XML, SOAP) in a big way, consumers expect similar benefits and access from healthcare too. Even within the same institution, in spite of an implemented EHR, a patient may have to repeatedly provide the same demographic and other administrative information when visiting different departments of the institution. Explaining these anomalies as routine business can be quite tricky, if not embarrassing.

Responding to customer needs, large information technology vendors have started to redesign their products around standards. This increased interest should have a domino effect in the healthcare market. Augmenting the private sector efforts, the federal government has demonstrated a willingness to assume the chore of regulating and mandating standards through entities such as HITSP and AHIC. Indirectly, the government is also encouraging institutions such as the VA, CDC, DHHS, NIH, NLM, and the Department of Defense to take a leadership role in framing the debate surrounding the role of standards in healthcare and advocate for them. Professional bodies such as AMIA and AHIMA are also advocating greater collaboration on a global scale in developing and implementing standards (32).

As the importance of the role standards play becomes more prominent in the discussions surrounding the development of an electronic healthcare infrastructure, the time for standards has arrived. With the debate shifting from *why* standards are needed to *what* standards are needed, there is clarity in the goals and a renewed sense of purpose to make it all work in a seamless manner.

References

1. Rector AL. Clinical terminology: why is it so hard? Methods Inf Med. 1999;38:239–52.
2. Standards for medical identifiers, codes, and messages needed to create an efficient computer-stored medical record. American Medical Informatics Association., J Am Med Inform Assoc 1994; 1: 1-7
3. http://www.iso.org (accessed on May 30, 2007)
4. http://www.ansi.org/hitsp (accessed on May 30, 2007)
5. http://www.cen.eu (accessed on May 30, 2007)
6. http://www.ansi.org (accessed on May 06 30, 2007)
7. http://www.astm.org (accessed on Jun 30, 2007)
8. http://www.ada.org (accessed on Jun 30, 2007)
9. http://www.ama.org (accessed on Jun 30, 2007)
10. http://www.amia.org (accessed on Jun 30, 2007)
11. http://www.himss.org (accessed on Jun 30, 2007)
12. http://www.cdc.gov/nchs/ICD-9.htm (accessed on Jun 30, 2007)
13. http://www.snomed.org (accessed on Jun 30, 2007)
14. http://www.regenstrief.org/medinformatics/loinc/ (accessed on Jun 30, 2007)
15. http://www.nlm.nih.gov/research/umls/rxnorm/index.html (accessed on Jun 30, 2007)

16. http://www.gene.ucl.ac.uk/nomenclature/aboutHGNC.html (accessed on Jun 30, 2007)
17. http://www.cms.hhs.gov (accessed on Jun 30, 2007)
18. Mayes R. The Origins, Development, and Passage of Medicare's Revolutionary Prospective Payment System. Journal of the History of Medicine and Allied Sciences. Oxford: Jan 2007. Vol. 62, Iss. 1; p. 21
19. http://dsmivtr.org/ (accessed on Jun 30, 2007)
20. Departments of Labor, Health and Human Services, Education, and Related Agencies Appropriations for 1986: Hearings Before the Subcommittee on the Departments of Labor, Health and Human Services, Education, and Related Agencies of the House Committee on Appropriations, 99th Cong., 1st Sess. Part 4B, (857) (1985)
21. http://www.nlm.nih.gov/research/umls/about_umls.html (accessed on Jun 30, 2007)
22. http://www.ama-assn.org/ama/pub/category/3113.html (accessed on Jun 30, 2007)
23. http://www.nanda.org/ (accessed on Jun 30, 2007)
24. http://www.omahasystem.org/ on Jun 30, 2007)
25. http://www.hl7.org (accessed on Jun 30, 2007)
26. http://www.x12.org/ (accessed on Jun 30, 2007)
27. http://medical.nema.org/ (accessed on Jun 30, 2007)
28. http://www.ncpdp.org/ (accessed on Jun 30, 2007)
29. http://www.w3.org/XML/ (accessed on Jun 30, 2007)
30. http://www.hl7.org/ehr/. Accessed on June 30, 2007.
31. http://content.healthaffairs.org/cgi/content/full/hlthaff.w5.10/DC1?maxtoshow=&HITS= 10&hits=10&RESULTFORMAT=&fulltext=electronic+medical+records+billion&and orexactfulltext=and&searchid=1108567041755_725&stored_search=&FIRSTINDEX= 0&resourcetype=1&journalcode=healthaff on Jun 30, 2007)
32. http://library.ahima.org/xpedio/groups/public/documents/ahima/bok1_032401.html (accessed on Apr 07, 2007)

7

Identifying and Understanding Business Processes in Clinical Practice

Blackford Middleton, MD, MPH, MSc
John J. Janas III, MD

A major problem that plagues many information systems projects is poor understanding of the underlying clinical and business/administrative processes that the systems are intended to support. This chapter addresses how one can identify and analyze important business/administrative processes and then use this information to evaluate and implement an appropriate supporting clinical information system. Particular attention is paid to those processes that occur in clinical environments—registration, schedule, clinical documentation, patient education, quality management, billing, and check-out—and require an interface to a clinical/EHR system to be maximally effective. Examples of how the computer may be used to support advanced business and clinical process re-engineering will also be given. A discussion of basic terms and concepts is presented along with a case-study example.

The "Business" of Clinical Practice Today

Business Pressures on Clinical Practice

In the contemporary practice of medicine, much has changed compared to the practice of medicine in years gone by. After World War II, the biomedical industry emerged as one of the fastest growth industries fueled by an extraordinary amount of research funding from the federal government, fee for service reimbursements in private practice settings, and cost plus accounting in hospital environments. With the advent of prospective payment in the mid-1980s, the emergence of managed-care and health maintenance organizations, and increasing regulatory pressures from the federal government, physicians often felt beleaguered by these new administrative pressures. Now, in a post-managed care world, the pressures are shifting from managing costs of care alone to managing both costs and quality of care. In some reimbursement schemes in different plans, physician compensation may be directly tied to pay for performance programs and other quality incentives. The vast majority of physicians remain in small to midsize medical group practices in a variety of organizational models (PPO, IPA, etc.). Whether it's affiliation with an independent practice association (IPA), preferred provider organization (PPO), or other organizational structure, the pressure is still on us all to run an efficient practice and deliver high quality care.

Critical Office Workflows

There are five critical office workflows in the clinical practice environment. These are the communication, documentation, scheduling and time management, knowledge management, and quality management workflows. Each is central to the practice of medicine, and integrating these well together leads to an efficient practice.

Communication

The practice of medicine is largely dependent upon effective communication between physician and patient, and between physician and the rest of the clinical and administrative staff. In the average clinical office, the sheer volume of communications between members of the staff and patients and through telephone calls, administrative work, and clinic visits is staggering. In fact, many clinics have difficulty keeping up with patient demand for communications with their physicians or nursing staff and access to the clinic. A typical primary care physician may receive more than a hundred calls to the office in a single day for everything from a prescription refill, insurance information request, billing issue, referrals and consultation requests, etc. Similarly, the mail volume for all of the above reasons and more can add up to dozens of pieces of mail for an individual doctor each day. In a typical clinic of three to five physicians in a small group, the number of calls and pieces of mail can quickly swamp all the ancillary staff and the physicians themselves. Recently, the phone and postal letter are being complemented, and in some cases exchanged for, email communication from patients or other providers, potentially adding to the communication burden. Clearly, this may then affect the efficiency of the clinic in seeing the patients on the schedule on any given day.

In response, many clinics have several ancillary administrative staff who may be dedicated to phone messages, email, and administrative support of the practice. Many clinics now have "practice management systems", which can help support the administrative component of the practice, such as pay-roll, accounts payable, scheduling, managed care coordination, and other administrative functions. Some clinics have established complicated phone triage systems to handle high call volume. Many physicians use dictation systems to communicate effectively with their colleagues, whether they are physicians referring from primary care settings or consultants providing specialty opinions or performing procedures. Lastly, clinical practices have state and federal reporting requirements for such things as communicable diseases and the like, and if they are participating in a managed care con-tract, they have reporting requirements to manage the contract. All of these communications needs may have some dependence on the clinical en-counter data derived from patient care.

Documentation

A second critical workflow that occurs continuously throughout the day in the clinical environment is the documentation workflow. The contemporary practice of medicine calls for comprehensive and accurate documentation of clinical encounters to support the practice of medicine but also, regret-fully, to provide appropriate documentation to ward off malpractice claims and ensure appropriate reimbursement for services rendered. The central documentation workflow for the physician is to record a progress note for each clinical encounter and, ideally, a note for each communication regard-ing patient care (telephone call with patient or patient's proxy, communi-cation with remote care givers, etc.). At the same time, however, physicians typically are communicating routinely with other office clinical and admin-istrative staff to get things done for the patient. Physicians may call upon their nursing support staff to assist with the clinical assessment of the pa-tient and in performing clinical procedures. Physicians may call upon the administrative staff less directly, but the clinical encounter documentation serves as a communication vehicle to the administrative staff for purposes of generating a bill, coordinating insurance, and scheduling future care en-counters or other procedures.

Recently, very detailed requirements for clinical documentation require-ments have emerged from the Health Care Financing Administration (HCFA) due to recurring fraud and abuse in claims for reimbursements from Medicare and Medicaid. These "evaluation and management" (E&M) docu-mentation requirements place an extraordinary burden on the clinicians to properly document multiple components of the clinical note to support the claim for a level of service. The E&M rules are arcane and difficult to re-member for every possible visit type. Generally, physicians are observed to "under code" defensively in routine practice. That is, a physician may indi-cate a level of service that is less than what was actually rendered due to the difficulties in documenting the visit appropriately for the appropriate service level. While these E&M rules are important, the most important as-pect of clinical documentation is to clearly document clinical findings and reasoning to support the claims for services generated, and defend against malpractice claims if untoward outcomes occur.

Another requirement of clinical documentation, however, in the world of electronic records, is to capture sufficient information from the clinical encounter to drive the decision-support and quality management capabilities of the EHR system in use. Typically, this implies maintaining an up-to-date problem list, using the system for electronic prescribing, and thus keeping the medication list up-to-date, at least for users of that EHR (other physicians may prescribe for a patient in other care settings, making the medication list in the EHR potentially incomplete). Other data may be particularly relevant to clinical decision support such as healthcare maintenance information, including preventive screening procedure information and care management data for chronic conditions. Awareness of these data within the system will allow it to appropriately alert and remind the physician about key clinical interventions for various problems and healthcare maintenance, as well as avoid untoward medication interactions or allergies. Lastly, these data are also useful with others to support the Quality Management workflow and provide essential feedback on the quality of care delivered to the healthcare provider.

Schedule Management

A third critical workflow in the clinical practice environment is that of time management or, more simply, scheduling. A busy practitioner may see anywhere from twenty-five to forty or more patients per day: some will be new patients, and some visits may be for procedures performed in the office. This clinical volume generates an extraordinary amount of primary and secondary scheduling requirements. Primary scheduling requirements refers to the need to schedule patients appropriately for new or follow-up visit appointments within a single clinic or related group of doctors. Secondary scheduling refers to scheduling needs for patients who will have tests or procedures in other settings or patients being referred to a colleague. Effective management of these scheduling tasks includes the ability to match the availability of clinicians and other resources with the clinical needs for acute or follow-up visits. A common difficulty in scheduling arises when the clinical groups do not have access to the office schedules of their colleagues, or the schedule of a radiology, or other, department where tests and procedures may be performed. The scheduling process, which is in effect at most offices today, therefore, is very inefficient because the patient often must be the "go-between" to manage actually scheduling a visit or procedure.

Knowledge Management

The fourth critical workflow in the clinical practice environment is that of knowledge management. Physicians are obligated to provide the highest quality of care possible to their patients. This means that physicians must pay critical attention to appropriately documenting the clinical care delivered for outcomes or practice analysis and they must remain current on the latest medical developments that may apply to their patients. Clearly, to remain licensed to practice, physicians must comply with continuing medical education (CME) requirements for states in which they are licensed to practice. Fulfilling annual CME requirements, however, does not always translate into applying the most recent insights from the medical literature to each and every clinical decision.

Certain aspects of practice require knowledge that is never obtained in medical school or CME settings. Knowing the various formularies for different insurance plans or who are the appropriate specialists or primary care practitioners in various referral networks are examples of knowledge that is critical to the daily practice of medicine but is difficult to learn and use appropriately. Other aspects of medical knowledge, like medication interaction assessment, is so complex that it is best suited to a computer that can monitor prescriptions written for potentially adverse medication interactions, or allergies, and alert the clinician when a problem exists.

All of these components of knowledge must be kept up to date in the minds of physicians and their clinic staff, but also often in the EHR system that is being used for clinical decision-support or quality management reporting. Whether it is the EHR vendor or the clinical practice itself that assumes the responsibility, the knowledge within clinical information systems must be kept periodically checked for currency, deleted if out of date, or modified in light of new knowledge or clinical practice standards. The CME activities described above now must apply to both man (or woman) and machine.

Quality Management

An emerging fifth critical workflow in clinical practice is quality management. This refers to routine clinical requirements and, potentially, financial requirements for monitoring and reporting on the quality of care delivered within a clinic and sometimes at the individual practitioner level. Ideally, routine clinical practice includes both a case-based review of clinical practice and a population-oriented review. In the former, physician groups in both ambulatory care and hospital-based practices typically get together to review difficult cases, discuss management strategies, and, on occasion, review bad outcomes. The "clinicopathologic conference", "tumor board", or simply daily or weekly case review sessions are examples of this process. Such conferences may figure prominently in the education of medical students and residents, of course, as well as the continuing education of experienced practitioners.

A new requirement is emerging from payers for health care services, however, to monitor the quality of care delivered not only for each individual patient but also for an entire cohort of patients. For example, pay-for-performance reimbursement contracts may have a significant portion of physician or group reimbursement withheld pending documented performance on certain benchmark criteria for care. Commonly, such benchmark criteria might include appropriate screening or preventive care for an identified population or demonstration of improved clinical outcomes on an accepted measure of care management such as the HbgA1c for diabetics.

In addition, some new payer contracts are now requiring demonstration of effective use of electronic medical record systems themselves to warrant return-of-withhold payment or potential bonus payments. Such measures of effective use may include the percentage of prescriptions being written using the EHR, the percentage of clinical encounters with a note documented in the EHR, and what clinical transactions are sent electronically, as well as administrative (billing) transactions. Such measures of effective use may not necessarily reflect the quality of care delivered, but they will be of great interest to clinicians when they are associated with differential reimbursement.

These emerging requirements affect the quality management workflow and may be well served by an EHR system with advanced reporting capabilities and workflow support for patient cohorts. Both academically developed and select commercial systems now have the ability to present various forms of reports to the end user clinician and may allow a clinician to act on behalf of an entire cohort of patients. For example, a stored report in an EHR might report on various clinical parameters for the cohort of diabetics cared for by an individual clinician or a medical group such as HgbA1c, LDL, BP, Weight, etc. Alternatively, certain EHR systems support ad hoc query capabilities so that if a medication were recalled from the market an end user could quickly search for all patients taking that medication and write a batch letter to the entire cohort to discontinue the medication and contact their doctor.

Basic Business Process Management

Given the five critical workflows described above, it is clear that effectively running a clinical practice requires attention to managing processes and managing information. The practice of medicine is one of the most information-intensive industries of the modern era. The number of pieces of information that may apply to an individual patient is enormous when one considers all of the administrative and clinical information gathered and used in the course of the clinical encounter and the knowledge-base of information that may apply to both administrative and clinical decision-making. Effectively managing basic business processes requires that the relevant information for each process be available for that process or function. Below, we describe the six essential business processes that operate within the clinical setting to support the critical workflows described above and give examples of how electronic patient records may be used to support these

Table 7-1

RELATIONSHIP BETWEEN CRITICAL WORKFLOWS AND BASIC BUSINESS PROCESSES IN THE CLINICAL ENVIRONMENT

	Communication	Documentation	Time	Knowledge	Quality
Registration/ check-in	√	√		√	
Schedule			√		
Clinical encounter	√	√	√	√	√
Patient education	√	√		√	√
Billing	√	√		√	
Patient check-out	√		√		

processes. Table 7-1 shows how these business processes support the critical workflows.

Registration

The process of registration in the clinical environment typically means acquiring from the patient all the relevant demographic information to reliably identify that patient to the clinic and indicate the nature of the complaint for the current visit. Critical information to be gathered in the registration process, of course, includes information pertaining to the patient's insurance program, or guarantor, in the fee-for-service reimbursement model or information identifying the patient as a member of a particular managed care plan in the capitated reimbursement model. In either case, good business process management includes the ability, at some level, of correlating real costs of providing care with the amount reimbursed so, ideally, the clinic managers can determine whether they are providing cost-effective care or providing a service in a managed care contract that is profitable. Also, if the patient has any co-payment obligation on their insurance plan, these fees are received during the registration and check-in process.

It is beyond the scope of this chapter to detail the information gathered by most clinics in the registration process or to detail what information should be stored in a practice management or clinical system during the registration process. Nevertheless, sufficient information regarding patient identity; demographics; primary and secondary insurance coverage; employer; and important personal contacts such as next-of-kin, family members, contact information, preferred pharmacy, and other providers of care are typically stored in most such systems.

Today, many clinics may have a practice management system that serves principally to support the administrative management of the clinic and a clinical system (or electronic medical record) that serves to support the clinical management of the clinic. Whether from a single vendor or from two vendors, these applications typically require a system's interface to allow sharing of the registration information gathered in one system with the other system. In this situation, one system is typically designated as the "master" system and the second as the "slave" system to allow information to be gathered once and shared as appropriate with the other application.

Scheduling

The clinical schedule, whether managed with a practice management system, a clinical system, or in paper determines the volume of patients seen in a day and thus the most important determinant of the amount of work to be done in the clinic. Scheduling can be accomplished utilizing either a group's practice management software or through the clinical system. In most settings, only one system serves as the "master" scheduler and the other system (whether it is practice management system, or electronic medical record) is "slaved" to the master scheduler, as is done with the registration information.

Critical issues in managing the business process of scheduling include: matching the appropriate resources and people with the clinical need, scheduling the appropriate amount of time for the clinical need, leveling scheduling requirements across resources or people, and monitoring the schedule to report on clinical productivity, appointment "no-shows", on-call schedule, etc. One advantage of scheduling through a clinical system is the ability to link clinical encounter types to specific documentation forms or templates. Some EHRs will automatically launch encounter specific information when the patient arrives, which can save time and improve quality.

Clinical Encounter

The clinical encounter is at the "heart" of the process of delivering healthcare and thus the key process that drives all the business processes of medicine. During the clinical encounter, information is exchanged between patient and practitioner, decisions are made regarding a therapeutic plan and possible clinical interventions and diagnostic testing, and, hopefully, a therapeutic result is achieved for the patient. It is often claimed that decisions made by the clinician during the clinical encounter are responsible for 80% of the costs attributed to the healthcare economy.

The practice of medicine requires documentation, at a summary level at least, of the information gathered by the clinical team and the decisions made regarding the assessment and plan for the patient. Historically, documenting the clinical encounter was primarily intended to serve as a memory jog for the clinician who maintained a medical record to chronicle the events, observations, decisions, and outcomes on the patient's behalf. Additionally, the medical record served as a repository of information which, with the patient's permission, could be reviewed for the purposes of medical research. Often, the medical record consisted of very abridged notes: abbreviations and code words that had meaning to the author but often not to anyone else.

In the modern practice of medicine, the medical record must serve all of the above functions, as well as be the source document to support claims for reimbursement, legal inquiry, disability assessment, outcomes analysis, and more. Often, a patient may have many different medical records, all maintained by different clinicians, each with a partial view of the patient's comprehensive health status and history. The E&M requirements, described above (see earlier section "Documentation"), place a considerable burden on the clinician to document all components of the clinical encounter appropriately to garner reimbursement for the claimed level of service.

Today, EHR systems support the clinical documentation process through a variety of techniques, and often in the process of supporting clinical documentation, create a rich clinical database to support quality management. Most EHR systems now allow data entry either through dictation and unstructured document import, free text data entry, facilitated data entry with templates, or structured data entry using electronic forms to guide the user. Increasingly, essential clinical data for decision-support or quality management must be gathered at the point of care to allow clinical decision support from the EHR to work effectively and to facilitate quality management and reporting. Documentation methods are described in more detail below in the section discussing critical clinical information system features to support business process re-engineering.

Patient Education

Another essential business process in clinical practice is patient education. Physicians are obligated, along with their professional nursing colleagues, to inform patients about their health status, tests and procedures, methods for primary prevention of disease, and medical therapy. Effective, high-quality care and patient engagement is often dependent on the patient being well informed about their health status, medical conditions, and medications. Regretfully, this process is often an after thought and is poorly addressed during the clinical encounter or any part of the clinic visit. Most clinics have a variety of handouts that may be given to the patient but often they are not comprehensive or do not address more unusual conditions. Information technology is well suited to managing such handouts, and patients themselves are searching the Internet in vast numbers to retrieve information about their medical conditions and well-being.

An EHR can automatically generate most of the handouts, letters, reminders, or reports to patients and health plans, which in the past had to be manually created. A few examples include: camp and school physical forms, worker's compensation reports, lab result letters, preventive care reminders, disability forms, and HEDIS (Health Plan Employer Data and Information Set; National Commission of Quality Assurance) compliance reports. The improved quality and patient satisfaction it generates only surpass the timesavings of utilizing the EHR's automation.

Billing

After the clinical encounter, the business process of billing is central, of course, to the financial health of a clinic. As described above, practice management systems are available to support all financial aspects of managing a clinical office. A clinical system can assist in billing issues on several levels. Utilizing E&M (HCFA Evaluation & Management) software available with some systems can increase revenue and decrease risks associated with audits through proper documentation and coding. Time spent coding is also reduced because the EHR may be configured to require that a coded diagnosis be entered at each visit, thus minimizing time spent looking up ICD-9 codes by providers or coders. The ultimate integration between an EHR and a practice management system is an interface that allows coding and diagnosis to be entered in the exam room by the provider and then to cross through an interface directly into the billing software, thereby eliminating the need for manual entry. This can decrease labor costs and shorten claim turn-around when properly implemented.

Patient Checkout

The last business process, which closes the clinical and administrative cycles in the clinic, is patient checkout. At checkout, a patient may be required to pay any fees beyond a co-pay that were not gathered during registration and check in. Many other activities typically must be coordinated at patient checkout: prescriptions, scheduling and coordination of diagnostic tests and procedures, additional therapy, consultations and referral, and more. Using a clinical information system, one can improve the process of checking out by saving time and improving compliance with appropriate coding and documentation. As a provider completes a visit in the exam room, several processes can be automated or included in the provider's encounter. Instead of writing on encounter sheets or going to staff and giving verbal instructions to schedule labs, diagnostics, referrals, or follow-up, these steps can be accomplished while in the exam room by the provider or at a sign-out area and automatically documented in the encounter note.

Using a clinical system, which includes order management, one can order labs, diagnostics, referrals, and follow-up appointments through point-

and-click technology. The orders are automatically entered into the provider's note and can then be printed, faxed, or electronically communicated for completion. Time is saved and errors reduced in ordering as codes required for billing ("CPT" [Common Procedural Terminology]) can be generated by the system automatically and duplicate forms or documentation by ancillary staff eliminated. Referrals can be printed and given to the patient before leaving, and/or bulk faxed: electronically transferred to the specialist and managed care companies if necessary for authorization. This process can be centralized and coordinated by one or many referral coordinators, thus reducing time and expense associated with managed care referral compliance.

In many clinics, the most common result of a clinical encounter is for a patient to receive a medication prescription. Another checkout time saver built into the EHR is prescription completion. Once entered in the exam room during the encounter, the clinical encounter note automatically charts medications and prescriptions completed, which can be printed and given to the patient, faxed, or electronically transmitted to the pharmacy. This saves time and the provider's hands, especially with multiple prescriptions or the frequent vendor changes associated with managed care.

The Role of the Computer in Process Re-Engineering

Most of what has been written on information technology in the past has focused on billing, coding, and practice management applications. Claims data derived from such systems is the basis for most HMOs and major insurers' Utilization Management (UM) and Quality Assurance (QA) programs. Because these systems rely on claims information, the granularity of the information often does not reflect the true clinical scenario, and one is limited to retrospective reviews. One can determine past utilization and track trends over a period of time, often combining a retrospective review with a concurrent review process to try to manipulate results. The same holds true for quality measurements and assessment. This form of information allows an organization to know how it has done over a period of time and compare trends, but, again, one is limited to retrospective, or, at best, concurrent and retrospective review.

Another limitation in utilizing claims information stems from inconsistencies in diagnosis and procedure coding. Some groups try to add another dimension to their UM & QA efforts with costly labor intensive chart audits or reviews. So what is an organization to do? Those with insight and an eye to being the most competitive while providing the highest quality of care must be willing to invest the time and expense on an EHR information system. This is an area of information technology that continues to evolve, but it is only implemented in a fraction of ambulatory practice settings (est. <25% of all clinics have an EHR). The EHR is often viewed as a luxury but, as we will demonstrate below, this technology is quickly becoming essential in clinical practice.

Critical Clinical Information System Features to Support Business Processing Re-Engineering

In order to be competitive and successful in today's changing health care delivery systems, careful evaluation, selection, and implementation of information technology is essential. There are many vendors of software, hardware, and support packages to choose from, which sometimes makes it harder to pick the right package for a particular clinic or medical group. Before making a decision, the clinic should know what information it wants to gather, what it intends to do with the information, and then find the system that can meet the clinic's needs with the most efficiency and lowest cost. Sounds simple enough, but many organizations rely on system vendors to tell them what they need instead of making an informed decision. What is important or works for one group may not for the next. Because of the rapidly changing needs and trends in healthcare, it is difficult to predict current, let alone future, needs of a system.

Unlike traditional paper charts, which limit information collection to free text, the EHR combines free text with data fields, which may record clinical findings in a database. Once information is entered in a chart as a data element, it can be retrieved for reporting, tracking, or quality-improvement initiatives. Just as there are many billing, coding, and practice management vendors vying for your business, there are several EHR options to choose from. Below are the minimum features you should expect from an EHR system when it comes to information gathering in order to optimize basic and advanced clinical and business processes. More specifics on what can be done or accomplished after picking and implementing an EHR and return of investment issues are highlighted in the examples and case study presented below. (Features of EHR systems that can be used to optimize business processes are summarized in Table 7-2.)

Clinical Findings and Clinical Data

The heart of effective business or clinical process management is data. In any business setting, if information cannot be measured, it cannot be assessed or improved. The same applies in the clinical setting. For information to be retrieved, it must be first entered into a computer in data fields, which represent various clinical findings. It is desirable to select a system that not only has a substantial number of structured data elements but also a vendor that is willing to create custom data fields for your organization's needs. Taking it one step further, the ability to custom-tailor clinical findings directly at your home site without the vendor would be ideal.

Efficiency or Ease of Data Entry

In order to gather information in an EHR, it first has to be entered. Any obstacle to data entry will diminish the ability to retrieve the information at a later date. A system should allow multiple ways of entering information

Table 7-2

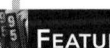

FEATURES OF AN EHR SYSTEM TO OPTIMIZE BUSINESS PROCESSES

- Sufficient number of structured data elements
- Efficiency or ease of data entry (e.g., preloaded or custom-made documentation forms, text templates, medication lists)
- Easy-to-read data display
- Demographics interface
- Lab interface with laboratory information system
- Interfaces with transcription system
- Internet-based system interfaces for e-commerce
- Quarterly updates provided by vendor
- Detailed start-up program (should be complete in all aspects of staff training, workflow re-engineering, and trouble-shooting)
- Decision-support capability for both clinical and administrative (workflow) decision making

with the least amount of effort either by physicians, providers, nursing and medical assistant staff, or administration. This may be accomplished utilizing either preloaded or custom-made documentation forms, text templates, data flow sheets, problem lists, medication lists, or a variety of methods to be discussed in more detail later.

Data Display or Retrieval

Once the information has been entered, it should be displayed in a format that is easy to read, prompts quality or utilization efforts, and can be gathered in easy-to-use reports. The system should have built-in protocols and allow customization to prompt for preventive care and quality care based on established guidelines either at the time of service or at a future date. Utilizing these features can proactively improve an organization's HEDIS compliance, ease in documenting compliance, and improve reimbursement from HMOs. You can also track internal compliance on a variety of disease-management or quality-improvement projects such as meeting American Diabetes Association guidelines for quality care of diabetics.

Interfaces

A system interface allows one computer to share or exchange information with another computer. Like language, there are many different ways for messages to be constructed and exchanged between computers. There are a variety of computer information interfaces commonly available, however, and those built on widely accepted informatics standards will be the most reliable. At a minimum, an EHR should have a demographics interface with

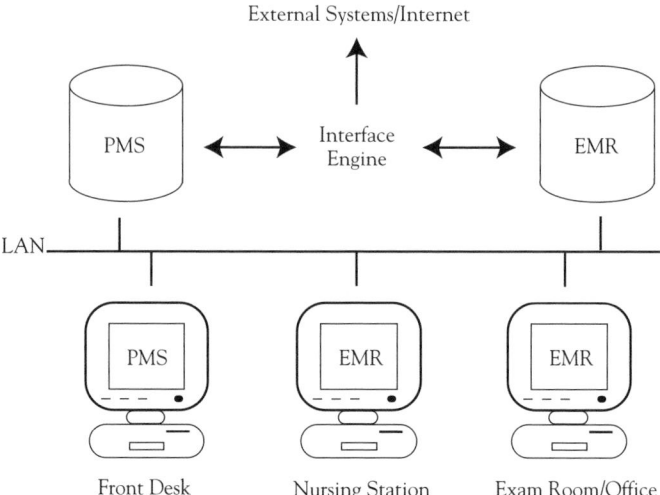

Figure 7-1   Schematic representation of basic clinic computing environment. PMS represents practice management system, EHR represents electronic medical record, and LAN signifies local area network. Other systems may be in place in some settings, such as laboratory systems, dictation systems, the Internet, etc. If not resident within the clinic, such external systems may exchange information with the PMS or EHR through an interface engine. The schematic does not depict all workstations in the case study. See text for details.

your practice management system, and a lab interface with the laboratory information system (Figure 7-1). The timesavings and enhancements in data entry that result from having automatic data flow from the practice management system and laboratory system to the EHR help defray the initial up-front costs of the system's interface. There are other interfaces that can improve productivity and decrease overhead: interfaces with a transcription system if dictation is to remain a data entry option; the hospital information system; and new Internet-based system interfaces for e-commerce in the healthcare arena. Healthcare e-commerce will soon include on-line eligibility determination, prescription fulfillment, referral authorization, and more. New order communication interfaces will allow orders to travel from the patient's EHR during the encounter directly to the laboratory or radiology department, decreasing errors and time required to complete requisitions. In the near future, this technology will be used to send referral requests electronically directly to insurers. Currently, internal tracking of referrals can be accomplished allowing organizations to provide internal UM without relying on data provided by the HMOs.

Support and Implementation Issues

A desirable EHR should have strong national and local support. Detailed training at implementation and start up, as well as ongoing support of your clinic, is essential. A minimum of quarterly updates provided by the vendor should be easily loaded with minimal disruption in day-to-day activities. It is important to have physician leadership in the initial and ongoing design of the EHR and support of the parent healthcare enterprise (if one exists) to ensure buy-in, quality control, and maximize the system's potential. The EHR vendor selected should provide a detailed start-up program, describing all the necessary steps in either a system conversion, or new start, before going live with the system. This program should be complete in all aspects of staff training, workflow re-engineering, and trouble shooting and should be geared to all levels of computer confidence of your organization's staff. Finally, the selected vendor should have a proven track record in the industry, and you must be confident they will be around to provide the above support. If their product has the above features, there is a good chance they will be around for the long haul.

Integrating Clinical and Business Processes for Advanced Business Process Management and Re-Engineering

Once an organization has a handle on the basic process improvements EHR affords, more advanced opportunities can be addressed. It is important to understand these opportunities early on in implementation so the proper data and information can be gathered. One cannot stress enough the importance of specific data collection to providers early on, even though a clinic may not utilize these features until later in the organization's growth. Failure to prepare in advance will delay your ability to maximize these opportunities.

Cost Accounting

Utilizing an EHR's reporting features can better account for and manage utilization of services and procedures provided by your group. An example is tracking and evaluating variations in budgetary items and practice patterns. Recently it was determined in the author's clinic (JJJ) that the cost for chargeable drugs was 25% higher than comparable family practices. Utilizing reporting capabilities of the EHR, the clinic was able to account for the variance by determining that because of a recent initiative utilizing protocols, the clinic's compliance rate for pneumovax, flu vaccine, adult and childhood immunizations were significantly greater, yet the budget was determined utilizing average practice costs. Since the clinic's compliance was greater than average, its cost was also greater than average. There is a price for improving quality, as this clinic was able to demonstrate. Theoretically, these costs should be recaptured by society overall, if not for this clinic, in the future through prevention of disease.

Clinical Profiling

As described above, An EHR can be used to do retrospective reporting on referral patterns, formulary compliance, diagnostic test utilization, and preventive care compliance for individuals or groups. The real value of an EHR, however, comes from the ability to be proactive.

Utilizing formulary decision-support functions built into an EHR, providers' prescribing patterns can be affected at the point of care. Done properly, providers still have ultimate control over prescribing but have more knowledge regarding costs and alternatives, which can reduce callbacks from patients, pharmacists, or managed care companies. For those organizations accepting risk on pharmacy costs, the savings can be significant. In the clinic of one of the authors (JJJ), working with a local HMO, an incentive program was implemented in an attempt to improve formulary compliance. Taking national statistics showing estimated savings of $0.30 pmpm for each 1% increase in generic or formulary compliance, an incentive program was developed whereby each provider would be credited $0.10 pmpm for every 1% increase in generic usage or formulary compliance. If this percent exceeds 5% in any given year, then $0.15 pmpm would be credited. The HMOs are interested in saving money, but the providers are more concerned about quality and minimal hassle. The formulary decision-support system allows for instant identification and notification of formulary compliance when a drug is ordered and also shows acceptable bio-equivalent alternatives. The provider does not have to search for alternatives, which often decreases compliance in formulary management. The provider can choose not to substitute if clinically indicated. By maximizing savings on cases where no significant clinical difference exists, non-formulary costs can be offset. Patients, providers, and insurers all win.

Utilizing preventive care protocols built into the EHR, provider compliance with HEDIS and other quality measures can be maximized. At each patient encounter, be it phone call, prescription refill request, or office visit, preventive care protocol reminders can be displayed and the necessary testing or service ordered. Using these capabilities, our group has been able to achieve and maintain compliance rates consistently above our peer groups. Quarterly reports are also generated for a variety of preventive care services such as adult and childhood immunizations, pap smears, mammograms, and annual diabetic eye exams. Patients are then notified either by phone or mailings generated by the EHR and the services ordered. This again improves quality but at a cost. Our group, following national guidelines established by the American Diabetes Association, has maximized compliance rates with a variety of recommended screenings, including number of visits, lab testing, and diabetes eye exams. This in turn has led, by word of mouth, to an increased number of diabetic patients transferring to our practice. Unfortunately one HMO recently tried to retain our withhold claiming over utilization. After meeting with the medical director of this HMO, armed with data showing a greater number of diabetics in our practice, greater compliance with quality measures, and decreased hospitalization and ER utilization rates, our withhold was returned and we received the maximum quality incentive bonus offered by this HMO. You should not be penalized for doing a good job, but if you are not aware of the possible consequences and armed with the data to support your claims, such blame can happen.

Quality Management

Utilizing built-in practice guidelines developed locally, or based on national standards, encounter forms, or note templates can automatically make available a variety of user-friendly practice parameters to improve quality and reduce variability. Examples include management of chronic disease states such as diabetes, asthma, COPD, and CHF through preventive care or recommended treatment protocols. Implementation of guidelines to assist in clinical decision-making can also be built into the EHR. Just a few topics developed and implemented in the author's (JJJ) clinic to date include the management of dyspepsia, utilization guidelines for x-rays in ankle and knee injuries, acute low back pain management, and asthma management, including acute and chronic management plans. A variety of nursing telephone triage protocols improves patient care and access for common problems such as UTI, sinusitis, pharyngitis, conjunctivitis, chest pain, and abdominal pain. Taking a proactive approach through teaching and implementation has proven to be more effective than retroactive manipulation of practice patterns based on utilization data.

Contract Management

Through the use of EHR, groups can take steps to improve quality and manage costs through formulary management, diagnostic and referral utilization guided by best clinical practices, reduced variation, and implementation of preventive care and disease state management protocols. Some impact and savings will be immediate, but many more may come from long-term patient management or not at all. Remember, there is often an inherent cost to quality. Adopting a value-oriented model is fundamental in looking at the quality of care provided by any clinic.

$$VALUE = QUALITY / COST$$

To maximize contract management, a clinic needs to be able to document its value to insurers (quality and cost measures) and the EHR gives you the tools to improve and measure quality through outcomes. Opportunities to explore and maximize in managed care contracts include:

1. Quality incentive bonuses based on measurable indicators that a clinic can maximize by taking a proactive approach.

2. Formulary costs: decisions within an organization need to be made on whether to take risk directly on health plan formularies or indirectly through incentives for formulary compliance.

3. Increased capitation rates or fee schedules based on continued documentation of quality, value, or reduced overhead costs for the HMO to manage an organization. The automation that EHR lends through interfaces can be used to decrease overhead expenses for the HMO in the areas of referrals, billing, pre-certification or prior authorization requests, and formulary management.

4. Self-insuring, direct marketing, or managed care partnerships with the HMOs become a viable option if the number of providers on the same EHR (or multiple EHRs if a central data repository is available and the products mutually have the above features) and the number of covered lives is large enough.

An Example of the Cost and Quality Benefits of an EHR

The following case study describes how the clinic of one of the authors (JJJ) used an EHR to support the business processes of the practice and begin clinical process re-engineering and workflow re-design.

Clinical Setting

Capital Region Healthcare (CRHC) is an evolving Integrated Delivery Network (IDN) located in central New Hampshire. It includes three acute care hospitals licensed for 450 beds, two visiting nurse associations performing 160,000 visits annually, an affiliation with a mental health system, and, under construction, a 100-bed assisted-living facility. In the mid-90s, CRHC embarked upon a strategy for acquiring primary care physicians and their practices. Today, there are twenty primary care practices comprised of seventy-five providers and a family practice residency/clinic composed of sixteen residents and eight faculty. Total revenue for the IDN is $175 million.

Recognizing the need to focus on the productivity of its primary care providers and the qualitative outcomes within those practices, CRHC began an information technology strategy that focused on implementing an EHR. The focus of this case study is on the cost reductions and qualitative benefits realized from the reengineered workflows implemented in conjunction with the EHR in CRHC's pilot clinic, Family Care of Concord (FCC).

FCC is located in Concord, NH. It is a member of Capital Region Physician Group, a subsidiary of CRHC. It consists of one board-certified family practitioner, one double board-certified internist/pediatrician, and two nurse practitioners. Support staff includes three registered nurses, two licensed practical nurses, and three medical assistants. The practice manages

7200 active patients and averages 1200 visits/month. The payer mix is approximately 42% managed care, 15% Medicare, 3% Medicaid, 5% self-pay, and 35% commercial insurance. The practice contracts with seven managed care companies.

FCC opened in April of 1996 using ClinicaLogic, a DOS-based EHR from MedicaLogic, Hillsboro, OR. In December of 1997, the practice converted to Logician, MedicaLogic's Windows-based EHR. The practice uses Medisense from Compusense for its practice management and scheduling needs.

EHR Implementation Overview

Project Implementation Challenges

An information technology project of this magnitude faced cultural, financial, and technical challenges.

As with any change, there are natural cultural resistances. Staff resistance to changes in traditional work roles and their readiness to use microcomputers had to be considered. Additionally, the team needed to be sensitive to the needs and concerns of the patients as they implemented this new technology.

The initial financial investment in 1997 of $87,000 for hardware, software, and implementation was significant. Annual support costs, which include software maintenance fees, upgrades, information technology support staff, and depreciation, are $37,000. Senior management endorsed the pilot of the EHR, despite the significant initial investment and the absence of relevant research about the benefits of an EHR.

There were technical challenges with the design and implementation of real time interfaces. Coordinating efforts between external vendors and information technology staff was time consuming yet critical. Room size, ergonomics, and patient-provider interactions all need to be taken into consideration when deciding where to place personal computers. Migration from the DOS-based product (ClinicaLogic) to the 32-bit windows product (Logician) required both an extensive data conversion, and a complete retraining effort.

Personnel Involved

To successfully implement the EHR, both clinical and technical expertise was required. Technical expertise included network, interface, and project management resources provided by the information technology department. The staff of FCC provided clinical expertise.

Responsibilities of the technical team included:

◆ Sizing of server based on number of concurrent providers to accommodate adequate data storage and acceptable response time

◆ Configuration and installation of server, network, software, and microcomputers

- Provision of customized training that integrated the newly designed workflows with the application software
- Establishment of a project timeline, coordination of project resources, and management of the budget

Responsibilities of the clinical design team included:

- Prioritization of feature implementation
- Creation of EHR-based workflows
- Establishment of clinical content for go-live
- Development of templates/encounter forms
- Testing of the system to verify functionality and integrity

Workflow Re-design

Productivity enhancements and quality improvements do not occur merely by implementing the EHR. A conscientious effort to reengineer workflows is necessary to optimize benefits. To support the newly created workflows and promote point-of-care documentation, microcomputers were placed in each exam room (8), each provider's office (4), and at each clinical workstation (7).

The following describes a patient's visit using the newly implemented workflows:

1. Support staff register and schedule patients in Medisense, which utilizes a one-way demographics interface to upload ADT information to Logician.

2. Upon arrival, patient checks in and is acknowledged in Medisense by support staff.

3. Fee slip is placed outside exam room door by support staff.

4. Nurse checks computer to confirm patient arrived.

5. Nurse brings patient into exam room. Customized encounter screens are assigned to the patient's electronic chart based on type of visit; vital signs are entered. Prior clinical results are automatically available.

6. Provider enters exam room. By accessing the encounter form the following information is readily available: applicable protocols, medications, current problems, allergies, and directives and vitals entered by nurse. Provider updates any necessary information at the point of care eliminating the need for transcription. Prescriptions and patient education handouts are generated and sent to the laser printer. Services, tests, and referrals are entered into the system.

7. Patient leaves exam room and checks out. Provider delivers prescriptions and patient education handouts. Support staff schedules any follow-up appointments. Fee slip is collected and forwarded to the central billing office.

8. All paper-based documents (consult notes, insurance correspondences, etc) are scanned. For medical/legal reasons, consent forms must be saved so the practice utilizes a day file system for tracking this information.

Benefits and Results

The benefits and results realized by implementing the electronic medical record system are as follows:

◆ Elimination of Transcription. The practice has eliminated all transcription costs by utilizing structured flow sheet views, note templates, and point-of-care documentation. The practice generates approximately 14,000 visits per year. The average CRHC practice generates approximately thirty-five lines of transcription per patient. At a cost of $0.11 per line, the practice estimates a savings of $53,900. However, it does take approximately one hour longer per week per provider to generate the documentation. That time at a blended rate of $55.00 per hour for four providers for 46 weeks equates to about $10,120. The net savings to the practice is $43,780.

◆ Eliminating Chart Pulls. At FCC, the traditional paper chart has been eliminated. Assuming one chart pull per visit at 6 minutes each and using the average salary for the practice's support staff of $17 per hour (including benefits), the practice estimates a savings of $24,500 annually.

◆ More Efficient Prescription Generation. New prescriptions and refills are generated as a by-product of the documentation process. Each prescription takes less than three minutes to complete. (Electronic steps include creation of prescription from the documentation, automatic allergy and interaction checking, flag to physician for review and signature, fax to pharmacy). Prior to the electronic record, the average time to complete a prescription was approximately 15 minutes. (A significant difference is that no chart pulls are necessary for prescription refills). The practice generates approximately 400 prescriptions per week, the majority of which are refills. Saving 12 minutes per prescription equates to a total savings of 4200 hours per year. Using the average salary for the practice's support, the practice estimates a savings of $71,400 annually. An ancillary benefit of electronic prescription data is the ability to easily regenerate patient prescriptions in the event of managed care company formulary changes, which has occurred eight times since the EHR was implemented.

◆ Reducing Time Spent Coding. By using the system, the practice has reduced time spent coding. When problems are documented in the EHR, ICD-9 diagnosis codes are automatically assigned. At 14,000 visits per year and an average of two codes per visit, the practice generates approximately 28,000 diagnosis codes. Assuming 15% of the codes needed to be researched, at an average of 5 minutes per code, 350 hours of coding time is saved per year. Using the practice's average support staff salary, $5950 has been saved. This feature also allows the practice to track and report their patient acuity to insurance companies. Insurance companies are beginning to use this information to calculate reimbursements and quality bonuses. In the future, through the use of MedicaLogic's enhanced Evaluation and Management Code module, FCC expects to accurately meet Medicare's coding compliance regulations.

◆ Lab Interface Reducing Data Entry and Filing Time. The practice utilizes a lab interface (HBOC Star Lab) to upload results into the EHR, thus reducing data entry and filing time. Results are sent every 20 minutes. The practice generates about 6500 laboratory tests annually. It took about one hour to file twenty results; therefore, the practice has saved approximately 325 hours of filing time. Using the practice's average support staff salary, it saved $5525 annually. In addition, the system generates letters notifying patients of their results. The average turnaround time has been reduced from two or three weeks to one week, thus improving patient satisfaction.

◆ Referrals More Efficiently Generated. The provider generates referrals during the clinical encounter, eliminating the need to manually fill out paper-based payer forms. The practice generates about 3600 referrals annually. Using the system, an estimated 7 minutes per referral is saved for a total of 420 hours per year. Using the practice's average salary, it has saved $7140 annually. Overall turnaround time for a referral has been reduced from one day to within one hour. Additionally, using the reporting tools and the documentation database, the practice has eliminated payer-based denials and can report provider referral patterns for payer utilization requirements.

◆ Qualitative Reporting. The practice uses the system to report their quality indicators to qualify for managed care payer's incentive bonus programs. Typical areas targeted include pap smears, mammograms, and diabetic eye exams. For one managed care company, the average compliance is approximately 60% for providing diabetics with annual eye exams. By capturing discrete data through the system, FCC was able to document that 199/200 patients received such exams. Compared to the average compliance estimate of 60%, the practice performed approximately 80 more eye exams. Nationally it is expected that about 40% of all diabetics tested will have a surgically correctable complication detected. Therefore, the practice estimates that it diagnosed and prevented complications in thirty-two patients that otherwise may have gone undetected. Based on these results, the practice has qualified for the maximum quality bonuses provided by this payer.

◆ Drug Recalls. The practice can utilize the system to generate patient letters in the event of drug recalls. Since opening the practice there have been four recalls effecting 45 patients. All patients received letters within one day of the drug recall alerts.

◆ Hospital Inpatients: EHR Accessibility to Hospitals Help Support Patient Care. FCC generates approximately 760 admissions per year. The EHR is accessible from within the hospital in the emergency room and on the inpatient floors. Instead of dictating discharge summaries and having them transcribed by the hospital's medical records department, the discharge summary is produced directly from the EHR and a hard copy is forwarded to the medical records department for filing. Having access to the patient's record in the hospital setting allows providers to have up-to-date patient information to support clinical decision-making.

◆ Patient Satisfaction. Throughout the project, concern for patient satisfaction was of paramount importance to the practice. CRHC began performing patient satisfaction surveys in the third quarter of 1997. Results are now available for the past year. The average patient satisfaction for the practices within Capital Region Physicians Group is 88.2%. FCC's average results are 88.9%. FCC concludes that the EHR did not negatively affect patient satisfaction and in fact may have contributed to improving patient satisfaction.

EHR Benefits and Results Summary

FCC, a group of four providers, has measured net annual cost reduction of approximately $121,300 for the practice or $30,300 per provider annually (Table 7-3). Another method for estimating cost reduction is to compare FCC's staff to provider ratio to the national average. FCC has a staff to

Table 7-3

FCC's DIRECT COSTS ANALYSIS

Direct Costs Analysis	Annual
Total benefits	$158,295
Total expense	$37,000
Net benefits	$121,295
Net benefits/provider	$30,324

Table 7-4

FCC's Staff/Provider Ratio Analysis

Staff/Provider Ratio Analysis	Annual
Total benefits	$198,000
Total expense	$37,000
Net beneftis	$161,000
Net benefits/provider	$40,250

provider ratio of 2.0. The industry average according to National MGMA survey data is 3.4. Based on a difference of 1.4 staff per provider, the practice is saving approximately 5.6 full-time equivalents annually. Using the support staff average salary of $17 per hour, the practice estimates a net savings $161,000 or $40,200 per provider annually (Table 7-4).

The implementation of the EHR has also made several quality improvements. FCC has been able to respond faster to prescription refill requests, alert patients to drug recalls, notify patients of laboratory results, and quickly initiate referrals. Through the documentation and reporting, the practice has demonstrated that it has exceeded the quality standards set forth by HEDIS and managed care companies.

Conclusion

In this chapter we presented a review of critical clinical office workflows and business processes to support them. We then discussed how computers may be used for business and clinical process re-engineering and workflow re-design. A case study was presented that detailed the costs and economic benefits arising after implementation of an EHR system. This study demonstrated that a well-implemented electronic medical record can create numerous savings and quality improvements.

In the overall integrated delivery network, CRHC will strive to duplicate the successful use of the EHR in each of its primary care practices. Cost savings of between 2.25 and 3 million dollars could be achieved if the EHR is successfully implemented in the CRHC practices (75 providers). In addition, and equally as important, it recognizes that numerous qualitative advantages are inherent in using an EHR. It also concludes that a successful implementation of an EHR need not negatively affect patient satisfaction ratings and may contribute to increased patient satisfaction. However, CRHC recognizes that successful implementation of the EHR is largely dependent on multiple factors such as provider belief the system will make a difference, provider willingness to promote and accept change, management commitment, technical competence of staff, and leadership and project management abilities. The challenge is to duplicate FCC's success.

References

1. Ziegler R, et al. Change Drivers: Information Systems for Managed Care, American Hospital Publishing. Chicago;1998.
2. Walton M. The Deming Management Method. The Putnam Publishing Group, New York;1986.
3. McLaughlin CP, Kaluzny AD. Continuous Quality Improvement in Health Care: Theory, Implementation, and Applications. Aspen Publishers, Inc. Gaithersburg, Maryland;1994.
4. Landholt MD, Thomas F, The Coker Group. Managing the Outpatient Medical Practice, American Hospital Publishing. Chicago;1999.
5. Donaldson MS, Lohr KA, eds. Health Data in the Information Age: Use, Disclosure, and Privacy. National Academy Press;1994.
6. Murphy GF, Hanken MA, Waters KA. Electronic Health Records: Changing the Vision. W.B. Saunders Company, Philadelphia; 1999.
7. Institute of Medicine. The Computer-Based Patient Record: An Essential Technology for Health Care. National Academy of Sciences. Washington DC;1991.

8

Identifying and Understanding Clinical Processes

Matthew Morgan, MD, MSc

The need for an electronic health record (EHR) can be justified on many fronts; however, one of the greatest benefits to both clinicians and patients is the EHR's ability to improve clinical care processes. The EHR is becoming the twenty-first century's version of the "physician's black bag". Ever present, reassuring, and useful, containing powerful instruments to assist in diagnostic and therapeutic decision-making, improving communication amongst clinicians and between clinicians and patients, resulting in more knowledgeable, compliant and satisfied patients and clinicians, and delivering safe care with less expense, less time and of higher quality. For those who are naysayers, remember the folly of the physician who declared "that it will ever come into general use not with-standing its value . . . is extremely doubtful; there is even something ludicrous in the picture . . . of . . . physicians using this device." This was reported in the London Times, not recently about the EHR, but in the 1860s about the stethoscope (1). Today the stethoscope remains an important instrument to the clinician. The challenge of the EHR is to clearly show how it can provide more value than the stethoscope to the clinician, patient, and health care system.

This chapter will focus on the EHR's ability to assist in the everyday activities and work flow of clinicians and offer guidance to the reader in identifying and analyzing clinical care processes for the ultimate purpose of selecting and specifying an EHR system to support them.

Historical Overview

Historically the paper medical record was the only medium for supporting clinical care processes. However, as clinical practice has evolved the paper medical record has not. Paper does not support the shift away from the solo physician to multi-disciplinary patient-centered care. Paper does not allow information to be shared in a timely manner and cannot adapt to the reality that the doctor's office is being replaced by multidisciplinary care teams. The paper-based medical record does not support efficient and safe communication amongst clinicians, real-time decision support, medico-legal protection, quality improvement and outcome analysis (2). Despite these limitations, clinicians find paper to be a fast, comfortable, and user-friendly mechanism for transaction-based clinical care processes such as documentation and test ordering. Although paper has caused a great deal of trouble and expense when it comes to storing, retrieving, and reviewing large amounts of data, administrative personnel have protected clinicians from many of the mundane information management activities. Simply put, paper is a fast medium for clinicians to use at a single point in time. It is analogous to the use of a paper day-timer compared to an electronic organizer. Those using a paper day timer will initially be faster than those using an electronic organizer at simple activities such as finding addresses, penciling in appointments, and entering new contacts and phone numbers. It is not until information management becomes more complex, of greater volume, and required by more than one user that the electronic organizer's advantages become clear. Clinical care processes have become more complex and now involve teams of professionals instead of the solo-practitioner. As a result there is an overwhelming need for EHR systems that recognize this complexity and are able to replace and improve upon the limitations of the paper medical record.

EHR systems have been under development for more than forty years. The classic EHR systems focused on integrating non-clinician-derived data such as diagnoses, laboratory results, and medication lists (2). Character-based user interfaces provided clinicians with the ability to view and trend simple results, but clinician data entry was difficult and time consuming. In the 1970s, several organizations were able to develop EHR systems that went beyond this limited functionality and included the ability to document clinician-patient encounters and enabled clinical alerting (3). The publication of the 1991 Institute of Medicine (IOM) report "The Computer-Based Patient Record: An Essential Technology for Change" served as a catalyst to move the EHR agenda forward and outlined 180 features divided into 12 key attributes (4). These are:

1. Supports problem lists

2. Measures health status and function levels

3. Documents clinical reasoning and rationale

4. Provides longitudinal and timely electronic linkages with other records on the patient

5. Guarantees confidentiality and audit trails

6. Provides continuous authorized user access

7. Supports simultaneous user views

8. Provides timely access to local or remote information resources

9. Facilitates clinical problem solving

10. Supports direct data entry by physicians

11. Supports practitioners in measuring and managing costs and improving quality

12. Provides flexibility to support existing and evolving clinical needs of each discipline

In 1997, the former director and senior staff officer of the IOM study described five key underpinnings (5):

1. Clinical data dictionary

2. Clinical data repository

3. Point-of-care facility

4. Ergonomic presentation facility

5. Anticipation of clinical processes

and nine clinical attributes:

1. Supports images, multimedia data

2. Links with other patient records

3. Supports multiple formulary lists based on each patient's plan of care

4. Checks and documents RBRVS (resource-based relative value scale) compliance

5. Supports multiple EDI (electronic data interchange) financial links with concurrent clinical link support

6. Supports automated history, physical

7. Supports icon-generated text

8. Supports SNOMED-III (Standardized Nomenclature of Medicine, 3rd ed.), UMLS (Unified Medical Language System) vocabularies

9. Supports other integrated or interfaced technology.

From 1997 to 2004 the IOM issued numerous reports that reconfirmed the essential need for EHRs in the delivery of safe, high-quality, efficient care (6-8). Since the publication of the first edition of this guide, the availability of commercial EHR systems that have the potential to provide the 12 attributes has expanded, and there is growing acceptance and adoption of the EHR as a tool to support best practice. Numerous resources are now available to help clinicians and administrators navigate the EHR vendor world, including the comprehensive and up-to-date resources from the Certification Commission for Healthcare Information Technology (CCHIT) as discussed in Chapter 16.

It is important that prospective buyers develop a practical and realistic strategy for the selection and implementation of the EHR. This strategy should clearly articulate and convince clinicians as well as other stakeholders that it will result in the improvement of care upon implementation and will have the ability to grow, mature, and provide additional value in the years to come. With this caution in mind, successful EHR selection and implementation today is possible and rapid and measurable improvements in clinical care processes can be achieved.

Clinical Processes

Identifying the clinical processes and understanding how the EHR system can improve patient care in the local environment must be clearly understood. Without applying this understanding, the selection, purchase, implementation, and utilization of the EHR will at best fall short of expectations and at worst result in clinician rebellion, front page headlines, and the abandonment of the EHR system (9).

The IOM's 180 features, 12 categories, 5 key underpinnings, and 9 additional clinical attributes are extensive. However, EHR systems can have over 2000 features and functions that directly or indirectly support the clinical care processes (10). In order to prevent the reader from becoming overwhelmed and to assist in a practical approach to the identification and selection of EHR systems that support clinical care processes, this chapter will focus on those processes or activities that consume the majority of clinicians' time. The proposed list is by no way exhaustive and serves merely as an introduction to the clinical benefits of EHRs. A more thorough approach to EHR selection is provided in Section 4 of this book.

In order to perform clinical processes, clinicians spend a great amount of time and energy retrieving, reviewing, tracking and trending, documenting, ordering, deciding, communicating, and educating. For the purpose of this chapter, the following 10 major clinical processes will be discussed:

1. Time management and scheduling

2. Reviewing diagnostic test results and clinical documents

3. Diagnostic test ordering

4. Patient encounter documentation

5. Electronic prescribing

6. Electronic signature

7. Clinical decision support

8. Disease management

9. Data analysis and report generation

10. Patient education

In evaluating EHR systems, it is helpful to prioritize which of the above clinical processes are of most importance and in most need of change. Table 8-1 can assist in this prioritization exercise when evaluating EHR systems. The check list can be used to assess each feature and major module of the EHR system and to assess the EHR overall.

Time Management and Scheduling

As discussed in the previous chapter, time management and scheduling is not by strict definition a clinical process but rather a business process that is essential to the care delivery and efficient running of a clinical practice. EHR systems should provide time management and patient scheduling

Table 8-1

CHECK LIST FOR EVALUATING EHR IMPACT ON CLINICAL PROCESSES (EXAMPLE: WILL THE EHR'S METHOD OF REVIEWING RESULTS PROVIDE . . .)		
	Yes	No
Greater chart availability		
Less time consuming care for the clinician		
Less time consuming care for the patient		
Better diagnosis		
Better therapy		
Better patient compliance		
Improved communication between clinicians		
Improved communication between clinician and patient		
Better clinician knowledge		
Better patient knowledge		
Less expensive care		
Safer and higher-quality care		

Adapted from Finley (11).

capabilities that are truly integrated into clinical processes. This type of solution, offered by many EHR vendors, has been termed the clinician's desktop. The desktop provides the clinician with a complete view of the day's activity, as well as providing quick and easy access to the most relevant sections of the EHR. From the desktop, the clinician can quickly access the charts of patients scheduled for the day, know the status of the patient encounter (i.e., "pending, arrived, cancelled"), and allow the clinician and support personnel to reserve protected time and to schedule new appointments. In addition, the desktop should serve as the gateway to all other required clinical information management tools such as email, the internet, and educational resources. The clinician's desktop should also be customizable to recognize the unique role of each member of the team and enhance workflow and efficiency. For example, the desktop of the physician, nurse, and office administrator should have a unique "look and feel" to support the unique role of each member of the team. A well-designed, easy-to-use functional and customizable clinician's desktop will improve patient flow and aid in the delivery of efficient, safe, high-quality patient care.

A relatively new trend in patient scheduling is "open access", where patients can access their provider's schedule and choose appointment times (12). Some emerging EHR systems can support "open access" by providing patients with secure internet access to the EHR scheduler and "self-schedule" an appointment.

Important point: *When evaluating EHR systems, the clinician's desktop should be easy to use, logical, comprehensive, and integrated with a scheduling and time management system that will meet the needs of all members of the care team. In addition, it should be customizable by clinical role and allow integration of other commonly used applications such as the internet. If "open access" is required or planned for, then the EHR's capabilities to support this process using web-based tools should be assessed.*

Reviewing Diagnostic Test Results and Clinical Documents

Clinicians spend a significant amount of time retrieving and reviewing patient results. It can account for up to 25% of a clinician's day (13). Without the dedicated support of health records personnel and clerical staff, this percentage would increase significantly. EHR systems have been successful at solving many of the problems associated with finding, retrieving, organizing, and reporting patient results that exist with paper medical records (14).

Unlike a paper medical record, which can only be used by one person at a time, EHR systems make it possible to quickly inform not only a single clinician but numerous clinicians of patient test results such as: critical patient lab results, previous ECGs, recent chest radiographs, and past hospital discharge summaries. Important clinical data is available 24 hours a day, seven days a week. EHR systems can greatly assist in providing the right information, to the right person, at the right place, at the right time.

The display of patient results should be well organized, easy to find, and clearly indicated as normal, abnormal, or critical. Results include numerical data, text, and images, and may also include audio and video files. **Structured** data such as laboratory results and vital signs and **unstructured** data such as word-processed documents should be indexed, searchable, and easily available to the clinician for review.

Data Input

The reader should be cautioned that EHR vendors will always demonstrate how impressive their system's result review functionality is from an output or viewing perspective. But it is essential to ask the question "How did that data or document get captured?" Without data input/entry there are no results to review. Data entry requires careful planning, willingness to change work flow, and a significant amount of effort to solve the technical and human issues of data entry. The good news is that there are a growing number of modalities to support data entry.

Most EHR systems utilize all of the above modalities for data input. However, **interfaces** with systems such as laboratories, pharmacy, diagnostic imaging, and point-of-care equipment can result in more efficient, less manual data entry. Interfaces allow for the communication of electronic data between systems. In order for this to work, systems must be able to understand each other or talk the same language: this requires message standards of data exchange. The most common message standards are **ASTM, HL7, and DICOM** (see Chapter 6 for details). In addition, although **point-to-point interfaces** are common, a more sophisticated method of interfacing involves the use of an **interface engine** that allows HL7 messages to be communicated amongst numerous systems.

An alternate approach is to utilize **scanning** to input documents into the EHR. Almost any piece of paper can be scanned, but this approach has many disadvantages and severely limits its usefulness. Specifically, scanned documents must be indexed to enable efficient retrieval. In addition, an illegible hand-written note will continue to be of little clinical use as a scanned document. More importantly, a scanned document remains a passive document, there is no opportunity for the EHR to interact and interpret its data, a prerequisite for clinical decision support and data analysis. At best, scanning should be reserved as an adjunct for the entry of clinical data that is either too difficult or too time consuming/expensive to capture electronically and for mailed correspondence that cannot be received electronically and is deemed of value to the longitudinal patient record.

Another useful approach for the electronic capture and storage of unstructured data is the automatic uploading of word-processed documents into the EHR. Since dictation and transcription of clinical notes contributes significantly to the medical record of most clinical practices, uploading these documents to the EHR is advantageous and replaces the need to store them as part of the paper medical record. Some EHR systems provide automatic upload capabilities that require indexing by the transcriptionist based on a unique patient identifier, the date of dictation, and type of report. However, like scanned documents, uploaded unstructured word-processed documents have minimal clinical decision-support capability.

Important point: *When evaluating EHR systems, determine the best modality for data entry for each type of data and document, realizing that a willingness to change current practices may be needed to take advantage of EHR capabilities. Ensure that vendors are able to provide required interfaces and the necessary data entry modalities. Consider all costs for data entry, including the development of interfaces, ongoing support of interfaces, scanners, voice recognition hardware and software, and labor.*

Results Reviewing

Once the data input issues have been solved, attention can be turned to the data output or viewing functionality of the EHR. Some of the required features are outlined in Table 8-2.

When reviewing results, the key goals are to save clinician time, prioritize the results to review, and ensure that critical information is not missed. In order to accomplish these goals results must be patient specific and easy to navigate within a patient's chart and from one patient chart to the next. Clinicians should be provided with a snapshot of patient results that provides "at a glance" views and clear visual cues that differentiate critical and abnormal results from those that are normal.

In addition, a summary of the results and further detailed information should be available to the clinician for review. Reference ranges for normal results should be provided, and abnormal results should be indicated. Critical results should be brought to the attention of the clinician immediately. Some EHR systems now utilize push technology such as auto-paging and auto-emailing of critical laboratory results, allowing clinicians to be informed of results as soon as they become available (16). Results review functionality should include the ability to quickly trend and graph a series of results, thereby enhancing interpretation and allowing important trends

Table 8-2

IMPORTANT FEATURES OF EHR RESULTS REVIEWING

Easy-to-Navigate	Patient-Centric	Summary and Details
Searchable	Reference ranges	Normal, abnormal, critical
Trending/graphing	Flagging	Acknowledge/sign
Copy and paste	Print	Email

to be identified. Results that require further action should be flagged and the ability to electronically acknowledge and sign results must be available. Finally, in order to improve communications with others, results in the form of reports should be available for copying and pasting to email and printing to paper. The ability of clinicians to customize results reviewing to meet their own personal workflow is also advantageous.

Important point: *When evaluating EHR systems, the results reviewing functionality should provide clinicians with flexible and customizable views of patient results. Results should be indexed and stored in a manner that is intuitive to the clinician and provides rapid access. Results should be clearly flagged as normal or abnormal and mechanisms to immediately alert clinicians of critical results should be available*

Diagnostic Test Ordering

One of the greatest attributes of EHR systems is the ability to perform direct order entry. The potential to improve diagnostic test utilization and improve care can be recognized through direct computerized physician (provider) order entry (CPOE). Yet one of the main reasons that EHR implementations have failed to live up to expectations has been the unwillingness of clinicians to embrace CPOE. The main reason for this reluctance has been the negative impact of CPOE on physicians' time. Order entry takes time and it takes longer to order an individual test electronically compared to ordering on paper, especially if support staff have completed all the necessary patient demographic information and simply hand a paper requisition to a physician for signature. However, EHR systems available on the market today have worked diligently to streamline order entry and provide additional added value. If properly designed, CPOE can be easy, quick, safe, and rewarding. The use of **order sets** and **order protocols** can be time saving and support best practices when compared to paper-based ordering. CPOE provides an opportunity to suggest or advise the ordering clinician on the choice of test at the time of order entry. In addition it must be recognized that all the benefits of reviewing results such as trending/graphing, clinical alerting, and flagging are not possible without someone assuming the role of order entry. Cost savings can be realized by the elimination of the production, processing, filing, and storage of paper requisitions. Finally errors in interpreting hand-written orders are eliminated with CPOE.

Important point: *When evaluating EHR systems, if there is an unwillingness to plan for and adopt CPOE, the return on investment from a cost and patient safety/quality of care perspective is questionable.*

Once CPOE is confirmed as a goal of the EHR implementation, the next step is to evaluate the order entry capabilities of the EHR system. Of paramount importance is the design of the graphical user interface (GUI) and order entry screens. In general, those EHR systems that are designed by clinicians for clinicians are more likely to succeed. Most EHR vendors utilize clinicians to assist in the development of the GUI. When evaluating EHR systems, the order entry process should be tested with several different types of simple orders (for example, INR daily x 5 then daily X 3 then weekly). Counting both the number of screens required to place an entire order and the number of seconds it takes will provide valuable information about the GUI design and the EHR's **online transaction processing** (OLTP) capacity. A simple order like the one above should require the clinician to navigate through only one or two screens and take only several seconds to complete. Moving from one screen to the next should be instantaneous in a production environment for simple transactions. The EHR vendor should guarantee acceptable response times to support CPOE.

Besides simple order entry, the ability to order groups of tests, known as **order sets** is an important feature of the EHR. This provides the opportunity to **build disease-specific order protocols** (for example, orders for atypical community-acquired pneumonia). Complete protocols require the ability to order not only diagnostic tests but medications and nursing/allied health orders as well.

Important point: *When evaluating EHR systems, diagnostic test ordering should be easy and fast. The vendor should guarantee adequate OLTP response times. Simple orders as well as order sets and disease-specific protocols should be available. It is strongly recommended that the entire process be thoroughly evaluated in a production environment similar to your own in order to clearly determine the impact on clinician time.*

Patient Encounter Documentation

Documentation of the patient encounter provides additional challenges for the EHR. Historically, clinicians who have adopted EHR systems have relied heavily on the use of dictation, transcription and uploading word-processed documents. Scanning of printed patient encounter documents is also possible. As mentioned, these two modalities support unstructured reports and do not take full advantage of the EHR's clinical decision-support potential.

The ultimate goal is to develop efficient mechanisms to convert unstructured patient encounter documents into structured electronic forms that can be completed before, during, and after the patient encounter by the clinician.

The ease of generating unstructured documents is significantly outweighed by the benefits of structured reports as long as the time required and effort involved in completing electronic forms is acceptable. EHR systems that truly understand this have designed electronic forms and tools to achieve this goal.

Electronic forms may contain both structured and free-text entries that can be rapidly completed using input devices such as the keyboard, mouse, pen, scanner, and voice recognition microphones. The structured data can be coded, allowing for real-time clinical alerting and retrospective data analysis and report generation. In addition, structured data is searchable and can be automatically sent to other systems that support patient care delivery such as coding and billing applications.

Electronic forms can be customized to display and capture required data such as those required to meet the Health Care Financing Administration Evaluation and Management guidelines (17). Electronic forms work well for encounters that can be easily standardized and are relatively brief in duration, such as office follow-up visits (i.e., hypertension), short procedures (i.e., colonoscopy), and progress notes. Electronic forms are also practical for problem list documentation. Problem lists that utilize structured codified data not only serve to describe important clinical conditions but also can be proactive in nature, initiating additional actions such as the launching of disease guidance, clinical alerts, and health maintenance reminders. Problem list documentation can also be used for billing and other administrative purposes.

The complexity of converting unstructured documents to structured reports increases significantly as the length of the document increases. For example, consultant letters, discharge summaries and surgical reports are often lengthy and complex. It may not be practical to try and convert these to electronic forms. However, the combination of electronic forms with word processing templates is another option to consider, not only does this decrease the need for transcription services, it provides an opportunity to provide high level coding to otherwise unstructured documents.

Patient encounter documents that are generated outside the organization such as consultants' reports or outside imaging study reports usually arrive on paper. The most practical option for including these reports within the EHR is scanning. Another possibility is to request that the reports be sent via secure email as word processing attachments and then indexed and uploaded into the EHR.

Important point: *When evaluating EHR systems, the ability to document patient encounters using structured data provides significant added value. These benefits must be balanced by the work required to convert unstructured data to structured data and the ability to provide a user friendly and efficient solution for data capture by clinicians. EHR systems should provide flexible encounter forms and tools to allow for easy customization and come preloaded with an inventory of useful clinical encounter forms.*

Electronic Prescribing (ePrescribing)

The deadliness of the pen and prescription pad is highlighted by the fact that each year prescription medication errors injure one and a half million Americans and contribute to the deaths of more than seven thousand people in the US (18). It is estimated that over half a million preventable drug-related injuries occur among Medicare recipients in outpatient clinics alone

(18, 19). Numerous organizations have called for direct EHR prescribing of medications by physicians, known as electronic prescribing (20). In July 2003 the IOM endorsed eprescribing and recommended that all physicians in the US adopt this technology by 2010 (8). Currently it is estimated between 5% and 18% of US physicians perform ePrescribing (21).

EHR systems have been shown to be an effective ePrescribing tool to decrease adverse drug events, decrease medication errors, decrease costs, and improve patient care (17,21,22).

Electronic prescribing with an EHR requires similar considerations as CPOE and documentation, as well as some unique considerations. In order to get physicians to buy in, it must be an easy, fast, user friendly process that can be successfully integrated into physician work flow. The added value must be clearly shown in the form of medication management that includes clinical alerting, medication tracking, automatic renewals, and printing and faxing capabilities. EHR systems should allow for quick and easy viewing of current and previous medications, dosages, and duration of therapy. Completing initial prescriptions and refills should be aided by drop down menus that contain medications listed on formularies. Suggested dosages, recommended duration of therapy, and additional physician and patient educational information should be easily accessible. Substitutions should be possible and the ability for prescriptions to be printed, sent electronically to in-house pharmacy systems or automatically faxed or emailed to outside pharmacies should be available.

One of the greatest advantages of ePrescribing using the EHR is the opportunity to guide and advise the clinician's therapeutic choices and alert clinicians about allergies and possible adverse interactions. Table 8-3 describes some of the common forms of medication clinical alerting that can be incorporated into EHR ePrescribing.

Clinical alerting consists of real-time alerting as the clinician is prescribing medications. In addition to informing the clinician of potential interactions, it may also suggest alternative medications for consideration. Automatic reference to therapeutic guidelines such as locally developed antimicrobial guidelines for common infections may be incorporated. Additional advice may include suggested dosage adjustments, duration of therapy, route of administration, cost of therapy, and substitutions where appropriate. Many EHR vendors utilize drug databases from commercial vendors. The extent of integration and advantages and disadvantages of such databases should be clearly explained and understood as part of EHR evaluation and selection.

The reader should be made aware that there are a number of stand-alone ePrescribing solutions on the market that do not substitute for a comprehensive EHR. The National ePrescribing Patient Safety Initiative (NEPSI) has developed one such solution that is being offered free of charge to all physicians in the US (23). The value of these stand-alone ePrescribing solutions is debatable. Although they have the potential to eliminate transcrip-

Table 8-3

MEDICATION CLINICAL ALERTING

Type of Alert	Description	Example
Drug-drug	Identifies drug combinations that may have serious adverse interactions	Warfarin and aspirin
Drug-lab	Identifies laboratory values that could effect drug dosages, commonly renal and liver abnormalities	Digoxin-potassium Aminoglycosides-creatinine Liver?
Drug-pregnancy	Identifies drugs contraindicated in pregnancy	Warfarin
Drug-condition	Identifies drugs that may be contraindicated with certain medical conditions	NSAIDS in peptic ulcer disease
Drug-pediatric	Identifies reduced drug dosing in children (BMI)	Antibiotics
Drug-duplication	Identifies co-administration of similar classes of drugs	Lorazepam and valium
Drug-food and drug-herb	Identifies common interactions that effect drug metabolism	Warfarin and vitamin K containing foods (i.e. brussel sprouts) Aspirin and gingko

tion errors, their ability to provide appropriate clinical alerting is dependent on the ability to access all of the pertinent data that would only be found in an EHR. Prescribing medications without access to all the pertinent patient data is just as dangerous with an EHR as it is with paper.

Important point: *When evaluating EHR systems, ePrescribing can provide many advantages over hand-written prescriptions and can significantly improve patient care and reduce costs. Medication clinical alerting software should be fully integrated into EHR systems. The emergence of stand-alone ePrescribing systems is a growing trend but does not substitute for an EHR solution.*

Electronic Signature

The EHR provides clinicians with the ability to review results, place orders, document encounters, and prescribe medications. Ensuring that these clinical processes are appropriately authorized and tracked is accomplished with electronic signature. Electronic signature allows the clinician to access information, handle action items, and place orders and requests from any location at which the EHR is available. Electronic signature can be achieved by simply clicking on the item's sign button or by entering a personal identification number or through the use of biometric devices such as finger print scanners. For viewing numerous results simultaneously, for example, a trend of INR values, summary electronic signature should be available, allowing all data points to be viewed and acknowledged. All items for signature may be kept in a queue similar to an email in-box, providing clinicians with an easy-to-use mechanism that ensures that important patient data to review is not overlooked. Once signed, items become a permanent part of the patient's EHR and are automatically removed from the clinician's in-box.

Provision of thoroughly integrated/multilevel securities within the EHR ensures that appropriate authorization occurs and audit trails can be performed.

Important point: *When evaluating EHR systems, electronic signature from authorized users allows items that require review or action to be easily tracked and signed from wherever the EHR is available. Items, along with signature acknowledgement, become a permanent part of the EHR that can be retrieved and audited at later dates.*

Clinical Decision Support

Defined broadly, clinical decision-support systems (CDS) "can be any automated tool that helps clinicians improve the delivery or management of patient care. In its ideal sense, CDS is a set of knowledge-based tools that are fully integrated with both the clinician workflow components of an EHR and a repository of complete and accurate clinical data" (24). Examples of CDS capabilities designed to improve clinical care processes are highlighted in Table 8-4. Many EHR vendors provide off-the-shelf CDS in the form of

Table 8-4

FUNCTIONS OF CDS SYSTEMS

Function	Example
Alerting	Highlighting a critical blood potassium level
Reminding	Annual flu vaccine reminder
Critiquing	Rejecting duplicate diagnostic test orders
Interpreting	Diagnosing atrial fibrillation on ECG
Predicting	Predicting mortality risk from a severity-of-illness score
Diagnosing	Listing a differential diagnosis for patient with chest pain
Assisting	Modifying antibiotic choice for patient with renal failure
Suggesting	Generate suggestions for mechanical ventilator weaning

Adapted from Randolph et al (25)

simple clinical alerting and reminders. The ability to provide online access to guidelines is also available in most EHR systems today. More complex CDS such as interpreting, diagnosis, and suggestions requires more sophisticated CDS logic.

The evidence of the benefits of EHR-integrated CDS continues to grow, both in terms of patient care improvements and cost savings (24,26,27). However there is also recognition that CDS capabilities within EHR systems are often turned off after implementation because of the negative impact on clinician work flow, inappropriateness of advice and what has become known as the "nuisance effect" (28).

In order to perform CDS operations EHR systems rely on the ability of the system to gather data, analyze data in relation to predefined rules, draw conclusions, and then send this information to the clinician in a predetermined manner. Simply put, it requires computer processing that can perform a series of "if this, do that" actions. The most successful EHR-integrated CDS systems have come into existence through decades of work by computer programmers and clinical informatics specialists who have taken advantage of home grown proprietary systems to build their own CDS systems using **rules engines** and **data dictionaries.** An example of this is LDS's Health Evaluation through Logical Processing system (HELP) (29). One of the greatest challenges and disappointments in clinical informatics has been the inability to replicate CDS successes in other institutions. One of the main reasons for this has been the proprietary nature of EHR systems. The languages used and resulting rules and logic operate within a single system and often cannot be applied outside the walls of the institution that developed the CDS system. The emergence of CDS standards and commercially available CDS content that can be integrated into EHR systems is resulting in greater adoption and benefit (30).

Important point: *Determine what if any standards the EHR CDS functionality supports and how easy it is to build, customize, maintain, and support existing and new CDS interventions. When evaluating EHR systems, a clear understanding of the tools used to build the system is needed in order to determine if they will meet your needs.*

Historically, one of the arguments made in opposition to EHR systems is the notion that CDS systems will dictate to clinicians the only course of action. The resulting disastrous consequences of clinicians being replaced by computers and patients falling prey to technology misadventures makes for good fiction but represents a hollow threat in the real world of clinical practice. CDS systems do not dictate policy; they simply disseminate information and expertise that can be heeded or ignored by clinicians. When implemented and adopted they represent powerful tools to assist the clinician in the gathering and analysis of clinical data and present information and expertise for consideration in real time at the point of clinical decision-making. CDS systems should be viewed as on-line advisors available 24 hours a day at the point of clinical decision-making.

There are many obstacles to the implementation of a successful EHR-CDS system. The following critical success factors have been offered to assist in achieving clinician acceptance (31).

1. Frequent direct contact between the clinician and computer. CDS interventions are most effective when the clinician is the one who is directly exposed to the intervention. Clinicians need to embrace the EHR as an essential tool for clinical practice.

2. The existence of a rich clinical database. CDS interventions require the analysis of data on many patient factors. An EHR that integrates or has ready access to all the required data necessary is more likely to succeed.

3. Leadership support. Clinical and administrative leadership must provide strong support for EHR-CDS initiatives. At budget time, these initiatives must not be seen as competing for scarce patient care dollars but rather as initiatives that are essential for efficient and effective care delivery.

4. Track record. Establishing early wins with basic CDS initiatives (i.e., drug allergy alerting) should make clinicians more willing to give additional more complex initiatives an opportunity to prove their worth.

5. Software quality review. Ensuring that the CDS software is performing in the manner that it is supposed to perform is critical for user acceptance. CDS interventions that result in poor advice or inaccurate advice must be avoided.

6. Impact assessment. Showing to clinicians that CDS interventions can improve patient care in their own clinical practice will assist in converting the reluctant volunteer to a committed supporter.

Although these critical success factors are offered for CDS initiatives, they are just as relevant and important for all aspects of EHR implementation. For a further discussion on the EHR and clinical decision support, see Chapter 9.

Important point: *When evaluating EHR systems, set modest goals for CDS at the outset. Early CDS interactions should be based on clinical priority, opportunities, and EHR functionality available. Implementing the entire spectrum of CDS requires expertise, experience, and a significant organizational commitment.*

Disease Management

Clinicians are inundated with clinical practice guidelines (CPGs), yet there exists a significant gap between recommended care and received care (32). Despite the publication of thousands of CPGs reflecting best evidence, most guidelines are never followed. In a survey of physician attitudes on CPGs only 52% reported using them at least once per month, citing difficulty integrating paper-based CPG into clinical practice and the lack of evidence about the impact on outcomes as reasons for infrequent use (33). It appears that in the busy world of clinical practice, guidelines won't be used if they are not believed or readily available when clinical decisions are being made. Recently there has been a growing interest in the use of EHR systems and other health information technologies to narrow the quality gap and improve disease management. Stand-alone disease management solutions exist in the market place and, like ePrescribing solutions, offer a more economical and faster implementation time but do not substitute for a comprehensive EHR solution (34).

In order to support disease management, EHR systems must help coordinate five clinical processes necessary for comprehensive disease management. These include:

1. Identification and enrollment of individual patients and populations of patients with specific diseases, commonly through a disease registry;

2. Ongoing assessment and diagnosis of the disease progress and complications;

3. Care planning and management;

4. Ongoing monitoring and feedback of the individual patient and disease population;

5. Patient education

Table 8-5 provides examples of common EHR features that support disease management clinical processes.

Table 8-5

EHR FEATURES TO SUPPORT DISEASE MANAGEMENT

Disease Management Process	Supporting EHR Features
1. Identification and enrollment	◆ Disease registry ◆ Problem list documentation
2. Assessment and diagnosis	◆ Disease specific encounter documentation ◆ Risk stratification
3. Care planning and management	◆ Health maintenance reminders (i.e. vaccines and screening frequencies) ◆ Disease specific care plans that incorporate CPGs ◆ Diagnostic and treatment protocols
4. Monitoring and feedback	◆ Quality indicator reporting ◆ Variance tracking
5. Patient education	◆ Self-management plans ◆ Personal health records

Most EHR vendors will provide pre-packaged guidelines, protocols, and pathways that have either been developed by the vendor or customer base or bought from third-party organizations. It is important that these "packages" be reviewed during the selection process and endorsed by local clinical leadership. In addition, disease management content must be updated and refined on a regular basis. EHR vendors should provide the necessary tools, training, and support to achieve this.

Important point: *When evaluating EHR systems, determine the capability of the system to support comprehensive disease management. Evaluate the extent to which the EHR can support individual patients with specific diseases and entire disease populations. Disease management content should be evidence-based and easily customizable to the local context.*

Data Analysis and Report Generation

This chapter has discussed how the EHR can assist in the day-to-day delivery of clinical care. The emphasis has been on how the clinician uses the EHR for **online transaction processing** (OLTP). However the EHR benefits also include enhanced analytical capabilities as discussed in Chapter 4. Transactional EHR data can be analyzed on a retrospective basis, known as **online analytical processing** (OLAP). The generation of reports based on OLAP can provide valuable information to clinicians, including the opportunity to evaluate their own practice patterns and benchmark against colleagues and external standards. It also allows clinicians to gain powerful insight into population-wide health conditions and trends. In addition, lists of patients requiring interventions, such as those who have missed their annual flu vaccines, can be easily generated and reminder letters sent out.

Data analyses designed to assist clinicians in the identification of opportunities for clinical care improvement requires access to a large amount of diverse data that often resides in multiple **databases, warehouses, and data repositories** (see Chapter 4). Unfortunately, merging of these data is often difficult and complicated. If the data is not stored electronically and resides only on paper, then OLAP is not possible. It is therefore important to determine prior to EHR selection not only how it will be used for transaction processing but also what data is critical for retrospective analysis and report generation. Table 8-6 lists some of the key clinical data required for this purpose. In most organizations today, if the data does exist electronically, it will be stored in numerous databases. This requires the creation of a **data warehouse** that stores and provides access to all the required data and allows analyses to be performed using standard analytical and **data mining** tools. A few examples of such tools are provided in Table 8-7. Technical infrastructure requirements for data warehousing solutions are complex and have been described elsewhere. (35, 36)

Important point: *When evaluating EHR systems, it is important to determine the organization's OLAP requirements prior to EHR selection. EHR*

Table 8-6

KEY CLINICAL DATA REQUIRED FOR OLAP

Data Element	Examples
Master patient index	Patient demographics
Admit discharge transfer (ADT)	Encounter data including length of stay, attending physician
Claims data	ICD-9, CPT-4, DRGs
Medication data	Drug, dose, route, duration of therapy
Diagnostic test utilization	Labs, diagnostic imaging, echos, PFTs
Procedures	Surgeries, endoscopies
Nursing and Allied Health	Workload
Outcomes	Morbidity, mortality, readmissions, quality of life
Costs	Diagnostics, therapeutics, physician, nursing

vendors should demonstrate how retrospective data analysis and report generation can be achieved and whether their solutions are proprietary or provide an open solution such as a analytical relational databases in which commercially available analytical software can be utilized.

Patient Education

An essential component of clinical care is ensuring that decisions made respect patient autonomy and are the result of informed and shared decision-making. Patient educational interventions take time, and time is a precious resource for both clinicians and patients. There is evidence that computer-based approaches to patient education improve patients' knowledge, more actively involve them in decision-making, and also may lead to better

Table 8-7

EXAMPLES OF ANALYTICAL AND DATA MINING SOFTWARE

Product	Category
Microsoft Access	SQL Queries
SAS/SPSS	Statistical analysis (some data mining)
Intelligent Miner (IBM)	Data mining
PowerPlay (Cognos)	Data mining (OLAP)
Business Miner (Business Objects)	Data mining (OLAP)
Oracle	Data mining (OLAP)

health outcomes (37). These approaches could be integrated into EHR systems.

Patient education handouts can be viewed on-line within the EHR and discussed with the patient and printed or saved to a disk for take home review. Some EHR vendors have created libraries of professionally written patient handouts that assist in making information easier to understand and cover a wide variety of conditions and procedures.

Electronic prescribing can be accompanied by the automatic printing of medication information sheets that provide important educational information such as administration details, drug interactions, and complications. In addition, patient educational interventions can be documented and tracked within the EHR for later review and to assist with reimbursement. EHR systems may also provide access to multi-media patient educational material such as the audio and video files, podcasts, and online decision aids.

The ability to easily launch internet applications and the internet from within the EHR allows clinicians access to a wealth of patient educational material. High-quality sites can be book-marked for later reference. Details on evaluating medical web sites for quality have been published to assist clinicians and patients (38). In addition numerous **super medical web sites** are now available, serving as portals to a wide range of patient and clinician information management resources.

A growing trend in patient education and improved patient-provider communication is the personal health record (PHR), which is a web-based extension of the EHR designed for and used by the patient to review relevant information such as historical results, medications, and self-management plans. PHRs can also be used to communicate with the patient and health care team to answer clinical questions, schedule appointments and update progress against agreed upon goals.

Important point: *When evaluating EHR systems determine what patient educational material is provided and whether it is possible to integrate additional patient educational material into the EHR. Assess the vendor's approach to PHRs and whether it is a stand-alone product or an extension of the EHR.*

Future Advances

Computer processing power continues to increase, and costs of data storage continue to fall. As a result, emerging technologies will offer exciting advances for the EHR. Several of the future advances referred to in the first edition of this guide have occurred. Commercially available web-based EHRs that can be hosted on-site or remotely are providing an attractive alternative to the traditional EHR. Knowledge management vendors are offering evidence-based content that can be incorporated into many EHRs and kept up to date. Handheld devices such as the BlackBerry are being used to extend the reach of the EHR, push critical laboratory results, and provide a way to better communicate amongst clinicians. Personal health records and patient portals are becoming mainstream, and the idea of an EHR for all has become a national priority. Adoption of voice recognition remains slower than anticipated but is still a main contender to replace expensive dictation and transcription services and provide EHR systems with a new modality for efficient and effective clinical documentation.

The improved design of graphical user interfaces (GUIs) is a major advance over former character-based user interfaces. However, for the most part, EHR GUIs require clinicians to actively search for and "pull" the clinical data for viewing. The introduction of email in-boxes and the ability to "push" critical data automatically to pagers, fax machines, and email addresses represents the first stage of **push technology** in clinical practice. Future advances will see the introduction of **intelligent agents** that will be able to anticipate clinicians' information management needs and push information to clinicians based on predefined choices, scheduled patient encounters, and other clinical care requirements. For example, intelligent GUIs will recognize that the core clinical data set for a follow-up chemotherapy patient visit is different than the core clinical data set for a patient with an emergency ruptured aortic aneurysm, pushing to the clinician the right information at the right time. These intelligent agents will not only be disease specific but will also be clinician and patient specific, and will result in significant efficiency gains for clinical care processes.

Conclusion

Successful EHR implementation requires a thorough understanding of the everyday activities and work habits of those providing care. The purpose of this chapter was to provide the reader with a practical approach to identify and analyze clinical processes for the ultimate purpose of selecting an EHR system. There is growing evidence that the theoretical promise of the EHR can be achieved in clinical practice. . . However, although the growing number of successes is encouraging, there continues to be a large number of EHR failures. The reader should be reminded of this, not to discourage beginning the journey (for not beginning has the potential to ultimately cost more in many ways) but rather to emphasize critical success factors for EHR selection and implementation. These factors include:

1. Ensuring clinicians play leading roles in the EHR selection, implementation and evaluation processes.

2. Identifying and prioritizing clinical care processes within the organization that could be positively affected by the implementation of an EHR.

3. Setting realistic expectations given the organization's technical infrastructure, ability to learn, leadership, and commitment to the EHR.

4. Evaluating EHR systems from a clinical care process perspective, as well as an administrative and financial perspective. EHR systems must first and foremost support clinicians and patient care delivery.

5. A willingness of clinicians and in particular physicians to change current practices and utilize the EHR in all aspects of clinical care including CPOE, documentation, and disease management.

Throughout the evaluation phase of an EHR selection process, it is important to revisit the checklist described in Table 8-1. If you cannot convince yourself that the EHR will have a positive impact on clinical practice, then the chance of a successful implementation is extremely doubtful. EHR systems are of no benefit if they are not being used.

EHR systems are improving the way care is delivered, providing clinicians with powerful new tools to assist in the delivery of safe, high-quality, cost-effective care. These promises are well founded, but to be realized they need to be clearly shown. The impact of these systems on clinical processes is an essential step in realizing those promises.

References

1. Forbes J. In Laennec RTH. A Treatise on the Diseases of the Chest. New York: Hafner Publishing; 1962: xix.
2. Kohane IS. Synopsis: computer-based patient records. Yearbook of Medical Informatics, 1998: Health Informatics and the Internet. IMIA:227-229.
3. Tange HJ, Hasman A, deVriesRobbe PF, Schouten HC. Medical narratives in electronic medical records. IMIA: Yearbook of Medical Informatics. 1998, 230-252.
4. Institute of Medicine. The Computer-Based Patient Record: An Essential Technology for Health Care. Washington DC: National Academy Press; 1991.
5. Dick RS, Andrew WF. Where we've been and where we're headed. Healthcare Informatics. 1997;Feb:52-56.
6. Institute of Medicine. The Computer-Based Patient Record: An Essential Technology for Health Care. Washington DC: National Academy Press; Revised edition, 1997.
7. Institute of Medicine, Committee on Data Standards for Patient safety. Key Capabilities of an Electronic Health Record. Washington, DC: National Academy Press; 2003.
8. Institute of Medicine, Committee on Data Standards for Patient safety. Achieving a New Standard for Care, Washington, DC: National Academy Press; 2004.
9. Williams LS. Microchips versus stethoscopes: Calgary hospital, MDs face off over controversial computer system. CMAJ. 1992;147:1534-47.
10. Rose JS, Gapinski M, Lum A, et al. The Colorado Kaiser Permenente Clinical Information System: a comprehensive review. Proceedings of the CPR Recognition Symposium, Fifth Annual Nicholas E. Davies Award. CPRI. 1999;13-75.
11. Finley SW. The electronic health record as a tool to improve patient care: hypothetical and practical opportunities. Journal of the Healthcare Information and Management Systems Society. 1997;4: 5-11.

12. Butcher L. More doctors tell patients, 'we'll see you today'. ACP Observer. American College of Physicians. November, 2006. www.acponline.org/journals/news/nov06/access.htm

13. Tonks A, Smith R. Information in practice. BMJ. 1996;313:438.

14. McDonald CJ, Tierney WM. Computer-stored medical records: their future role in medical practice. JAMA. 1988;23:3433-40.

15. Overhage M, McDonald CJ. Medical records systems for office practice. Computers in Clinical Practice. ACP: 1995;19-36.

16. Teich JM, Wrinn MM. Clinical decision support systems come of age. MD Computing 2000;1:43-8.

17. Evans RS, Pestotnik SL, Classen DC, et al. A computer-assisted management program for antibiotics and other antiinfective agents. N Eng J Med. 1998;338:232-8.

18. Institute of Medicine, Committee on Quality in Healthcare in America. To err is human: building a safer health system. Washington, DC, National Academy Press; 1999.

19. Lazarou J, Pomeranz BH, Corey PN. Incidence of adverse drug reactions in hospitalized patients. JAMA. 1998;279:1200-5.

20. Schiff GD, Rucker TD. Computer prescribing: building the electronic infrastructure for better medication usage. JAMA. 1998;279:1024-9.

21. Electronic Prescribing: Towards Maximum Value and Rapid Adoption, A Report of the Electronic Prescribing Initiative eHealth Initiative Washington, D.C. April 14, 2004. www.ehealthinitiative.org/initiatives/erx/.

22. Bates DW, Leape LL, Cullen DJ, et al. Effect of computerized physician order entry and a team intervention on prevention of serious medication errors. JAMA. 1998;280: 1311-6.

23. National ePrescribing Patient Safety Initiative (NEPSI) www.nationalerx.com.

24. Perreault LE, Metzger JB. A pragmatic framework for understanding clinical decision support. Journal of the Healthcare Information and Management systems Society. 1999;2:5-21.

25. Randolph A, Haynes RB, Wyatt JC, et al. Users' guides to the medical literature XVIII. How to use an article evaluating the clinical impact of a computer-based clinical decision support system. JAMA. 1999;282: 67-74

26. Davis DD, Moriyama R, Tiwanak G, et al. Clinical performance improvement with an advanced clinical information system at the Queen's Medical Center. Proceedings of the CPR Recognition Symposium, Fifth Annual Nicholas E. Davies Award, CPRI. 1999, 77-120.

27. Hunt DL, Haynes RB, Hanna SE, Smith K. Effects of computer-based clinical decision support systems on physician performance and patient outcomes. JAMA. 1998;280:133946.

28. Kilbridge PM, Welebob EM, Classen DC. Development of the Leapfrog methodology for evaluating hospital implemented inpatient computerized physician order entry systems Qual Saf Health Care. 2006;15:81-4

29. Miller RA, Geissbuhler A. Clinical decision support systems: an overview. In E.S. Berner, ed. Clinical Decision Support Systems: Theory and Practice. New York: Springer-Verlag, 1998.

30. Broverman CA. Standards for clinical decision support systems. Journal of the Healthcare Information and Management Systems Society. 1999;2:23-31.

31. Teich JM, Kuperman GJ, Bates DW. Clinical decision support: making the transition from the hospital to the community network. Journal of the Healthcare Information and Management systems Society. 1997;4:27-37.

32. McGlynn, EA, Asch SM, Adams J, et al. The quality of health care delivered to adults in the United States. New Engl J Med. 2003;348:2635–45.

33. Hayward RS, Guyatt GH, Moore KA, et al. Canadian physicians' attitudes about and preferences regarding clinical practice guidelines. CMAJ. 1997;12:1715-23.

34. Metzger J. Using computerized registries in chronic disease care. California Healthcare Foundation, 2004.
35. Nussbaum GM, Ault SP. The best little data warehouse. Journal of the Healthcare Information and Management Systems Society. 1998;4:79-93.
36. Ledbetter CS, Morgan MW. Toward best practice: leveraging the electronic patient record as a clinical data warehouse. Journal of Healthcare Information Management. Summer 2001
37. Lewis D. Computer-based approaches to patient education: a review of the literature. Journal of the American Medical Informatics Association. 1999;4:272-82.
38. Silberg WM, Lundberg GD, Musacchio RA. Accessing, controlling, and assuring the quality of medical information on the internet: Caveant lector et viewor: let the reader and viewer beware.

9

Clinical Decision Support

Bruce Slater, MD
Jerome A. Osheroff, MD

This is a chapter about making the right thing to do the easy thing to do. That is the essence of clinical decision support (CDS). Shortliffe et al (1) makes the point that medical care *is* decision making and defines CDS as a computer program designed to help healthcare professionals make clinical decisions. Robert Greenes, in his book on the subject, defines CDS as the use of the computer to bring relevant knowledge to bear on the health care and well being of a patient (2). Eta Berner, in the second edition of her review of the subject, defines it as computer systems designed to affect clinical decision-making about individual patients at the point of time that these decisions are made (3). The broadest definition of CDS is taken from a guidebook published by Health Information Management Systems Society (HIMSS) (4). CDS is clinical knowledge or patient-related information, filtered or presented at appropriate times to enhance patient care. Because this, the broadest definition, is also the most specific, this chapter will work from this definition. It is instructive to take this definition apart and examine all the elements.

- **Clinical knowledge** is the best available evidence on the topic, supplemented with authoritative guidelines where available, and with expert opinion as appropriate. Occasionally the clinical knowledge that can help may be traditional medical textbook contents related to diseases and pathophysiology or normal anatomy or physiology. More valuable in many cases but often less readily available are results of a meta-analysis of randomized clinical trials showing an advantage of a treatment or diagnostic modality.

- **Patient-related information** is taken from a patient's medication list, problem list, lab results, coded interpretations of imaging studies, or other recorded patient data.

- **Filtered** means gathering and presenting data that is directly pertinent to one or more specific clinical management decisions, and therefore does not distract the provider with extraneous information. For example, a diabetes data flowsheet culls out data particularly important for managing diabetic patients from the full array of the patient's lab results.

- **Presented at appropriate times** means being responsive to the current context of the workflow. In other words, presented at a time that the provider is able and ready to act on the information.

- To **enhance patient care** covers all aspects of error prevention, quality improvement, and enhancing value to the patient by creating improved process and outcomes of care and/or better cost-effectiveness.

The "5 rights" paradigm sums this up: 1) right information (evidence-based and context sensitive), in the 2) right intervention format (guideline, order set, reference, alert, relevant data display, or documentation tool), to the 3) right stakeholder (including patients), through the 4) right channel (Computer Provider Order Entry (CPOE), EHR, or mobile device), 5) at the right point in workflow to drive improved outcome (4).

All medical care is prospective. Patients are not treated in the past. The simplest CDS intervention is providing reference information, ideally in the context of the current patient. When a provider discovers an information need, the answer, customized for this patient, should be a click or two away. On the other hand, when a need is not recognized, a type of support is desirable that does not require an active quest for information. As described later, specific types of CDS apply to these circumstances and can be inserted seamlessly into the workflow.

Evidence-Based Medicine and Clinical Decision Support

Evidence-based medicine (EBM) has gained prominence as issues related to medical errors and unmet information needs have become more appreciated. A widely used definition comes from the work of Haynes and Sackett: "Evidence-based medicine is the conscientious, explicit and judicious use of current best evidence in making decisions about the care of individual patients" (5,6). Ideally, EBM utilizes high-quality randomized controlled clinical trials and meta-analyses to create useful information. Evidence can be graded by the quality of the studies referenced and the strength of the results. The best CDS is based on high-quality findings from the medical literature. Weaker forms of evidence and expert opinion are used when studies are not available and not likely to become available (7).

The science of grading evidence strength and stability is new. Published articles have characteristics that when combined create a body of evidence. Many interventions accepted as standard practice (e.g., giving oxygen to heart attack patients) are not based on formal studies. In addition, some interventions can be shown to have a statistically significant benefit without any significant clinical effect. Treadwell et al (8), reviewed several evidence grading systems and proposed a system to address perceived deficiencies in current systems. Their approach stresses 1) the distinction between quantitative (How well does it work? What is the size of the effect?) and qualitative (Does it work? What is the direction of the effect?); 2) a priori criteria for judgments; and 3) the impact of meta-analysis and sensitivity analysis on the ratings. It is a complex new system and its ultimate utility remains to be determined.

Why Do Clinical Decision Support?

As mentioned above, providers periodically recognize the need for additional information while taking care of patients. Recognition that physicians frequently have important unanswered questions or unmet information needs during patient care resulted from publication of a study by Covell (9) with follow-up and amplification by Osheroff (10), Gorman (11), Ely (12), and others. These studies confirmed that physicians have many questions that, if answered, would potentially change a patient's care. This supported the premise that it is not possible to make physicians perfect information processors and that they are subject to the inevitable mistakes of all humans (13). Follow-up studies documented that physicians either do not think it important or do not have time to actually answer a substantial portion of their recognized questions. Gorman demonstrated the futility of trying to know all the information necessary for medical practice. Studies suggest that more than half of all primary care encounters involve an unsatisfied information need and that it takes 43 minutes on average to answer each question (14).

While the difficulties in addressing recognized information needs are great, unrecognized information needs may present an even worse problem. Studies using participant observation in training settings readily demonstrate unrecognized information needs by physicians-in-training. Similarly, practicing clinicians are just as likely to have unrecognized information gaps that could be a major contributing factor to quality and safety problems. These unrecognized needs may never be addressed unless and until they are pointed out to the provider. Since any inquiry into information needs is very resource intensive and limited to the specific situation and context, a solution is needed that is generalizable and works whether the provider recognizes the need or not. Proactive CDS interventions such as alerts and reminders can help address this need.

Based on reports pointing to tens of thousands of unnecessary deaths due to medical mistakes, the IOM convened a committee in 1998 to make recommendations to reduce that number over the next 10 years. The report "To Err is Human" (15) is a call to action to set national goals for safety, enable effective reporting of errors and protect these disclosures, set safety standards, and make continually improved patient safety a declared and serious aim for health care organizations and providers. In the follow-up report, "Crossing the Quality Chasm" (16), the committee recommended ways to close the gap by proposing an agenda focused on producing the highest quality outcomes.

These IOM reports received widespread coverage and broadly raised awareness that many patients die due to healthcare adverse events, many of which are unnecessary and due to preventable errors by providers and others.

Basic science, clinical science, and health services researchers have been prolific in the last quarter century in creating new knowledge. Journals are full of evidence waiting to be applied to clinical care. Unfortunately healthcare operations have not been very swift in applying these discoveries. On average, it takes 17 years for research evidence published and accepted in the literature to come into evidence-based practice for a majority of providers (17). CDS exists to satisfy information needs and has been specifically shown to be efficient and efficacious when made available in CPOE and EHR applications. Chaudhry et al performed a meta-analysis that included CDS systems in addition to applications such as CPOE. They found publications from four benchmark institutions that offered evidence for improved quality in preventive medicine due to guideline adherence, better disease surveillance, and decreasing medication errors (18). In a systematic review focused on CDS and its effect on practitioner performance and outcomes, Garg et al reported improvements in performance, but patient outcomes were mixed and not well studied (19). The IOM and other influential groups have recommended implementing EHRs, including CPOE and CDS functionality, to help address many of the problems outlined above.

Improved adherence to quality measures, surveillance for adverse health care events, reduced medication errors, and improved efficiency are benefits of information system use that are well documented. In some cases these benefits require additional investments in clinician time, while in other settings they are net time saving. As with any intervention, some may not produce the expected result. Ash et al studied information technology implementations in health care from a sociological perspective and found unintended negative effects on the actual entering and retrieving of data, as well as the communication and coordination of care supported by the IT intervention (20). Campbell et al reported on an expert panel looking specifically at unintended consequences of CPOE (21).

The best CDS occurs as a by-product of the usual flow of care and does not intrude into normal events unless a dangerous or unusual situation has developed. Properly designed CDS makes the care process easier because information is offered in the context of normal workflow. With well-executed CDS, providers may not even notice that knowledge is being brought to bear.

Types of Clinical Decision Support

There are different ways to classify CDS. Perhaps the most comprehensive is a taxonomy related to functional application. This was proposed in a 2005 HIMSS book on CDS (Figure 9-1) (4).

---

1. Documentation forms/templates

   Benefits: provide complete documentation for quality/continuity of care, reimbursement, legal; reduce errors of omission by displaying items for selection; provide coded data for other data-driven CDS

Subtypes	Examples
1.1 Patient self-assessment forms	Pre-visit questionnaires Health Risk appraisals
1.2 Nursing patient assessment forms	Inpatient admission assessment Kardex
1.3 Clinician encounter documentation forms	Structured history and physical template Problem-specific assessment template Intelligent referral form
1.4 Departmental/multidisciplinary clinical documentation forms	Emergency department documentation Ambulatory care documentation Combinations of the above
1.5 Data flowsheets (usually a mixture of data entry form and relevant data display, see below)	Immunization flowsheet Health maintenance/disease management form Pay-for-performance (e.g., quality measure tracking) form

2. Relevant data presentation

   Benefits: optimize decision making by ensuring all pertinent data are considered; organize complex data collections to promote understanding of overall picture and to highlight needed actions

Subtypes	Examples
2.1 Relevant data for ordering or documentation	Display of relevant lab tests when ordering a medication Display of current hematocrit and status of crossmatch when ordering blood products
2.2 Choice lists	Suggested dose choice lists, possibly modified by patient's renal function and age On-formulary display for a drug class
2.3 Practice status display	OR scheduling and status display Emergency department tracking display
2.4 Retrospective/aggregate reporting or filtering	Physician practice audit and feedback Physician "report cards" List of all patients overdue for a key preventive care intervention List of all patients in disease management program with abnormal results

---

Figure 9-1   Clinical decision support intervention types. With permission from Publisher. Improving Outcomes with Clinical Decision Support: An Implementer's Guide. Chicago: HIMSS; 2005.

Continued on next page

2.5 Environmental parameter reporting	Recent hospital antibiotic sensitivities

3. **Order creation facilitators**
   Benefits: Promote adherence to standards of care by making the right thing the easiest to do

Subtypes	Examples
3.1 Single-order completers including consequent orders	Prompts for appropriate orders and documentation (e.g., for specific sub-tests when ordering toxic screen), or for reasons when ordering certain tests
	Suggested dose choice lists, possibly modified by patient's renal function and age
	Consequent order suggestions (e.g., for drug levels when ordering certain antibiotics or pre-medication when ordering blood products)
3.2 Order sets	General order sets (e.g., for hospital admission)
	Condition-specific orders sets (e.g., for heart attack)
	Post-op order sets
	Order sets containing orders that are fully specified, contain parameter choices, have "fill-in-the-blank" fields, or a combination of the three
	Active Guidelines
3.3 Tools for complex ordering	Guided dose algorithms
	TPN ordering forms with built-in calculators

4. **Time-based checking and protocol/pathway support**
   Benefits: Provide support for multi-step care plans, pathways, and protocols that extend over time

Subtypes	Examples
4.1 Stepwise processing of multi-step protocol or guideline	Tools for monitoring and supporting inpatient clinical pathways (e.g., for pneumonia admissions) and multi-day chemotherapy protocols
4.2 Support for managing clinical problems over long periods and many encounters	Computer-assisted management algorithm for treating hyperlipidemia over many outpatient visits

5. **Reference information and guidance**
   Benefits: Address recognized information needs of patients and clinicians

Subtypes	Examples
5.1 Context-insensitive	General link from EMR or clinical portal to a reference program (at table of contents or general-search level)

Figure 9-1 *Continued.*

5.2 Context-sensitive	Direct links to specific, pertinent reference needed (via infobuttons, knowledge links); e.g., link from medication order screen to display of side effects for that medication; link from problem-list entry to recent reviews of treatment for that problem
	Link from immunization flowsheet to table of standard immunization intervals
	Link in patient-messaging application to relevant patient information leaflets
	Calculators/nomograms
	Diagnostic decision support driven by patient-specific data

6. **Reactive alerts and reminders (i.e., unsolicited by patient or clinician recipient)**
   Benefits: Provide immediate notification of errors and hazards related to new data or orders entered by CIS user or the CIS itself (e.g., when abnormal lab result is posted), or passage of a time interval during which a critical event should occur; help enforce standards of care

Subtypes	Examples
6.1 Alerts to prevent potential errors or hazards	Drug allergy alert
	Drug interaction alert (e.g., with drugs, food)
	Under/overdose alert (single dose, total dose, frequency, etc.; general or specific for age, weight, laboratory results)
	Wrong drug route alert
	Patient specific contraindication for clinical intervention
	Inappropriate therapeutic duplication or medication administration route
	Incorrect test or study for an indication or inappropriate testing interval
	Critical lab test result notification
	User-requested notification when lab result is available or other key event has occurred

Figure 9-1   *Continued.*

Documentation Tools

Forms and templates are usually thought of as just another artifact of using computers. Yet well-designed order forms support sound decision-making by ensuring that required fields are completed and the proper information is reviewed. Computer-based forms and templates should have a logical order corresponding to the order in which a clinician elicits information. Poorly designed data input or confusing display formats can be cumbersome to use and impede workflow.

Computerized flow sheets, disease maintenance forms, and other quality measure tracking documents can be designed to enhance patient care by supplying information as they record data (for example including recommended intervals and ages for important preventive healthcare interventions).

Patient self-assessments conducted prior to provider visits as well as health risk appraisals are also tools useful for supplementing provider data collection and thus improving patient care. These CDS interventions are useful in the inpatient as well as outpatient settings and for nurses and other clinicians. Well-designed documentation systems aid in reducing unnecessary variation that occurs as a by-product of common care delivery activities.

Relevant Data Presentation

Patient data can have great decision support value to providers, especially when filtered to address the needs of particular circumstance. CPOE display of pertinent results during order-entry makes sense and has been shown to reduce orders for unnecessary tests (22,23). Medication order-entry that depends on certain lab values also benefits from results display. Display of relevant formulary information, including costs, in CPOE can have a beneficial effect on the bottom line while supporting quality care and patient safety.

Reports containing relevant data from a provider's practice in the form of a feedback audit or "report card" can be instructive. Reports of patient data also find widespread use in prevention and disease management programs. Hospital antibiotic sensitivities updated frequently and incorporated into treatment selection lists and prioritization algorithms in CPOE can mold generalist provider behavior into the patterns of the infectious disease specialists. Documentation tools and relevant data presentation represent a form of embedded CDS. They can be of value for unrecognized information needs because the user benefits without having to change their workflow or even recognize the information need.

Order Creation Facilitators

Much of what makes an EHR valuable has to do with facilitating order creation in the CPOE component. Making provider orders safe is of paramount importance in correcting the epidemic of errors that plague healthcare. As documented in the IOM reports, CPOE can add additional value by making the right thing to do the easy thing to do. Certain orders should trigger consequent orders. For example, a gentamicin order should trigger a gentamicin level after a few half-lives. Overhage described these as corollary orders (24). Some orders, such as imaging, must be placed with adequate information for the radiologist to determine whether the procedure ordered is going to answer the clinical question that triggered it, as well as guide the interpretation of the result. Offering orders that provide patient-appropriate doses of medication based on inferences from renal, hepatic, and electrolyte values can avoid injury to patients and increase efficacy. Order sets are an excellent means of supporting both provider efficiency and best practices.

One of the downsides to CPOE is it can take more time than simply writing orders if each order must be created individually. Using order sets created by a consensus committees of experts and end-users based on clinical evidence from the literature efficiently brings expertise of the specialists to bear on clinical problems faced by generalists, frequently saving them time. General medical admission order sets ensure that all required elements are included in a standard sequence and format for safe execution by nurses. Pre-op, post-op and procedure-specific orders do the same for surgical patients. When faced with complex interacting patient parameters, offering the provider guided dose algorithms, such as for total parenteral nutrition orders (TPN), is often the best way to ensure clear, accurate orders.

Protocol and Pathway Support

Many best practices, especially for disease management, include procedures executed over prolonged periods of time. Determining where a patient is in a management protocol, for example, for diabetes, hypertension, or hyperlipidemia, takes precious minutes during brief primary care encounters. If a patient is followed using a computerized pathway, providers can easily track progress and devote more time to patient interaction. In the inpatient setting, computerized protocols can ensure that required tests and treatments are executed in the proper sequence for ideal management (e.g., pneumonia pathway and many multi-day chemotherapy protocols).

Reference Information

Drug, disease, laboratory, and other reference materials delivered into workflow via EHRs and their component systems (CPOE, eMAR, etc.) can provide important benefits to care processes and outcomes. Interfaces that provide information with the fewest clicks permit quicker access, saved time, and more satisfied clinicians. More advanced systems place links to drug information on the specific drug name or attach disease references to problem list entries (25). These pre-configured links, called "infobuttons", are readily integrated into EHRs and can deliver content that is either locally developed or acquired from an external knowledge source. Having a link to patient education or patient prep information from the appropriate place in CPOE or EHR increases the ease of doing the right thing in informing and educating patients. Calculators and nomograms that are "smart" in that they "know" the patient's appropriate clinical data provide additional value to providers who may wish to explore "what-if" scenarios.

Reactive Alerts and Reminders

CPOE is a common place where implementers use alerts and reminders. Alerts and reminders are generally triggered in the background by patient data and user data entry. They can provide immediate notification of errors and hazards (potential errors) related to incoming new patient data or orders entered by the user. In addition, the lack of an order can also trigger a reminder if an action should take place consequent to a previous event or result. For example, an alert may fire in response to orders for a drug for which the patient should, but doesn't, have a drug level also ordered. Duplicating an existing drug or test, or prescribing a drug known to interact with another drug or food the patient is exposed to, are other situations for which alerts are often used. Drugs dosed under or over certain limits can trigger alerts as well as drugs ordered by the wrong route.

Alerts may also warn of serious issues such as contraindications to a procedure based on a previous procedure in the past. Laboratory tests at critical high or low values can be brought to the immediate attention of the user. Knowing that a result is back for review, even if normal, can be helpful for a provider waiting to complete orders. As a result of background checking, reminders may be used for a wide variety of situations such as disease management, cost-effective medication substitutions, health maintenance, and even identifying potential clinical trials subjects.

Modes of Advice Delivery

How advice is delivered to the provider is often described in potentially confusing terms. Although it is tempting to use "active" and "passive" to describe the way CDS offers advice, they are not particularly helpful because these terms can be understood in very different ways. "Passive" could mean it is intrinsic in the way the intervention is designed. For example, the location of data on a page or screen, location of data input areas, or relation of data display to data input could be considered passive. However, the term "passive decision support" also refers to CDS that must be sought by the user to be activated. So, the use of the term "passive decision support" is not helpful and will not be utilized further. Instead CDS that requires user activation will be referred to as "embedded". Links to referential texts on the page the user is viewing is an example of embedded CDS. Links may lead to an index, table of contents, or a search window, or go directly to the appropriate place in the reference based on provider workflow. This latter mode is called "context-specific help" and is more valuable than taking the user to the table of contents.

The concept of the infobutton has been popularized as a generic way to describe getting context-specific help. Several clinical information system and CDS vendors have technology to enable these context-specific reference links. Infobuttons are an excellent vehicle for the delivery of evidence-based reference materials into the workflow via clinical information systems. They can be particularly useful when embedded in various displays and data entry forms.

Buttons, empty fields, or pick lists in a display offer an opportunity to click them, fill them in, or choose them. This delivery of information is called an "affordance" and is defined as the attributes of objects that enable individuals to know how to use them (26). This is a great concept to apply to CDS. The presence of something raises the question "What is that for?" A pot with a handle gives a clue and a suggestion. The clue is "This is meant to be picked up!" The suggestion is "Pick it up here!" Even if the hinges of a door are hidden, someone approaching intrinsically expects it to open from the side with the knob and pivot from the other side. Similarly the presence of a data entry field in a well-designed form suggests that asking the patient about that data item or examining that body part might be a good idea. This is specifically called a "perceived affordance", as referred to by Norman (27). In the medical realm, it may also trigger an "Ah Ha!" in which the user remembers the related classroom material from many years ago. This recognition can make the user feel comfortable collecting and thinking about the suggested data. An affordance prompts the user to recall something previously learned and reminds them to collect it. Embedded decision support can be a perceived affordance.

Active decision support should be fairly unambiguous. Because passive CDS has been confusing, we will refer to things that happen without human intervention as unsolicited, rather than active CDS. Events in the workflow or events from the patient's results trigger actions without provider initiation. These conditions are covered by CDS that is said to execute or "fire" when the events are detected. As the provider enters orders in CPOE, many different actions can be triggered. Corollary orders can be suggested or queued. Orders may be compared to the problem list or lab results and advice given concerning potential problems or better choices of orders.

Sometimes events develop that require intervention outside of the providers' awareness. For example, a lab result may indicate a need for a therapeutic intervention such as replacing low potassium. A patient's heart monitor could indicate an arrhythmia or other abnormality. This brings up the question of how these events are made known because they are unlikely to occur while the user is logged in and viewing the particular patient with the abnormal result. Occasionally results must be transmitted immediately. In that case, pagers or network-connected devices are the best way to enable a quick response to an urgent condition. Flagging a provider on log-in or alerting them while they are viewing a different patient is possible but raises the issue of intrusiveness.

Intrusiveness

One of the potentially irritating features of clinical information system installations is inappropriate intrusiveness of unsolicited CDS. The alert has to be matched to the importance and timeliness of the threat. While it is easy to see that a critical time-sensitive alert must be brought to the attention of someone who can intervene appropriately, the dangers of over-alerting cannot be minimized. The EHR or the CPOE system is frequently designed to be one of several systems to manage abnormal conditions. Unnoticed alerts may be re-programmed to be more assertive while back-up systems that were in place before the alert was created should continue to provide a failsafe function.

The opposite can be, in some ways, a worse problem. If a frequent set of multiple alerts are fired for minor conditions, providers may reject a high percent of alerts. Users become fatigued with alerts and do not attend to them. Alerts that do not take into consideration basic pertinent patient data such as age or gender and thereby fire inappropriately also add to the alert overload problem. Installations with experience in managing CDS alert rejection frequency generally try to minimize the number of alerts that are rejected by using available data to optimize the relevance of the alert.

To providers suffering from alert fatigue, however, that critical alert may not appear different from others that can be and usually are rejected without any deleterious consequences. The excessive frequency of unimportant alerts can be particularly damaging to the EHR initiative because the users quickly develop a negative feeling about the EHR as a whole and are at risk of rejecting it due to a poorly designed CDS component. Unsolicited alerts should be reserved for only the most important and severe warnings. A group of clinical leaders, informaticists, and computer programmers can then decide on stepwise activation of additional important alerts as users develop more confidence and enthusiasm for the system.

When an alert is fired the result can either be a hard stop to the action in progress or a warning in some less intrusive way. The hard stop is the most severe intervention and should be used sparingly. Users do not want to stop and go back and correct the action, even if they "know" the right thing to do. Making the easy thing the right thing, whenever possible, is still the goal. In CPOE, only in the most serious situation should the user have to completely back out of a proposed order. When it is not clear algorithmically exactly what the provider might want to do in response to an alert, if there are several good alternatives queued up as complete orders, it is better than a hard stop without recourse.

In most cases it will be obvious what the provider is trying to do and an alternative can be offered. If a medication ordered is one the patient is allergic to and if the situation is well defined, a therapeutic alternative can be offered. The suggestion in these situations should be already dosed appropriately and expressed as an alternative order that can immediately be executed without further intervention by the provider. These alerts, while easy to use, are hard to design. The appropriate information must be gathered in a coded fashion since the computer cannot easily use human knowledge unless rigorously encoded. The complexity of the decision-making otherwise may exceed the capability of the system.

Real-Time Consultant or Critique After the Fact

Another way to think about CDS is whether the system functions in a consultant mode, helping the provider along the way, or as a final critique, offering an opinion of the users' actions after-the-fact. The consultant mode is the most interactive and potentially most powerful. Suggestions or corrections are offered in real-time during data entry.

In critiquing mode, the CDS is applied to the coded findings from the history and physical compared with the coded assessment of the provider. The assistive information may be similar to that outlined for the consultative method, only delivered all together later in the process. There is less CDS value to critiquing since the timing does not affect the selected interventions. It is sometimes used in a teaching mode for students or in difficult cases after the patient has left to inform the subsequent visits.

Technical Foundations of Clinical Decision Support Systems

At a foundational level, the techniques that are used to build CDS are important to mention. Because this book is focusing on practical applications of CDS, the following will only touch on these aspects.

Bayes theorem plays a large part in the design of some types of decision support systems. The ability to take a prior probability and transform it mathematically to get a posterior probability made it possible to apply computers to CDS in more effective ways (28). Clinical prediction rules, derived from logistic regression equations, have been applied with great success to many areas, including chest pain triage in the "Goldman rule" (29). Rule-based CDS systems built using simple "if-then" rules are most commonly applied for deciding when to activate or fire alerts and reminders. For example, an EHR could use chief complaint entries to populate the workflow with specific order sets.

When building rule-based systems, separation of the rules function into a rules base and a rule execution engine (computational routine) allows for systems that are easier to maintain, expand, and possibly share. The engine compares the patient's data to the rule to see if it should fire. This separation potentially allows the rules to be exported to other systems and shared. Some progress has been realized on making rules shareable across implementations, but there is much work to be done in this area.

Algorithms-based systems are more sophisticated than rule-based CDS. In an algorithm, branching logic is used to execute a guideline and keep it on-track over time or to assist with other complex, multi-step decisions.

In the early days of computers in medicine, before clinical information systems were widespread, pioneers built stand-alone applications to assist physicians with diagnostic decisions. They yielded interesting results in some studies but did not evolve into a must-have application. They were grounded in the Oracle at Delphi model in which a complete problem was described to the priestesses at the Oracle and a complete answer was returned to the seeker (30). This approach used artificial intelligence techniques to simulate human cognition and has generally been abandoned as too difficult to get good performing systems with current techniques. Though there remains academic and commercial interest in supporting diagnostic decisions, stand-alone systems still have not gained widespread popularity among physicians.

One area in which stand-alone programs have done well is prescription support. Drug information is available on a PDA as well as web-based references from several vendors (31). They have good usability, are fast, and present simple but important information to providers as they are writing prescriptions. Drug information has rapidly succeeded when careful attention is paid to design factors and because providing referential drug-prescribing information is a more tractable information delivery problem than robust diagnostic support.

Clinical Decision Support: Begin with the End in Mind

A central goal of CDS is an alteration in behavior that results in an alteration in outcome. During CDS intervention design, process and outcome measurements must be built in so that managers can tell if they are reaching their goals. Usually the ultimate goal is slowly changing and the final outcomes cannot be used to tune the system. Choosing an interim measure that is directly linked to the desired outcome can make it easier to follow and manage progress. Interim measures are helpful because it is easier to change the system and see their numbers improve long before the expected clinical outcome is apparent. For example, if the ultimate goal is reduction in breast cancer, a logical interim measure would be mammography rates.

A tightly integrated CDS design phase brings in all the stakeholders to discuss what the outcomes and process variables are for a particular high-level strategic goal. Data collection or documentation design is much easier if done from the beginning rather than going back and retrofitting. For example, if JCAHO hospital quality measures are a goal (32), implementing a function in CPOE to suggest aspirin for acute myocardial infarction patients (e.g., by inclusion as a pre-checked item in an order set), works best when data collection allows for alternatives that providers may use when they wish to reject the advice but complete the data entry. A simple drop down box with reasons such as 1) Allergy, 2) Bleeding diathesis, 3) Other _____ , will help providers conform to expectations for high compliance with this quality measure and eliminate inappropriate patients from the measurement set.

An evidence-based approach to care should be basic to all CDS activities. If a simple intervention is planned but no published evidence shows its value, then local data collection can "prove" its value to the benefits realization team. In any case, outcomes should be measured for all interventions. A before and after snapshot may be all that is possible if the intervention removes the problem. In other cases performance measures can be followed over time and the intervention adjusted to continually improve the measure against an ideal clinical objective. For example, if excessive vancomycin use is identified as an adverse economic and clinical concern, a combination of order sets in CPOE, alerts, and infobuttons for culture results might be targeted to decrease the unnecessary part of this use.

The usage rates of the order sets, acceptance rates of the alerts, and click-rates of the infobutton will provide an idea of the relative use of each type of intervention. CDS interventions should be designed so that it is possible to determine which type of intervention results in the most effective behavior alteration. The important message is to continue to measure the effectiveness of each intervention and refine it over time.

All of the complex steps in gaining maximum effect of CDS must be applied to each intervention with care and completeness. It becomes a body of work crossing all specialties but centered on the nexus of clinical information systems, patient care, and process improvement. This is the work of clinical informaticists working with clinical experts and leaders in each subfield of the enterprise as well as the computer programmers and analysts.

Legal Issues

When building interventions, CDS implementers must be aware of an important difference in the legal treatment of medical interventions. Devices such as implantable defibrillators are not CDS. As a device, malpractice standards view it under a legal definition of strict product liability. This means, in simple terms, that if the device is used and a bad outcome occurs as a result, then the device is defective and the manufacturer is liable for claims of damages from patients harmed. This is a simpler standard to reach for plaintiff's attorneys than medical malpractice. In the realm of the EHR and CPOE, CDS is a software service that must be used by a provider to deliver care to a patient. If the software is properly designed, the provider can override any malfunction of the software. This lightens the burden on the software developer and transfers it to the provider. There is more discussion of legal issues in CDS in the HIMSS guidebook (33).

Terminology and Standards

It would be beneficial if CDS rules could be commonly developed or shared between institutions. A major issue in the sharing of rules is the vocabulary of the EHR or CPOE system. A vocabulary is an accepted standard way of naming things such as laboratory values and history or examination findings. Concepts must be represented identically in the CDS rule or application as in

CPOE and the rest of the EHR. Since computers cannot understand that a "CBC with differential" is functionally the same as a "hemogram with differential", designers must either convert all the names to a common system or create a mapping table that shows what each term means. Otherwise each rule must be translated for every installation of the software. Even if the software is the same, a site can adopt a different clinical vocabulary and make implementation of CDS rules problematic. Either task is labor intensive and prone to mistakes or gradual changes over time. Work is on-going to make CDS knowledge and interventions more interoperable.

Sources of Clinical Decision Support Content

In the early days of EHRs and CDS, systems were built piece by piece over decades by large development teams at centers such as the Regenstrief Institute in Indianapolis, the Harvard-affiliated hospitals, the Veterans Administration Hospitals (VA), the University of Utah, Vanderbilt and Duke Universities, and others. These informatics initiatives were frequently funded by National Library of Medicine Integrated Advanced Information Management Systems (IAIMS) grants and demonstration projects. In the case of the VA system, it was developed over many years also with government funding. Many of the benchmark statistics about CDS supporting care quality, safety, and efficiency came from these organizations.

However, healthcare has been slow to replicate these successes elsewhere. There are a variety of reasons for this, primarily related to the complex process of care delivery and CDS evolving from basically a cottage industry of local, hand-crafted solutions to a more industrialized set of processes. More widespread availability of actionable, best practice knowledge to drive CDS and the systems for delivering that knowledge efficiently to end users is helping accelerate change. Nonetheless, the painstaking attention to workflow integration, culture change, and user adoption that characterize the pioneering efforts are still critical success factors.

Categorizing the content delivery marketplace is not straightforward because of the wide range of products (stand-alone and embedded) available from a variety of sources. EHR or CPOE installations frequently rely on a mixture of the CDS content from multiple sources.

There are high-quality, free resources that can underpin some types of CDS interventions; examples include www.guidelines.gov and www.medlineplus.gov. Drug and allergy interaction databases are typically purchased from commercial vendors. Many clinical information system vendors and collaboratives (e.g., University HealthSystem Consortium; www.uhc.com) allow customers and participants to share content. Web sites that offer information concerning CDS content include www.medicalcomputing.com and www.openclinical.org.

There can be useful synergies between CDS and CME. CDS systems could leverage the unique view of a specific providers' strengths and weaknesses that could be inferred from their usage data. This "educational audit" of their practice could be used to design a personal CME curriculum. If the CDS system simply recorded the alerts and reminders that fired or the infobuttons clicked in a patient's record, that could provide a useful index of what that specific provider needs to learn (i.e., both recognized and unrecognized information needs). Educational specialists could then help design tools to offer learning modules that would correspond to each type of need. Such a personalized, needs-driven approach to CME could be a major advance in efficiency and effectiveness over traditional didactic CME activities that constitute the bulk of current CME activities.

Conclusion

Although there is some absolute value to EHRs as a repository of a patient's information, the goals of quality improvement, improved safety, and increased efficiency are all accomplished to a great extent by the CDS capabilities of these systems. CPOE or an EHR with CDS are not magic bullets and will not automatically improve the quality of care within an institution, reduce patient care errors, or make providers' work go faster. These advanced systems do motivate organizations to rethink information flows and decision-making processes that may be suboptimal. Implementing CDS-enabled systems help to promote better care by empowering all members of the care team with the information needed to make the right thing to do the easy thing to do.

Case Study

Elsewhere General is a 300-bed community hospital that did not do as well as they wanted on their recent Joint Commission survey. Specifically, they performed poorly on the heart failure measures of discharge instructions, ejection fraction measurement, ACEI/ARB treatment of left ventricular systolic dysfunction (LVSD), and documentation of smoking cessation counseling. Happily they have just completed roll-out of a CPOE system to complement their clinical data repository (CDR) containing their lab results and computer-based pharmacy system with bar-coded medication administration and electronic medication administration record (eMAR).

Currently, they are working the bugs out of their new systems and planning to implement the rest of the EHR over the next few years. The political situation with the survey is complicated. The hospital cardiology group is not optimally cohesive, but they just recruited a new chief to drive a cardiology quality improvement initiative.

Taking all of this into consideration, the CEO and COO have brought the cardiology chief, CIO and the Medical Director for Clinical Decision

Support (MD-CDS) together to kick off a heart failure quality improvement initiative. The MD-CDS takes this opportunity to get agreement from the CIO for an inventory of all clinical systems with names of technical and clinical contacts so that each system can be evaluated for potential CDS applicability.

The stakeholders have identified the high-level goal of improving cardiac care for their patients and narrowed that down to four specific clinical goals representing each of the four JCAHO hospital measures as listed in Table 9-1. (Readers should note in the following table that the percentage for compliance refers to patients for whom the intervention is appropriate.) In practice, separating out the patients for whom the intervention is contraindicated, for example, patients allergic to the drug, is a challenge.

Next they consult the inventory of clinical systems, meet with the contacts, and select specific systems to use. As they do this, they are mindful of the workflow and how the interventions will fit in without disruption or taking excessive time. The outline of their work is shown in the Table 9-2.

A workflow analysis is the next step. During this phase, the specific workflow point at which the intervention should occur is determined. Another critical but easily overlooked step is determining if any informatics standard or vocabulary conflict will occur when messages are shared between systems. Although it looks like we are done, now the actual work begins! Programmers must put together the specific clinical intervention

Table 9-1

CLINICAL GOALS MATCHED TO JCAHO MEASURES

High-Level CDS Goal	Specific Clinical Goal	Specific Clinical Objective
Improve care of patients with heart failure (HF).	Improve delivery of discharge instructions for HF.	100% compliance with docmentation of discharge instructions concerning activity level, diet, discharge medications, follow-up appointment, weight monitoring and what to do if symptoms worsen.
	Improve measurement of cardiac ejection fraction (EF).	100% documentation of results of cardiac ECHO including results of left ventricular ejection fraction.
	Improve prescribing of ACEI/ARB for LVSD.	100% compliance with prescribing or recording valid reason for withholding ACEI/ARB.
	Improve counseling of smokers to quit.	100% compliance with documentation of smoking cessation for smokers who have smoked in the last year.

Table 9-2

GOALS MATCHED TO SYSTEMS

Specific Clinical Objective	Specific Clinical System	Specific Clinical Intervention
100% compliance with documentation of discharge instructions concerning activity level, diet, discharge medications, follow-up appointment, weight monitoring, and what to do if symptoms worsen	CPOE	HF discharge order set with summary face sheet bringing documentation of all instructions to one electronic report
	eMAR	List of medications
	Electronic scheduling system	Date, time of follow-up appointment, and follow-up provider name
	Electronic reporting system	Report covering all 6 aspects of discharge instructions that must be covered
100% documentation of results of cardiac ECHO including results of left ventricular ejection	CDR	EF results from before hospitalization or during hospitalization
	CPOE	Pending order for cardiac ECHO to be done on discharge.
	Electronic reporting system	Report showing either result or EF evaluation or order for cardiac ECHO
100% compliance with prescribing or recording valid reason for withholding ACEI/ARB.	CPOE	Order set with option for ACEI or ARB plus optional drop-down list of codified reasons if neither prescribed (allergy, aortic stenosis, history of patient intolerance)
	Electronic reporting system	Report showing order for ACEI or ARB or reason neither prescribed
100% compliance with documentation of smoking cessation for smokers who have smoked in the last year.	Self-assessment forms, nursing intake forms, provider history forms	Add or confirm questions about current smoking status are available in forms to prompt users to ask.
	Nursing pathways or flow sheets	Add or confirm pathway or flow sheet steps include counseling appropriate to smoking status and ability to document completion of counseling.
General CDS support for care of HF patients,	CPOE	Order set contains links to evidence summary concerning all interventions. Individual medication orders contain links to drug information about each drug. Nursing order for smoking cessation contains link to materials to use and handout to patient to help stop smoking.
	Alert and reminder engine	Upon encountering discharge order or order set in patient with HF look for result or EF evaluation or order for ECHO Monitor potassium level and fire alert if level low, patient on diuretic and no replacement ordered

designs that have been requested (this is called the "build phase"). When an intervention is finished, it is presented to a group of clinicians to validate that it works as expected. This completes the design, build, and validate phases of creating CDS.

After final approval, interventions are tested both by technical personnel and clinical personnel using simulated patient scenarios prior to being embedded into "live" systems. When testing is completed, the trainers will be called on to design and deliver training to end-users before launch.

Typically a relatively straightforward set of interventions such as these could be brought live all at once in a "big bang" rollout. In some cases of complex interventions or large groups of related interventions, a pilot project would be used for a few weeks to be sure they work as we expect.

All CDS interventions should be formally evaluated. The intervention design should include mechanisms for generating reports that provide information on outcomes, e.g., when/how the intervention is used and its intended and unintended effects. If some steps will benefit from more emphasis on an individual provider basis, a "dashboard" (set of visual color-coded simple iconic displays showing good, adequate, and poor compliance with each of our interventions) of indicators can be created for personal use or hospital-wide reporting.

After a several-month development and deployment period, Elsewhere General is able to see gradual and incremental improvement in their dashboard indicators for heart failure. Its success was ensured by starting with stakeholders and specific goals, working with an inventory of clinical systems, selecting interventions based on systems available, designing the interventions, building them, and validating them carefully with the target users before final functional testing and deployment. Now the hospital is in the enviable position of being able to monitor its improvements and use these successes to encourage other departments to undertake quality improvements of their own and energize the push to finish the EHR at their hospital.

References

1. Shortliffe E, ed. Biomedical Informatics: Computer Applications in Health Care and Biomedicine, 3rd ed. New York: Springer Science; 2006.
2. Greenes RA, ed. Clinical Decision Support: The Road Ahead. Boston: Elsevier; 2006.
3. Berner ES, ed. Clinical Decision Support Systems: Theory and Practice, 2nd ed. New York: Springer Science; 2006.
4. Osheroff JA, et al. Improving Outcomes with Clinical Decision Support: An Implementer's Guide. Chicago: HIMSS; 2005.
5. http://www.cebm.net/ebm_is_isnt.asp. Accessed 2/6/08.
6. Sackett DL, et al. Evidence-based Medicine: How to Practice and Teach EBM, 2nd ed. New York: Churchill Livingstone; 2000. Accessed 2/6/08.
7. http://www.cebm.net/levels_of_evidence.asp.
8. http://www.pubmedcentral.nih.gov/articlerender.fcgi?artid=1624842 accessed 1/26/2007. Accessed 2/6/08.

9. Covell DG. Information needs in office practice: are they being met?. Ann Intern Med. 1985;103:596-9.

10. Osheroff JA. Physician's information needs: an analysis of questions posed during clinical teaching. Ann Intern Med. 1991;114:576-81.

11. Gorman PN. Information seeking in primary care: how physicians choose which clinical question to pursue and which to leave unanswered. Medical Decision Making. 1995;15:113-9.

12. Ely JW. Analysis of questions asked by family doctors regarding patient care. BMJ. 1999; 319:358-61.

13. McDonald CJ. Protocol-based computer reminders, the quality of care and the non-perfectability of man. N Engl J Med. 1976;295:1351-5.

14. Gorman PN, Ash J, Wykoff L. Can primary care physicians' questions be answered using the medical journal literature? Bull Med Libr Assoc. 1994;82:140-6.

15. Institute of Medicine. To Err is Human: Building a Safer Health System. Washington, DC: National Academy Press; 2000.

16. Institute of Medicine. Crossing the Quality Chasm: A New Health System for the 21st Century. Washington, DC: National Academy Press; 2001.

17. Institute of Medicine. Crossing the Quality Chasm: A New Health System for the 21st Century. Washington, DC: National Academy Press; 2001: 13.

18. Chaudhry B, Wang J, Wu S, et al. Systematic review: impact of health information technology on quality, efficiency, and costs of medical care. Ann Intern Med. 2006; 144:742-52.

19. Garg AX, Adhikari NK, McDonald H, et al. Effects of computerized clinical decision support systems on practitioner performance and patient outcomes: a systematic review. JAMA. 2005;293:1223-38.

20. Ash JS, Berg M, Coiera E. Some unintended consequences of information technology in health care: the nature of patient care information system-related errors. J Am Med Inform Assoc. 2004;11:104-12.

21. Campbell EM, Sittig DF, Ash JS, et al. Types of unintended consequences related to computerized provider order entry. J Am Med Inform Assoc. 2006;13:547-56.

22. Tierney WM, McDonald CJ, Martin DK, Rogers MP. Computerized display of past test results. Effect on outpatient testing. Ann Intern Med. 1987;107:569-74.

23. Tierney WM, Miller ME, McDonald CJ. The effect on test ordering of informing physicians of the charges for outpatient diagnostic tests [see comments]. New Engl J Med. 1990;322:1499-1504.

24. Overhage JM, Tierney WM, Zhou XH, McDonald CJ. A randomized trial of "corollary orders" to prevent errors of omission. J Am Med Inform Assoc. 1997;4:364-75.

25. Maviglia SM, Yoon CS, Bates DW, Kuperman G. KnowledgeLink: impact of context-sensitive information retrieval on clinicians' information needs. J Am Med Inform Assoc. 2006;13:67-73.

26. Rogers Y. New theoretical approaches for human-computer interaction. Annual Review of Information Science and Technology. 2004;38:87-143.

27. Norman DA. The Psychology of Everyday Things. New York: Basic Books; 1988.

28. Shortliffe E, ed. Biomedical Informatics: Computer Applications in Health Care and Biomedicine, 3rd ed. New York: Springer Science; 2006: 99.

29. Lee TH, Juarez G, Cook EF, et al. Ruling out acute myocardial infarction. A prospective multicenter validation of a 12-hour strategy for patients at low risk. N Engl J Med. 1991;324:1239-46.

30. http://en.wikipedia.org/wiki/Delphi accessed 2/6/08.

31. Perkins NA, Murphy JE, Malone DC, Armstrong EP. Performance of drug-drug interaction software for personal digital assistants. Ann Pharmacother. 2006;40:850-5.

32. http://www.jointcommission.org/ accessed 1/20/2007. Accessed 2/6/08.

33. Osheroff JA. Improving Outcomes with Clinical Decision Support: An Implementer's Guide. Chicago: HIMSS; 2005: Appendix B, 117.

10

Quality Improvement and the Electronic Health Record: Concepts and Methods

Feliciano B. Yu, MD, MSHI, MSPH
Jeroan J. Allison, MD, MS
Thomas K. Houston, MD, MPH

Health information technology (IT) is rapidly transforming healthcare. Many believe health IT, through decision support mechanisms, can help improve the effectiveness, safety, and quality of healthcare (1,2). Tremendous amounts of data are amassed with the exponential growth of electronic health record systems (EHR), making this digitized health information available for administrative and operational purposes as well as for quality measurement and continuous process improvement (3).

Until recently, providers and payers used claims data to facilitate billing and reimbursement related transactions. Today, private, public, and academic institutions are utilizing electronically stored administrative and clinical information for epidemiologic, performance measurement, benchmarking, and other forms of predictive analyses for use in healthcare management, policy, and research. Although information systems such as EHR systems play a significant role in measuring and enhancing the quality of patient care (4), its adoption and use has been limited (5).

The healthcare industry's recent focus on measuring and reporting on provider quality and performance will make the adoption of the EHR more imperative and pragmatic. For instance, the recent move to align reimbursement of healthcare services to reporting of and performance on predetermined quality indicators rely mostly on resource extensive medical chart abstraction, data entry, and data submission. For healthcare practitioners, one thing is certain; their performance on measurable indicators of quality care will be assessed, and incentive mechanisms will be linked to certain performance thresholds. Therefore, it is imperative that healthcare practitioners be knowledgeable about quality measurement and its role in improving care and about EHR systems and how they can be utilized to meet this purpose.

The first half of this chapter is an overview that introduces the reader to the main principles of quality and the framework of healthcare QI (QI). Readers with prior knowledge of quality may wish to proceed to the second half of the chapter, which starts with the section Using Quality Improvement to Change Clinical Practice, and describes how EHR systems can be leveraged as a tool for QI activities. It also provides explicit examples on how EHR systems have been used for improving quality and an overview of the issues surrounding QI functionality of the EHR.

Overview of Quality Improvement in Healthcare

According to Don Berwick, *"every system is perfectly designed to achieve exactly the results that it achieves"*. As the central law of QI, it states that the product of every system is the direct expression of how the system works. QI views the healthcare system as a series of dependent micro-systems that must work together. As a result of healthcare's diverse services, silos of care must work in harmony to deliver quality of care. QI aims to identify faulty and redundant processes that often plague undesirable systems and replace them with processes that are recognized to improve outcomes. The underlying theme for quality improving strategies is the systematic use of the scientific method (i.e., data driven) for process improvement.

History of Quality Improvement in Healthcare

Over the past three decades, the advances in medicine, changes in federal regulations, rise in consumer empowerment, and shifts in payment systems dominated the healthcare arena. Navigating through the healthcare delivery system has become very complex. Healthcare services have become more diverse and often disconnected, leading to multiple silos of care. This complexity often led to gaps in quality and an increase in unnecessary healthcare costs. As a result, the healthcare industry began to look at QI concepts used in the manufacturing industry as a possible mechanism to improve the quality of care and contain costs.

Quality control and measurement has its roots in physics and in the advancements in the management of the manufacturing processes as long ago as the early 1900s. Walter Shewhart, W. Edward Deming, and Joseph Juran were among the prominent proponents of controlling quality (6,7). Consequently, the creation of the Malcolm Baldrige National Quality Improvement Act of 1987 marked the period when QI has taken root in the US (8).

Among those who were influenced by Deming's philosophy was a pediatrician named Paul Batalden. Following Deming's philosophy, Dr. Batalden believed that the patients are the "customers" and quality stems from well-designed workplace systems. He applied this management philosophy in the clinical setting and promoted continuous measurement and feedback mechanisms as vital to the improvement of the care delivery process. In 1991, Batalden and his colleague, Dr. Donald Berwick, formed the Institute for Quality Improvement, which later became the Institute for Healthcare Improvement (www.ihi.org).

Today, attention to quality is in the forefront of healthcare redesign. On the national level, organizations such as the Joint Commission for Accreditation of Healthcare Organizations (JCAHO), the Agency for Healthcare Research and Quality (AHRQ), the Institute of Medicine (IOM), National Quality forum (NQF), National Committee for Quality Assurance (NCQA), and the more recent Alliance for Pediatric Quality (APQ), among others, have all focused the spotlight on the standards of the quality of healthcare delivery. The public has also been very interested in the quality of care that they receive. As a response, publicly available rankings of institutional quality of care are now posted though sites such as HealthGrades.com, Hospital Compare initiative (www.hospitalcompare.gov), America's Best Doctors, and America's Best Hospitals, to name a few.

What is Healthcare Quality?

The IOM's definition of quality is *"the degree to which health services for individuals and populations increase the likelihood of desired health outcomes and are consistent with current professional knowledge"* (2). There are a lot of assumptions in that statement. One of the assumptions is that in order to achieve quality, one must know *what* needs to be improved, the type of *outcome* that one expects to achieve, *who* the recipient/s is/are, and *how* one will go about achieving quality or improving the process (e.g., best practices, evidence-based medicine, etc).

How Can Quality Be Measured?

Achieving the best possible health outcomes has always been the focus of medicine. However, it is not always easy to define what the "best" outcome is for a certain healthcare activity or service. Hence, a need for defining quality is very important. Although QI is a recent phenomenon in healthcare, evaluating quality has been practiced in healthcare since the 1970s. Today, quality evaluation is commonly approached in two distinct ways: quality assessment and quality measurement.

Quality assessment (QA) is best exemplified by Avedis Donabedian's work. QA is often associated with quality assurance. In essence, QA is *"a judgment concerning the process of care, based on the extent to which that care contributes to valued outcomes"* (9). QA is an effort to evaluate certain healthcare practices or health outcomes based on a predetermined standard or quality. It has been traditionally used by hospitals and other healthcare organizations (e.g., payors, accreditations, compliance, etc) to improve or maintain quality. Donabedian's principle for evaluating quality focuses around the structure, process, and outcome of healthcare delivery. His principle for assessing quality (also known as Donabedian's triad) provided a framework upon which quality can be measured (10).

Quality measurement (QM) is best represented by the tools that are being used in QI. As the name "measurement" implies, this manner of evaluating quality relies heavily on the use of data in collection, analysis, and problem-solving activities in QI (11).

What Are Quality Measures?

Healthcare quality measures are quantitative indicators that are utilized to evaluate the quality of specific healthcare activities (12). Quality measures are developed by certain healthcare stakeholders for a variety of uses such as support for operations, resource utilization, and performance improvement. The measures, which are often called "indicators", serve to inform the stakeholders or guide certain actions that will help improve performance or quality of healthcare delivery process or service. In some cases, the measures serve to enforce accountability for certain healthcare activities that are known to impact quality. Given the magnitude of the reliance on quality measures for health policy and provider accountability, these measures must be *"meaningful, scientifically sound, and interpretable"* to all the stakeholders (13,14).

The current sets of quality measures are commonly derived from Donabedian's triad for assessing quality (15). At its core, measures are composed of discrete data elements. Data elements often include a numerator and a denominator and are often reported as rates or proportions.

Structural data refers to the attributes of the setting or system where health care is provided. Examples of structural measures include hospital teaching status, ownership, presence of modern technologies, credentials or qualifications of medical staff or facility attributes such as patient volume and nurse-to-bed ratios, among others (16,17). Implementing sophisticated clinical information systems such as EHRs fall into this category. Although EHRs can be used to assess certain structural measures (i.e., nurse-to-bed ratio, patient volume, etc), a number of structural measures are not immediately "actionable" (i.e., hospital characteristics such as ownership, teaching status, etc) (18).

Process data refers to attributes of the interaction or activity between the healthcare provider and the patient. Examples of process measures include the use of beta blockers, aspirin, ACE inhibitors, and reperfusion medications for patients with heart failure or myocardial infarction (19). The advantages of process measures are that they are very responsive to detecting quality problems without waiting for poor outcomes to become evident (20). The healthcare activities that are often used as process measures can also provide the best opportunities where EHRs can provide support for QI activities (21,22).

Outcome data refers to the consequent health state of the patient as a result of healthcare. Outcome measures are often in the form of mortality, morbidity, and patient satisfaction (9). Examples of outcome measures include mortality after cardiac surgery, co-morbidities following cardiopulmonary bypass surgery, or quality of life among patients after cardiac surgical procedures (9,23,24).

Although process measures are more sensitive to variations on the quality of care, outcome measures are more specific to the end result of care (Figure 10-1). For example, a poorly designed process may not necessarily lead to an adverse outcome. However, the absence of an adverse event does not imply quality. Over time, poorly designed processes may eventually lead to or contribute to the development of an adverse event (2,25).

Risk adjustment deals with the probability of developing undesirable health outcomes depending on the susceptibility of the patient (i.e., patient's health status), random variation, and the quality of care delivery. For example, the susceptibility can be influenced by the patient's severity of the illness, age, and associated co-morbidities (26). Risk adjustment is often performed using epidemiological tools to address the confounding effects brought by these external factors.

Outcome measures often require risk adjustment because of the multitude of factors that can influence the health outcome of the patient. The complexity of risk adjustment and the numerous confounding possibilities render using outcomes measures controversial indicators for QI (27). In contrast, most process measures may not require risk adjustment. Since process measures require a well-defined population that is suitable to receive the measure, process-based measures already contain intrinsic adjustments for the differences among patients under study (21,22).

Health Issue: Diabetes Mellitus type II
Outcome Measure: Diabetic Nephropathy
Process Measure: Assessing for Nephropathy (i.e., proteinuria)

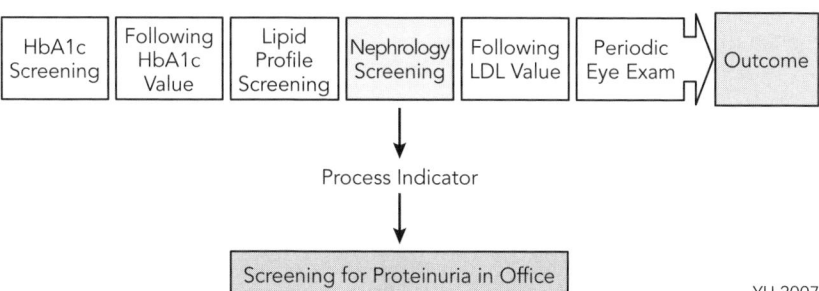

Figure 10-1 Illustration of process and outcome measures that are applicable for diabetes care.

Limitations of Quality Assessment Approach to Improving Quality

Solely focusing on the structure, process, and outcomes of care may not be enough. Healthcare providers must also possess the most updated information as well as the skills necessary to deliver quality care. Fihn asserts that, *"knowledge, in and of itself, is neither a structure nor a process"* (28). This new information about the process must be operationalized back into the system in order to yield a better outcome. Knowledge about the structure, process, and outcome is important, but the infusion of new knowledge about the current system, maintenance of up-to-date medical information, best practices and updating skills can increase the chances of success for achieving quality. Berwick notes that quality programs using the QA approach can have limitations (11). Methods that rely only on inspection and judgment (i.e., not complying with standards) can be counter-productive and do not often lead to genuine improvement of quality. It is vital to learn from what was done. The knowledge about one's performance, how it affected the system as a whole, and how this new information can be used to improve the current process comprise the crux of QI.

Over the past decade, the science and practice of healthcare QI have become more developed. Recent advances in its methodology have made it more simple and relevant, often incorporating evidence-based medicine into the healthcare QI philosophy (29). Systems are designed to *iteratively* produce the desired outcomes. If the outcome is undesirable, the system needs to be changed or improved *incrementally* to yield better results, always keeping in mind the needs of the beneficiary of the process or outcome that one is trying to improve.

In healthcare, the patient is the most important beneficiary, but staff or physicians can be the beneficiaries as well. For example, when the problem involves prolonged waiting time in the doctor's office, improving waiting time can benefit the patient; however, in some ways, the physician also can benefit from the improvement. Team work is essential for effecting change in the system. More importantly, and this is where the EHR can be of great help, accurate data provides the crucial information required for evaluating the processes, identifying the issues, and measuring the performance of the system.

Conducting a Quality Improvement Activity

QI activities are not only geared towards well-validated measures (e.g., acute myocardial infarction, congestive heart failure, asthma measures) but can also be used for day-to-day problems that plague the underlying system. For example, throughput and service turn-around times, patient satisfaction, and even improving documentation for appropriate coding of services can be targets for improvement. The next section gives an overview of the essential components for conducting a QI activity.

Methods of Data Collection

One can collect data for QI in a number of ways. Depending on your organization, data can be collected from incident reports, medical record screening or reviews (i.e., screening for certain criteria such as adverse events), medical record audits, surveillance systems, outbreak investigations, or even patient satisfaction surveys. Data for QI can be obtained from a combination of paper and electronic sources. For practices with advanced EHR systems, this step can often be automated and performed using queries to the database.

Methods of Data Validation

Accuracy of the data: Data used in QI can come from a variety of sources and are stored in different formats (e.g., paper, electronic). In the paper environment, data are usually disorganized, illegible, and unstructured. Data coming from different electronic sources (e.g., clinical information systems, biomedical machines, etc) also suffer the same fate. Most are not integrated and are often not interoperable (30). In any case, whether in paper or electronic format, the data derived from various sources are complex, and validating the data is crucial to the accuracy of the measurement process. When data are collected as a byproduct of delivering care, extra attention must be given so that the results are meaningful and actionable.

Validity of the measure: An equally important aspect of QI is the validity of the measure or the performance indicator. It is important to establish the association of the outcome and the process one is measuring. For instance, if one is following the global measure for diabetic heath outcomes (i.e., diabetic patients with renal manifestations), then we need to be convinced that the process measure, *"Rate of diabetic patients screened for proteinuria"*, can identify substandard care and can help identify patients at risk for early renal disease, thereby addressing or preventing complications early in the disease process.

Reliability of the measure: An appropriate measure or indicator must also be reliable. Measurements are often taken at different times, performed by different observers, and performed at different clinical settings, so care must be taken to minimize observation and or selection bias and ensure consistent results. For instance, using our example above, when determining the *"Rate of diabetic patients screened for proteinuria"*, it is important to decide whether to include only the diabetic patients without pre-existing kidney disease or to include all diabetic patients in your practice regardless of any renal manifestations.

Recordability of the data: Finally, the data required for the measure must be readily available. An effort must be made to decrease the barriers for capturing, storing and retrieving of the data required for the analysis, because this can impact the QI process.

Ethical Considerations and Study Designs

Performing QI seems to contain aspects of research. Data gathering and analysis as well as the problem-solving processes are methods common to research. However, it is important to distinguish QI from clinical research because for any activities that involve risks to patients, ethical considerations must be in place (i.e., informed consent) to protect the patient's rights (31).

QI projects are often initiated to evaluate clinical processes and outcomes, with the end goal of improving the outcome or process under study. Just like research, QI involves looking at the current process (concurrent) or the past (retrospective) or even following processes in the future (prospective). Research aims to generate new knowledge and is often designed to address or answer a formalized hypothesis. A clearly defined methodology for data collection and analysis is the standard, and an adequate sample must first be satisfied.

In contrast to research, QI involves frequent modifications, smaller samples, condensed documentation, and often use performance indicators or measures to inform stakeholders about the progress. These measures drive the analysis, which in turn is used to correct the problem or improve the process, often in an iterative, incremental fashion.

It is important to establish at the onset of any QI activity the risk and benefits of the project to the patients. Any foreseeable risk to patient safety necessitates an oversight and review from qualified persons (i.e., institutional review boards or IRBs) to ensure the project is conducted with the utmost ethical considerations (32).

Tools for Problem and Data Analysis

There are a number of tools that are useful for QI. Table 10-1 lists some of the more common techniques used for problem solving.

Statistical process control for healthcare QI: Statistical process control (SPC) is a method that uses a set of statistical tools to detect whether the process being observed falls within acceptable distribution or is statistically under "control". SPC charts allows one to represent information about a process in a simple and unambiguous manner. Control charts are used to see if there are non-random influences that exist within the given data or set of observation. For example, a simple *run chart* provides an easy way to look at a specific process, especially if the data gathered is from a time-ordered manner (Figure 10-2). A run chart, however, cannot tell you whether the process is under statistical "control". It can only test for the existence of a *special-cause* variation. In order to test whether the process is in control, the use of control charts with statistically derived limits are needed (Figure 10-3).

Applying SPC concepts to the workflow process: There are a number of uses for SPC control charts within the healthcare organization. Its use

Table 10-1

TOOLS FOR PROBLEM AND DATA ANALYSIS

Brainstorming	Used to generate ideas and rank them according to predetermined priorities (33)
Nominal group technique	Used to generate ideas about possible causes of problem. Team members list their ideas, and ideas are then collated and voted on (34)
Process flow charts	Used to analyze and describe processes; allows process or system to be graphically dissected into smaller sub-processes (35)
Cause-effect or Fishbone diagram	Graphic tool used to help describe primary and secondary causes of the problem
Pareto, histogram, bar charts	Used to depict relative frequency of events or distribution of data using bar graphs (33)
Run and Control charts	Used to visually represent chronologic trends and patterns of data or events (33) (see Figure 10-2)

can range from administrative to clinical applications. In most cases, each workflow process has a quantifiable activity or outcome that can be observation or measured. These observations, assuming that there are enough numbers collected and plotted on a curve, often follow a normal distribution, where the majority of the data gather around the mean. The distance from the mean is determined by the sample's standard deviation. What this

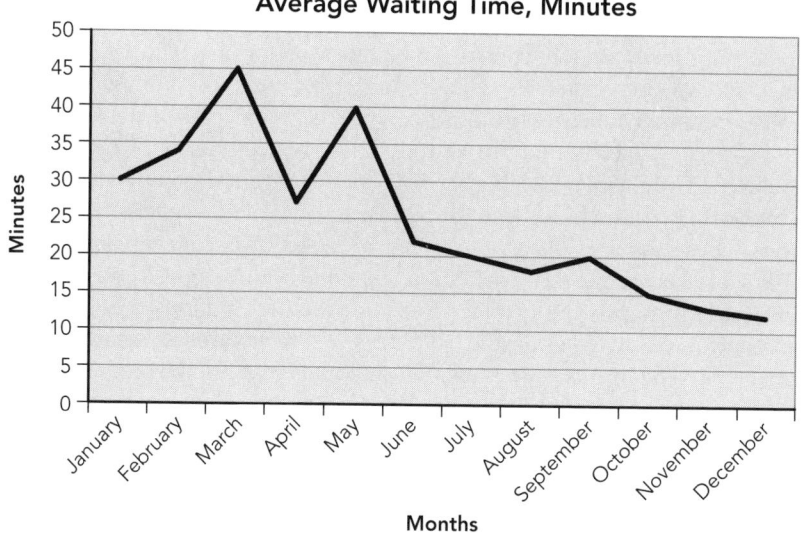

Figure 10-2 Example of a run chart.

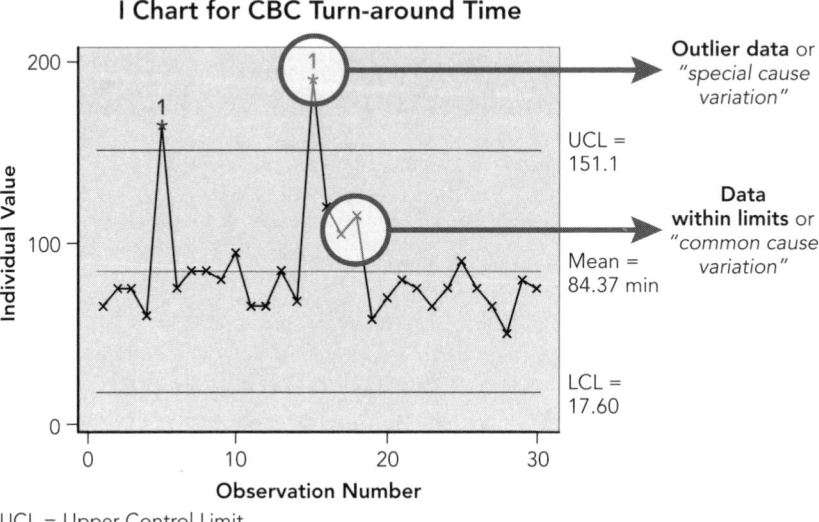

Figure 10-3 Example of data points that fall within and outside specified limits.

all means is that, inherent in each process, there exists a degree of variability among the data. By providing statistically valid assessments on the set of observations, a specific outcome measurement can be classified whether it belongs to a *"common-cause" variation* or whether they belong to a *"special-cause" variation*. Common-cause variation is a result of the normal variation intrinsic to the process. On the other hand, special-cause variation is an aberration of the process and does not reflect the capability of the process. A group of data or observations that exhibit common-cause variation is statistically under "control", whereas a set of observations that contain a special-cause variation is NOT under "control". A process that is in control does not mean that the process is acceptable. All it means is that the process is stable enough to produce a predictable set of measurable outcomes. The process can be controversial or of good quality and still be in control. The same holds true for processes that exhibit special-cause variations. These atypical observations can be good or bad. It just means that they exhibit outcomes or observations that are not inherent to the process.

In order to improve a certain process, these observations must be identified and assessed whether the outcomes are acceptable or unacceptable. Management often reacts to events or outcomes that are deemed unacceptable. The goal of management then is to identify whether the common-cause and special-cause variations are acceptable or unacceptable outcomes of a specific process. Reacting to common-cause variations and changing a process because of a special-cause variation can result to misuse of management resources. The proper use of resources would be to eliminate unacceptable special-cause variation and to change undesirable processes that exhibit common-cause variation (36) (see Figure 10-3).

Quality Improvement Methodology

QI follows distinct steps that may be very familiar to the healthcare practitioner (37,38) (Table 10-2).

Step 1: Identifying the Problem

Improvement opportunities in our healthcare delivery system are in abundance, and identifying what needs to be improved is a key step in QI. The problems can be anything from a faulty process to an undesirable outcome. For example, one may look at improving the patient waiting times in a physician's office or the emergency department. Alternatively, perhaps one may want to improve the compliance to following guidelines for asthma treatment among physicians or even decreasing certain types of medication prescribing errors. After the problem has been identified, one needs to further determine the extent of the problem. How often does the problem occur? What are the consequences of the problem if left unsolved?

Choosing the problem: There are a number of QI tools that help determine the problem (see Table 10-2). For instance, brainstorming activities, as mentioned above, involve having stakeholders independently suggest the problem/s of the current system. This method encourages creative thinking, and ideas are recorded then shared with everyone on the team.

Forming a team: The size of the team will depend on the size of the organization or the problem under study. In small practices, it can simply consist of a physician and/or a nurse. What is important is the selection of the process owner, the leader or stakeholder of the project. Using the tools described above, the team may vote or rank each of the problems according to its importance or priority. For example, Nominal group technique or the Delphi method (see Table 10-1) can be used to help the team come up with a consensus (42).

Table 10-2

QUALITY IMPROVEMENT METHODOLOGY (BATALDEN AND STOLTZ, 1993)

Steps	Detail
Identify	Determine what problem to improve.
Analyze	Understand the problem to be addressed.
Develop	Hypothesize what changes will improve the problem.
Test/Implement	Test the hypothesized solution to see if it yields improvement. Based on the outcome, decide if it necessary to stop, modify or implement the solution.

Investigating the extent of the problem: The extent of the problem often needs to be further articulated. A frequently used QI tool for this activity is the Cause-Effect diagram, also known as the Fishbone or Ishikawa diagram (43). It helps the team focus on the processes that lead to the outcome in a more visual format. By identifying all the processes that influence the performance of the system, one can then make an appropriate recommendation to improve the system.

How Can An EHR Help at This Stage?

The EHR can be an essential tool for identifying areas for improvement. Whether you are responding to external pressures to improve (e.g., payors, managed care organizations, government, etc) or internally, it is important to first determine, at a higher level, what your goals are, and then proceed to narrowing the scope of the problem, up to a point where one can effectively make a positive change. For instance, a high-level goal would be to "Improve the overall care and safety of my patients". This, in turn, can be narrowed down to "Improve preventative services for diseases that are common in my practice", which can be further narrowed down to specific diseases that exist in your practice. Using the EHR, you may then run a query or report that looks at, for instance, the "Top 10 most common diagnoses", and then review the illnesses and determine which is the most urgent or practical disease to begin to address. For instance, your query may come out with a report suggesting that a significant portion of your patients are suffering from renal complications from diabetes. Then perhaps the goal can be reframed as "Improve the preventative services for my patients with diabetes, especially those at risk for renal complications". A more specific clinical process objective, "Increase the number of diabetic patients that receive annual screening for proteinuria" can then be put in place.

Step 2: Analyzing the Problem

This step involves an in-depth analysis of the problem in the context of a bigger process or system. In this stage, one may try to understand the existence of the problem as it relates to an existing workflow or process. Measuring the current state of affairs is performed at this stage. In other improvement models, this is often known as the *"gap analysis"* stage, where you are trying to explicitly document the current system's capability. Here, data collection is crucial for providing baseline information about the process or system one is trying to improve. A variety of ethnographic (e.g., observation, time-motion series, etc) and qualitative (e.g., interview, focus groups, survey, etc) techniques can be employed to determine the people, place/s, event/s, time, and precursor/s of the problem. For example, if one is trying to improve the waiting time for patients in the emergency department, an in-depth workflow analysis of the waiting room can be performed at this stage. Interviews, direct observation, and/or surveys can be performed on the emergency department staff to understand why this is happening.

Evaluating the current system: Visually representing the current process capability often helps in explicitly describing the issue that is being addressed. Using flowcharts often helps in clearly depicting the workflow or the thought-process involved on the problem/s at hand. With a flowchart, one can chronologically describe the flow of activities, information, logic, or algorithm for any healthcare process or system.

Examining the cause of the problem: It is common to identify multiple faulty processes that contribute to a problem. A common QI tool employed to facilitate the prioritization of improvement efforts is the Pareto chart. Data regarding the relative frequency of the faulty processes can be graphically represented in decreasing importance. The data can often be represented in a series of bar graphs or histograms.

How Can An EHR Help at This Stage?

Following the case above, once we have identified the problem, then the next step would be to understand the extent of the problem. Using the EHR's reporting tool, a query of all patients with diabetes with renal manifestations (e.g., ICD9-CM codes 250.xx, 250.4, 583.81, 581.81) and identifying those patients for whom a urinalysis was performed (e.g., CPT codes 81002, 81003, 81007) given a time period, can be performed. This can give you a starting point for reviewing the medical records of those patients with the problem of interest. Similarly, you may be able to get a baseline rate of diabetic patients with kidney complications (number of diabetic patients with nephropathy divided by the number of patient with diabetes), baseline rate of diabetic patients for whom a urinalysis was performed (number of diabetic patients with diabetes with urinalysis divided by the number of patients with diabetes), and so on. This baseline rate can, in essence, become the *performance indicator* for which one can follow during the QI activity. For highly advanced EHRs, the data points that rely on time stamps (e.g., turn-around times, time-series, etc) or service fulfillments (e.g., ordering tests, reporting results, etc) can be collected electronically, without the need for chart review or manual prospective monitoring.

Step 3: Developing a Solution

After getting a good sense of the baseline problem, one may develop a hypothesis on how to improve or solve the issue. There are no wrong solutions at this point, only hypotheses. The best sources of the possible solutions are the people who are directly part of the process or system under study. One may use the Fishbone diagram to illustrate the solution/s from the perspective of the system under study. For example, for the emergency department waiting room problems above, one might interview the staff from the emergency department and discuss possible solutions to the delay. One solution that may come up during one of the sessions for decreasing patient waiting time in the emergency department might be having a satellite laboratory for routine laboratory tests.

HOW CAN AN EHR HELP AT THIS STAGE?

A solution can be suggested once the extent of the problem has been identified. One of the advantages of a well-designed EHR is its ability to act as an event monitor that senses changes in the database level of EHR system. Reminder systems can be designed or built so that when patients come in with a diagnosis of diabetes (e.g., ICD9-CM 250.xx or an applicable health issue), then perhaps an alerting prompt or mechanism will be displayed to remind the clinician to check for proteinuria. The electronic reminders can be incorporated to the clinician's workflow, designed to remind the nurse or physician to screen for proteinuria before the patient is discharged from the clinic.

Step 4: Testing and Implementation

Once the possible resolution to the problem is identified, the solution is "tested" in the system's native environment. Similar to the "rapid prototyping" technique in computer software development, this method is sometimes referred to as "rapid cycle improvement" in healthcare QI, where the solution is implemented and then analyzed to see if it is effective or has produced the desirable outcome. If the results are unsatisfactory, then another solution can be put in place and then retested to see if it is effective. There is really no room for failure here because the goal is to test and retest until the desired results are achieved. The goal is small increments of change, rather than overnight system-wide improvements.

Shewhart and Deming's Plan-Do-Study-Act Cycle

In QI, the testing and implementation stage is operationalized through a series of steps that form a feedback loop. The Shewhart and Deming's "Plan-Do-Study-Act" (PDSA) cycle of improvement is the most often used feedback mechanism for healthcare QI (44) (Figure 10-4). Problem solving is achieved through continuous iterations of one or more PDSA cycles.

How Can An EHR Help at This Stage?

Once a query has been performed, the same report can be generated on demand, giving the practice an updated measurement of the process at any given period. It is important to understand that the reminder system must be supported by policy and procedures in the practice. The alert system

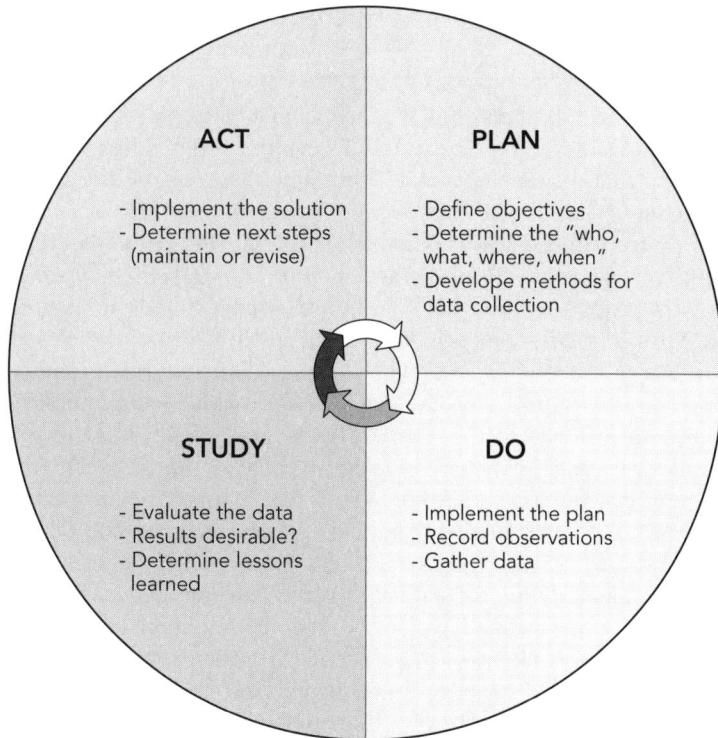

Source: Adapted from the Institute of Healthcare Improvement, www.ihi.org

Figure 10-4   The plan-do-study-act (PDSA) cycle of improvement. Adapted from the Institute of Healthcare Improvement, www.ihi.org. From W. Edwards Deming, THE NEW ECONOMICS FOR INDUSTRY, GOVERNMENT, EDUCATION, figure 13, page 132, ©1994 The W. Edwards Deming Foundation, by permission of The MIT Press.

will not work if it is not followed through by workflow redesign. For instance, prior to implementing the reminder to "check for proteinuria" for patients with diabetes, workflow must be adapted to facilitate the process (e.g., nurse to have urine cup ready, physician to ask patient about screening for proteinuria, nurse to check previous urinalysis, etc). Using the example above, the solution is "prototyped" at the clinic, and, assuming that it did improve the screening rates, it is implemented as a permanent service in the clinic.

The QI methods depicted here can be applied to simple and complex environments, from small solo practitioner's offices to a multi-specialty clinics and multi-hospital facilities. The problems and solutions can be simple or complex, involve one or more people, or can be costly or not. It all depends on the nature of the process being evaluated, the number of interdependencies within the system, and the urgency of the problem.

Using Quality Improvement Data to Change Clinical Practice

We can now begin to apply the QI concepts in clinical practice and describe how one can use the QI concepts to improve the way we treat patients.

Assuming that we have a goal of *"Improving the preventative services for diabetic patients who are at risk for renal complications"*. First, we need the baseline performance that was described in the previous example. Using our performance indicator, *"Proteinuria Screening for patients with diabetes"*, we are now ready to collect the data by either paper medical chart or EHR review. For our performance indicator, we need to know the *numerator*, which is the number of patients with diabetes that have been screened for proteinuria in the sample, and the *denominator*, which is the number of eligible diabetic patients in the sample. For paper-based recording systems, one may opt to "tag" diabetic patients prospectively for a specified period (e.g., one or two months), and then collect the "tagged" medical records for review to get the baseline data. Alternatively, one may use the billing software to look up patients with the ICD-9 CM codes for diabetes and then pick a convenient sample of patients for the baseline data. As mentioned above, for EHR systems that have query capabilities, patient selection can be automated and, most likely, one can get all the patients in the practice with diabetes for use for the baseline performance data.

The next step would be to plot the result of the data collection to describe the current capability or process. Using our clinical example above, one may find that for the past several months, only three out of ten patients coming to the practice has been screened for proteinuria. Therefore, the baseline performance indicator is 30%. We can now set up a goal to increase the rate to 100% over the next year.

It is important to make the most out of this baseline performance indicator by using the QI techniques above (e.g., brainstorming, cause-effect diagram, etc) to determine the processes that may have led to this baseline rate. Perhaps, collectively, the team may have identified faulty process and come up with a consensus on a specific solution to improve the process. For example, after several brainstorming sessions, the team may have come up with some workflow changes to improve the identification of patients who may benefit from the screening service. The team suggested that for patients with an existing diagnosis of diabetes the clerk or secretary "tags" the patient chart with a yellow sticker as they come for a visit in order to alert the physician or nurse to order a urinalysis. For newly diagnosed patients with diabetes, the nurse or physician tags "tag" the patient chart with the sticker. And at discharge, the clerk will check to see if a urinalysis was performed for those charts with yellow stickers and alerts the clinicians if this was not performed.

The workflow recommendations are put in place and the performance indicators are followed through time. Perhaps a quarterly review is performed and the results are disseminated and discussed among the team members. If the target performance level has not been reached, the current process is re-evaluated and workflow redesigns instituted and then monitored until the target performance level is achieved. Blame and retribution has no place here as setbacks are expected. It is important to note that incremental change and process evaluation is the key message in this activity.

How Can an EHR Help at This Stage?

In EHR systems capable of supporting clinical decision (CDS) support systems, the "tagging" of the patients can be automated by way of using alerts, reminders, or visual cues so that the clinicians are informed before, during, or after seeing the patient, while the patient is still in the clinic.

Using Quality Improvement Data to Guide Policy

It is recognized that the current focus on service-oriented reimbursement has done little to improve the quality of healthcare for patients (45). Realigning financial incentives towards quality of care and better patient outcomes seem to offer a better alternative. A number of institutions have used concepts derived from QI to enforce or guide policy and healthcare delivery and to influence the practice of medicine to delivery of cost-effective and quality healthcare. Emerging trends adopted by public and private organizations are aligning incentive mechanisms with compliance to reporting of data and performance on certain quality measures. Among the more recent initiatives towards this end are best exemplified by inceptive programs such as pay-for-reporting and pay-for-performance plans.

Pay for reporting (P4R) offers monetary rewards to institutions or providers that report certain data elements and/or performance measures that can be used as the receiving party for benchmarking and other reporting standards. For example, Medicare launched the Physician Quality Reporting Initiative (PQRI) under Title I of the Tax Relief and Health Care Act of 2006, Public Law 109-432. This project links physician payment to reporting of claims data to CMS that can be used later for assessing provider performance. Providers who have successfully met reporting criteria are awarded up to a 1.5% bonus payment above their CMS charges for a given time period. Providers will also be given a performance report based on their data submission after each designated reporting period.

Pay for performance (P4P) offers financial incentives for institutions or providers that achieve a certain threshold of quality of care or performance. Quality measures (i.e. outcomes of care or processes of care) are often used as the standard by which performance is evaluated against. A good example of a P4P program is the California P4P program sponsored by the Integrated Health Association (IHA). In this effort, participating providers receive financial rewards for meeting certain performance thresholds, as well as those who have made incremental improvement in performance measures over time (46). Providers received an average of 1.5% of total compensation as incentive during the reporting periods. Similar P4P initiatives are also being implemented by CMS that impact hospitals and physicians (47).

Future Challenges for Quality Measurement

Information technology has always been an essential aspect of quality measurement. Although mostly utilized by hospitals and large healthcare institutions, electronic transactions and analyses of administrative and clinical data has been in practice for a number of years. For example, large health care organizations like Health Corporation of America, utilize data gathered from routine clinical practices for use in quality measurement. Health insurance companies like Blue-Cross Blue Shield, collect clinical and administrative data to inform clinicians regarding their prescribing and health services utilization practices. Healthcare universities report clinical and administrative data to a central organization, such as University Health System Consortium (UHC), for benchmarking purposes and to inform participating institutions about their performance as compared to their peers. Pediatric hospitals across the nation contribute administrative and clinical information to central organizations (e.g., CHCA, NACHRI), and use aggregate information for benchmarking and QI purposes.

The federal government is also making use of administrative data to inform the public regarding the relative performance of healthcare providers in a given geographic area. HealthCompare.gov is an example of a publicly accessible Internet website that compares hospitals based on predetermined performance or quality measures. Other publicly available websites are run by private enterprises and rank or rate providers based on certain measures of quality (e.g., Healthgrades.com, Leapfrog.com). The success of electronic reporting as well the advances made in the development of stan-

---

Table 10-3

EXAMPLE OF INSTITUTIONS PROMOTING QUALITY MEASUREMENT

1. Agency for Healthcare Research and Quality (AHRQ), http://www.ahrq.gov/
2. American Medical Association (AMA), http://www.ama-assn.org/ama/pub/category/2946.html
3. National Quality Forum (NQF), http://www.qualityforum.org/
4. Joint Commission on Accreditation of Healthcare Organizations (JCAHO), http://www.jointcommission.org/
5. National Quality Measures Clearinghouse (NQMC), http://www.qualitymeasures.ahrq.gov/
6. National Committee for Quality Assurance (NCQA), http://www.ncqa.org/index.htm
7. The Alliance for Pediatric Quality (Alliance), www.kidsquality.org

dards for electronic health records sets the foundation for the future of quality measurement.

Institutions that are among those pushing for the development and adoption of quality measures are shown in Table 10-3.

Quality Improvement and the Electronic Health Record

The Institute of Medicine has recognized that health information technology plays a major role in the modern healthcare delivery system (49). EHR systems offer unique opportunities for evaluating and improving the quality of healthcare. An EHR system can be a very useful tool for applying QI methodology to the routine practice of medicine (Figure 10-5).

How Can An EHR Help at This Stage?

To maximize the use of EHR for performance measurement, one must first make sure that the data elements needed to determine the measures are captured, stored, and, most importantly, reported out by the EHR system.

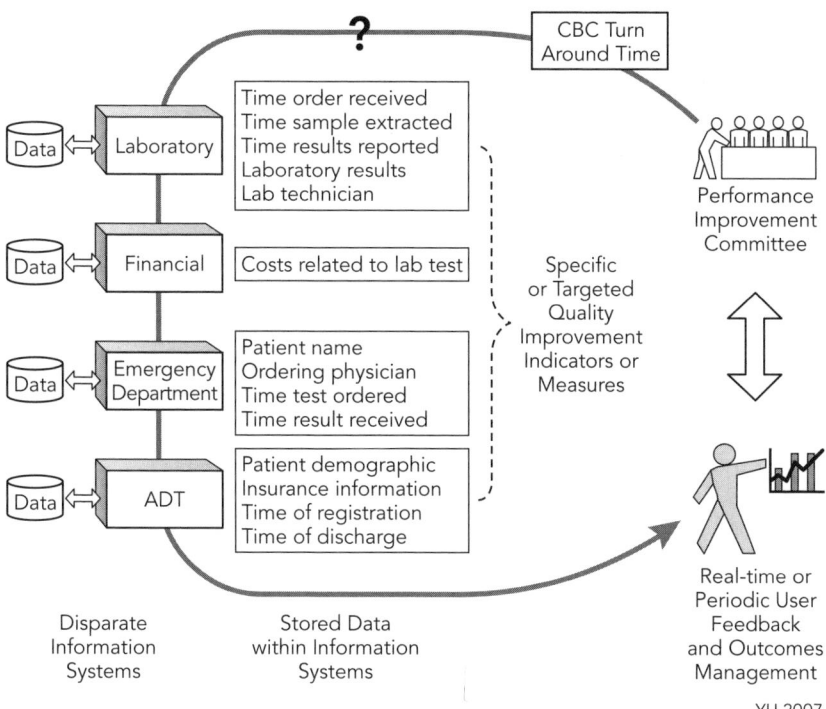

Figure 10-5 Embedding quality measurement into existing information systems.

Using the clinical scenario above, if one is trying to automate the collection of data for the performance indicator, "*Screening for proteinuria for patient with diabetes*", then one needs to find out if the EHR system is able to collect procedures or medical services performed at the clinic (i.e., urinalysis), as well as the diagnoses (i.e., ICD-9 codes) documented by the clinicians. More importantly, one needs to make sure that the EHR system can produce a report or run a query for the numerator and the denominator.

Development of EHR Standards and Quality Improvement

The recent release of the Health Level 7 (HL7) Electronic Health Record System Functional Model (EHR-S FM) supports process measurement as an essential function of the electronic health record (50-53). The main EHR functions described relating to quality measurement include:

1. The ability to "provide audit capabilities for system access and usage", providing the EHR the capability to audit records for security, data usage and exchange, as well as reporting activities.

2. The ability to "capture and manage patient clinical measures (physiologic and physical) as discrete patient data".

3. The ability to provide support for measurement, analysis, and research.

4. The ability to "support the capture and later export or retrieval of data necessary to provide quality, performance, and accountability measurements".

The Certification Commission for Healthcare Information Technology (CCHIT, http://www. cchit.org) is among the early adopters of the EHR functional model. In July 2004, CCHIT was launched as a private-sector led initiative to certify health IT products serving both the ambulatory and inpatient settings (54,55). The specific conditions for certifying health IT products that may relate to quality measurement include:

1. The ability to provide access control, audit, documentation and authentication for patient care in a secure and reliable manner.

2. The ability to receive, send, query, and publish reports in all aspects of patient care.

3. The ability to use clinical data for secondary uses such as public health surveillance and reporting, utilization review, and QI reporting.

Among the notable moves towards integrating quality measurement with health IT is the Doctor's Office Quality Information Technology project (DOQ-IT, http://www. qualitynet.org) (56,57). Sponsored by CMS, this initiative focuses on the adoption of EHR systems in the ambulatory setting. Providers participating in the DOQ-IT project would implement EHR systems that are able to capture and submit data that later can be used for quality measurement. The data are transmitted electronically via HL7 messaging standards to a central regional location such as a QI organization's data warehouse, where the aggregate measures are calculated and then reported back to the provider to support QI activities.

Recent initiatives in the health IT community continued the relentless pursuit to automating quality measurement. For example, the Collaborative for Performance Measure Integration with EHR Systems (www.ama-assn.org/ama1/pub/upload/mm/472/description-activity.pdf) led by the American Medical Association, CMS, and NCQA, seeks to "create a process to communicate the data necessary for EHR vendors to implement performance measure reporting functionality within their products and to develop standards for performance measure reporting". In addition, developments within the proponents of the healthcare IT standard such as the American Health Information Community (AHIC, www.hhs.gov/healthit/ahic.html) and the Healthcare Information Technology Standards Panel (HITSP, www.ansi.org/hitsp) have also promoted the automation of quality reporting, as well as the standard terminologies that are required to communicate elements of quality measurement. As a response to the industry need, Health Level Seven (HL7, www.hl7.org) and the Integrating the Healthcare Enterprise (IHE, www.ihe. net/quality) project have set forth early programs that will address the communication of quality measurement information across information systems.

Electronic Health Record Functions That Support Quality Improvement

EHR systems are particularly suited for collecting data that come as a byproduct of routine care. When data are captured automatically during the course of care, measurement becomes more practical as it removes the need for extra documentation (22) (Figure 10-7). We have learned that in QA or in traditional QI activities, changing provider behavior is achieved through feedback mechanisms. Often the provider receives a summary of the measures indicating whether he or she is not in compliance. While this form of feedback is important, the reality is that the feedback is retrospective, and that the opportune moment to affect quality has passed (Figure 10-6). EHR systems offer a more efficient mechanism to affect provider behavior. Real-time knowledge transfer (i.e., information retrieval, education) and feedback mechanisms at the point of care can usually be deployed

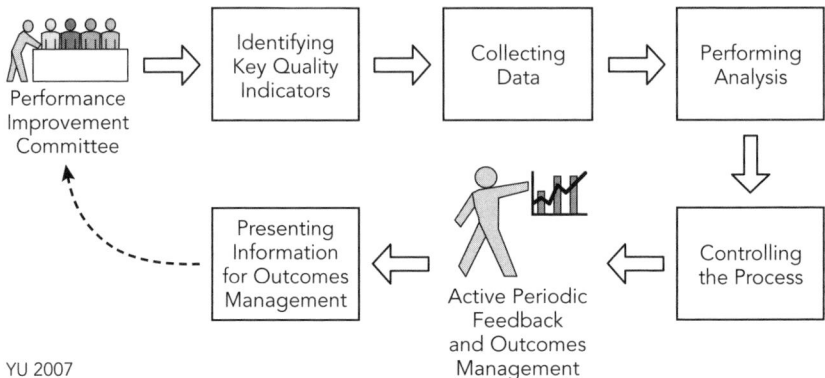

Figure 10-6   Traditional quality improvement process.

using CDS tools (58,59). And, if done in conjunction with QI strategies, the implementation of CDS increases the chances of processes to be successful (60) (Figure 10-8). Integrating measurement functionality into information systems can greatly reduce the burden of conducting quality and performance improvement projects, disseminating the findings, and maintaining and tracking the progress (61). To reiterate, the EHR cannot be deployed in vacuum. It is essential that the workflow (e.g., organization, clinic, physician's workflow, etc) must be redesigned to support the decision support

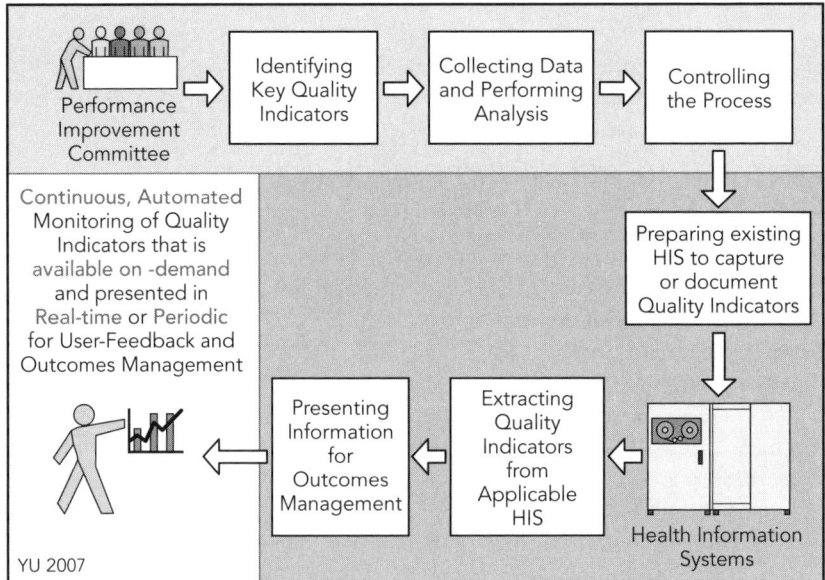

Figure 10-7   Automating the quality improvement process using existing health information systems.

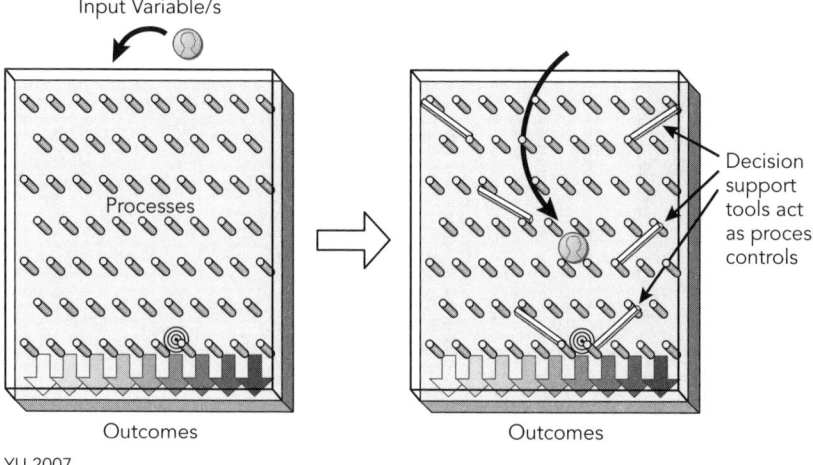

Input Variable/s

Processes

Outcomes

Decision
support
tools act
as process
controls

Outcomes

YU 2007

Figure 10-8   How EHR systems utilize decision support to guide clinicians in a quality improvement initiative.

prompts from the EHR (62). Table 10-4 lists real-world applications where the EHR was employed for QI activities.

Barriers to Using Electronic Health Records for Quality Improvement

EHR systems are effective tools for providing knowledge about a patient; however, most EHRs currently are designed to specifically support clinical operations but not healthcare process improvement initiatives. In addition, data elements required to calculate the performance measures are not readily available. If one is using the EHR to automate capture and collection of standardized quality measures (e.g., HEDIS, JCAHO core measures), then the EHR must be adapted for this purpose. Most of the data required for measuring performance are already captured in clinical and financial information systems (e.g., laboratory, pharmacy, radiology, admit-discharge-transfer systems, etc) (see Figure 10-5). However, the difficulties in integrating disparate data sources remain a challenge even in the most sophisticated healthcare systems (87).

The bottom line is that EHRs, at this time, may not come out of the box fully adapted for use in QI. Having an EHR installed does not mean that one can automatically reap its benefits. It has to be customized before it can be used to enhance performance. This means that extending its use beyond clinical operations has human capital, management, technical support, and governance implications. Barriers to using EHR systems for QI are listed and described in Table 10-5.

Table 10-4

ELECTRONIC HEALTH RECORD FUNCTIONS THAT ENABLE QUALITY IMPROVEMENT AND REAL-WORLD EXAMPLES

Activity	EHR Function	Real-World Application
Quality measurement	EHRs offer a rich source of data that can be used for assessing rocesses and outcomes of quality. Since clinical information is already stored electronically, it can be also be used for quality improvement. For instance, using the EHR, it will be more efficient to query the system for patients with specific conditions, follow up on their clinical information, and identify those who were at risk for certain undesirable outcomes (i.e., adverse events) (63,64). For routine quality measurement to be sustainable, some form of automation must be in place (65). Once the EHR system is configured, the query can be run automatically, thereby avoiding the tedious task of manual record review. With this degree of automation, healthcare can be transformed with easy access to data that can be utilized for process improvement activities. Using internet technologies, one can also reuse the data captured within the EHR to allow for automating reporting and submission of core measures mandated by external agencies such as JCAHO or CMS for accreditation, compliance, or benchmarking purposes. Using the data from the EHR, one can improve the quality of data and increase the cycle time for feedback of information used in QI initiatives. Some institutions have even used the data from the EHR to populate real-time information via executive or clinician dashboards (66).	In one academic institution, an EHR system was successfully used to measure the use of ß-blockers after myocardial infarction instead of manual chart review, offering the capability to provide timely and automated performance measurement. For this activity, they used electronic data that contained vital signs, ICD-9 CM codes, laboratory test results, and medication orders to assess the use of ß-blockers. They were able to successfully automate the extraction of the AMI measures, ß-blocker administration within 24 hours of arrival and ß-blocker prescription at discharge (61).

Analyze aggregate clinical information	The EHR system can greatly improve the quality of clinical information that is accessible to the clinician. By providing easy and organized view of laboratory results, medications, allergies, past health history, and diagnoses, patient information becomes more accessible, legible, and organized for easy retrieval (5).	In order to improve the care for children with pharyngitis, one pediatric practice used the EHR to assess prescribing patterns and the use of diagnostic interventions. Using data from the EHR system, they searched for patients diagnosed with pharyngitis and then determined the proportion of those who received a test for group A streptococci as well as those who had received antibiotics (71).
Adhere to clinical guidelines	For EHRs with order-entry capability, the quality the medication ordering process can be greatly enhanced. Providers can enter data at the point of care; this reduces the chances of error (e.g., no legibility problems, fewer drug-to-drug, allergy, or diagnosis interactions, etc). It can also potentially provide efficiency gains in the whole medication ordering process as well as adherence to appropriate formulary prescribing practices (68,69).	In one primary care clinic, the EHR system was designed to remind the clinicians to provide preventive care services and follow recommended care guidelines for common children and adults. With the help of the EHR system, the providers were presented with automated "prompts" to remind them that the medical interventions or services were due. Because of this, the practice was able to improve their rates for mammogram screening, immunization for varicella and influenza, monitoring for glycosylated hemoglobin for diabetic patients (67).
Enhance provider communication	One of the key features of the EHR is to facilitate communication among the members of the care team or even to the patient. Through electronic-based messaging, timely access to information, whether online, web-based communications or email, can be an adjunct to regular (e.g., phone, mail, etc) provider-to-provider and provider-to-patient communication can be enhanced (72).	In an effort to improve osteoporotic care after a fracture among geriatric patients, a health maintenance organization used the EHR to transmit reminders via email to primary care providers and patients regarding the need for bone density screening and potential need for osteoporosis medications. They noted an improvement in bone density screening and adherence to osteoporosis treatment guidelines after the reminder system as implemented (73).

Continued on next page

Table 10-4

ELECTRONIC HEALTH RECORD FUNCTIONS THAT ENABLE QUALITY IMPROVEMENT AND REAL-WORLD EXAMPLES (CONT'D)

Activity	EHR Function	Real-World Application
Improve patient care documentation	By using an EHR, patient care documentation is dramatically improved. Most obvious benefit is that illegibility is virtually eliminated. Also, by using user-defined templates and coded or structured data entry, patient care documentation is then made accessible, readable as well as organized. Once customized to the practice, the EHR can help standardize care and documentation especially for those patients that require specialized care.	In one busy pediatric office, they used the EHR to promote proper documentation for health pediatric check-ups, provide targeted patient educational information as well as targeted screening services for lead toxicity. After deployment of the EHR, they noted an increase in adherence to their lead screening, patient educational handouts and immunization rates during well-child check ups (74).
Improve reporting capability	Dramatic improvements in the ease of extracting reports about the clinical practice are among the advantages of the EHR. By being able to view basic information such as patient lists between visits, most common diagnoses or procedures, provider performance reports (e.g., tracking of services rendered, feedback, etc). All these information can be very useful in quality improvement activities.	Using the institutions' EHR, the need for better follow-up care patients was identified after a quality improvement initiative to assess the quality of preventive care services. The investigators evaluated the quality of the colonic cancer screenings that are being performed at the institution's primary care clinics. They used elements found in the medical records (e.g., age, gender, race, ICD-9 and CPT codes) to determine the patients that were screened for colon cancer (i.e., fecal occult blood test) and then used this information to assess the patients who were positive for the screening test, received follow-up diagnostic testing (e.g., barium enema, colonoscopy, etc). They found that, although the physicians were screening patients for colon cancer, a significant portion of the patients who are at risk for cancer did not receive any follow-up studies (79).

Table 10-5

BARRIERS TO USING EHR SYSTEMS FOR QUALITY IMPROVEMENT

Barrier	Comments
Cost	EHR systems are currently still priced beyond perceived benefit (89). Costs include hardware, software and training to cover IT support and users, additional costs for add-in functionalities (e.g., modules, enhancements), maintenance, and upgrades (83).
Learning curve for adopting EHR for QI use	Initial provider time costs can be high for deployment and successful use for QI; may ultimately depend on managing complex communications, decision-making structures and responding to internal conflicts (96,97).
Return on investment	Clinical benefits are often difficult to quantify and financial benefits vary and are not immediate (100). Too much emphasis on system's return on investment can stifle EHR adoption (99).
Lack of technical support	Shortage of health IT support is common, especially if current system is not robust enough for QI use (89).
Lack of communication standards	There is a lack of industry-wide data exchange standards for EHR QI functions.
Impact of EHR on workflow	A poorly designed EHR can be perceived to impede workflow or possibly even negatively impact patient care (103-106).
Lack of incentives	Need for additional support, especially for smaller practices (108). Current financial incentives benefit mostly payers and purchasers of healthcare (109).
Complexity of aggregate electronic data	Digitized information suffers from unstructured data, lack of standard terminologies, inadequate vocabularies; need to further understand the complexity of the data collected in routine patient care (107).

Unintended Consequences of Electronic Health Record Systems

Finally, implementing EHR systems is not without risk. Recent studies show that deploying EHR systems has its own pitfalls, with consequences that affect end-users negatively, and some resulting adverse patient outcomes. For instance, Ash et al showed that organizations deploying computerized physician order entry systems encountered unfavorable workflow and communication problems, changes in the organizational power structure, persistence of paper (as compared to paperless!), and strong, often downbeat, sentiments from the end-users (110,111).

Weiner et al has also described "e-iatrogenesis", an adverse consequence to patients during health IT deployments (112), usually as a result of error-prone system designs (e.g., faulty data presentation, unclear selection of orderable items) and end-user workflow discrepancies (113). This is an emerging issue that providers need to know when they implement EHR systems.

Conclusion

Quality measurement, reporting, and subsequent performance evaluation will become routine practice in the near term, a reality with which health-care practitioners must come to terms. Alignment of incentives and reward mechanisms on quality will predominate in the debate in the foreseeable future. Due to the rapid changes in the healthcare industry, healthcare providers will have to, at some point in time, adopt EHR systems to efficiently comply with documentation, reporting, and data submission requirements needed to provide patient care.

However, EHR diffusion is still low among physicians despite the industry's emphasis on health IT (88). Adoption is mostly seen on large, networked physicians than smaller and independent providers (89-91). Among those who have adopted the EHR, successful adoption and realized benefits have not been generelizable across institutions (92). Deployment of EHR is difficult because the system must be seamlessly integrated within the clinician's workflow for it to be successfully implemented and accepted (5,93). Because of the cost, complexity, and trepidations in adoption, it has

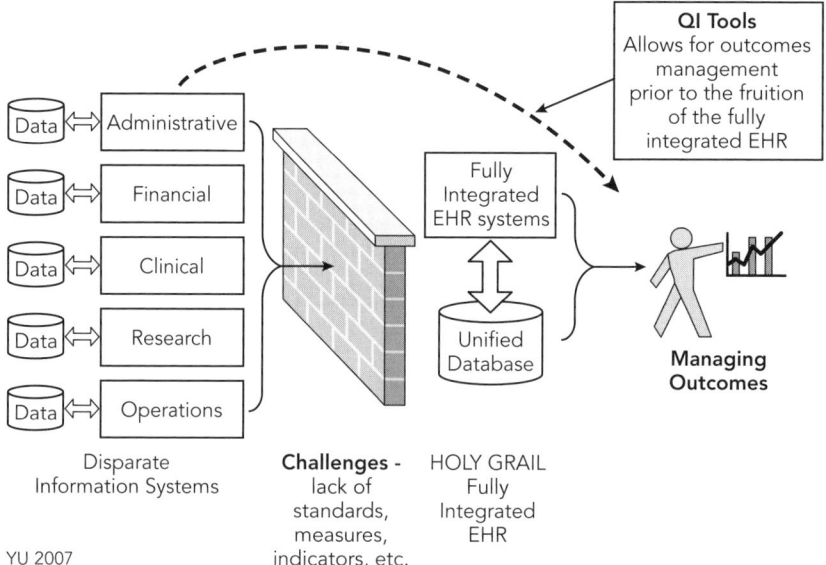

Figure 10-9 Employing health information technology for quality improvement.

been estimated that in a best-case scenario, full adoption of EHR will be around the year 2024, at least a decade beyond ONCHIT's goal of 2014 (94). Recent activities in both the legislative and private sectors is a reflection of the intense support for advancing health IT and the role of EHR systems in quality measurement (95).

Full adoption of interoperable EHRs can potentially save the healthcare industry over $300 billion annually due to efficiency and patient safety (114). The real value for EHR systems will be made through the ease of collection and analysis of data that can be used to transform the current healthcare delivery process (84) (Figure 10-9). The EHR presents a rich field of valuable information that can be utilized not only for operational and clinical applications, but also for process improvement. By understanding the capabilities of the EHR and its use within the QI framework, it allows one to utilize data effectively for improving patient care. QI tools offer simple but scientifically sound methods that one can employ to gather, measure, analyze, and, most importantly, supply feedback for incremental process improvement, one small step at a time.

References

1. Kohn LT, Corrigan J, Donaldson MS. To err is human : building a safer health system. Washington, D.C.: National Academy Press; 2000.
2. Institute of Medicine (U.S.). Committee on Quality of Health Care in America. Crossing the quality chasm : a new health system for the 21st century. Washington, D.C.: National Academy Press; 2001.
3. Hannan TJ. Variation in health care: the roles of the electronic medical record. Int J Med Inform. 1999;54:127-36.
4. Bates DW, Pappius E, Kuperman GJ, et al. Using information systems to measure and improve quality. Int J Med Inform. 1999;53:115-24.
5. Miller RH, Sim I. Physicians' use of electronic medical records: barriers and solutions. Health Aff (Millwood). 2004;23:116-26.
6. Berwick DM. Controlling variation in health care: a consultation from Walter Shewhart. Med Care. 1991;29:1212-25.
7. Beatty JR. The quality journey: historical and workforce perspectives and assessment of commmittment to quality. International Journal of Productivity and Quality Management. 2006;1:139-67.
8. Gaucher E, Kratochwill E. The Malcolm Baldrige National quality Award: implications and uses for healthcare organizations. Infect Control Hosp Epidemiol. 1995;16:302-7.
9. Donabedian A. The criteria and standards of quality. Ann Arbor, MI: Health Administration Press; 1981.
10. Institute of Medicine (U.S.). Committee on the National Quality Report on Health Care Delivery., Hurtado MP, Swift EK, Corrigan J, United States. Agency for Healthcare Research and Quality. Envisioning the national health care quality report. Washington, D.C.: National Academy Press; 2001.
11. Berwick DM. A primer on leading the improvement of systems. BMJ. 1996;312:619-22.
12. Decker MD. The development of indicators. Infect Control Hosp Epidemiol. 1991;12:490-2.
13. McGlynn EA. Choosing and evaluating clinical performance measures. Jt Comm J Qual Improv. 1998;24:470-9.

14. McGlynn EA. Selecting common measures of quality and system performance. Med Care. 2003;41(1 Suppl):I39-47.

15. Bernstein SJ, Hilborne LH. Clinical indicators: the road to quality care? J Comm J Qual Improv. 1993;19:501-9.

16. Brennan TA, Hebert LE, Laird NM, et al. Hospital characteristics associated with adverse events and substandard care. JAMA. 1991;265:3265-9.

17. Donabedian A. Evaluating the quality of medical care. 1966. Milbank Q. 2005;83: 691-729.

18. Shojania KG, Showstack J, Wachter RM. Assessing hospital quality: a review for clinicians. Eff Clin Pract. 2001;4:82-90.

19. Marciniak TA, Ellerbeck EF, Radford MJ, et al. Improving the quality of care for Medicare patients with acute myocardial infarction: results from the Cooperative Cardiovascular Project. JAMA. 1998;279:1351-7.

20. Mant J, Hicks N. Detecting differences in quality of care: the sensitivity of measures of process and outcome in treating acute myocardial infarction. BMJ. 1995;311:793-6.

21. Palmer RH. Process-based measures of quality: the need for detailed clinical data in large health care databases. Ann Intern Med. 1997;127(8 Pt 2):733-8.

22. Rubin HR, Pronovost P, Diette GB. The advantages and disadvantages of process-based measures of health care quality. Int J Qual Health Care. 2001;13:469-74.

23. Trowbridge CC, Stammers AH, Wood GC, et al. Improved outcomes during cardiac surgery: a multifactorial enhancement of cardiopulmonary bypass techniques. J Extra Corpor Technol. 2005;37:165-72.

24. Norris CM, Saunders LD, Ghali WA, et al. Health-related quality of life outcomes of patients with coronary artery disease treated with cardiac surgery, percutaneous coronary intervention or medical management. Can J Cardiol. 2004;20:1259-66.

25. Bates DW, Cullen DJ, Laird N, et al. Incidence of adverse drug events and potential adverse drug events. Implications for prevention. ADE Prevention Study Group. JAMA. 1995;274:29-34.

26. Iezzoni LI, Shwartz M, Ash AS, et al. Risk adjustment methods can affect perceptions of outcomes. Am J Med Qual. 1994;9:43-8.

27. Kuttner R. The risk-adjustment debate. N Engl J Med. 1998;339:1952-6.

28. Fihn SD. The quest to quantify quality. JAMA. 2000;283:1740-2.

29. Plsek PE. Quality improvement methods in clinical medicine. Pediatrics. 1999;103 (1 Suppl E):203-14.

30. Bates DW. The quality case for information technology in healthcare. BMC Med Inform Decis Mak. 2002;2:7.

31. Lynn J. When does QI count as research? Human subject protection and theories of knowledge. Qual Saf Health Care. 2004;13:67-70.

32. Lo B, Groman M. Oversight of QI: focusing on benefits and risks. Arch Intern Med. 2003;163:1481-86.

33. Brassard M, GOAL/QPC. The Memory Jogger Plus+ : featuring the seven management and planning tools. 1st ed. Methuen, Mass.: GOAL/QPC; 1989.

34. Gallagher M, Hares T, Spencer J, et al. The nominal group technique: a research tool for general practice? Fam Pract. Mar 1993;10:76-81.

35. Corbett MW. Flow chart to benchmark. Best Pract Benchmarking Healthc. 1996; 1:161-6.

36. Carey RG, Lloyd RC. Measuring QI in healthcare : a guide to statistical process control applications. New York: Quality Resources; 1995.

37. Batalden PB, Stoltz PK. A framework for the continual improvement of health care: building and applying professional and improvement knowledge to test changes in daily work. Jt Comm J Qual Improv. 1993;19:424-47; discussion 448-52.

38. Batalden PB, Mohr JJ, Nelson EC, et al. Continually improving the health and value of health care for a population of patients: the panel management process. Qual Manag Health Care. Spring 1997;5:41-51.

39. Berwick DM, Enthoven A, Bunker JP. Quality management in the NHS: the doctor's role—II. BMJ. 1992;304:304-8.

40. Berwick DM, Enthoven A, Bunker JP. Quality management in the NHS: the doctor's role—I. BMJ. 1992;304:235-9.

41. Headrick LA, Richardson A, Priebe GP. Continuous improvement learning for residents. Pediatrics. 1998;101:768-73; discussion 773-74.

42. Kaluzny AD, McLaughlin CP, Simpson K. Applying total quality management concepts to public health organizations. Public Health Rep. 1992;107:257-64.

43. Ishikawa diagrams help managers sort out facts, correct problems. Hosp Food Nutr Focus. 1996;12:2.

44. Batalden PB, Mohr J, Strosberg M, Baker GR. A conceptual framework for learning continual improvement in health administration education programs. J Health Adm Educ. 1995;13:67-90.

45. Institute of Medicine recommends new P4P system for Medicare. Healthcare Benchmarks Qual Improv. 2006;13:133-7.

46. Damberg CL, Raube K, Williams T, Shortell SM. Paying for performance: implementing a statewide project in California. Qual Manag Health Care. 2005;14:66-79.

47. Hagland M. Rewarding good behavior. With medicare as a major proponent, pay-for-performance programs are gaining traction across the country. Healthc Inform. 2007; 24:36,38.

48 Tierney WM, Rotich JK, Smith FE, et al. Crossing the "digital divide:" implementing an electronic medical record system in a rural Kenyan health center to support clinical care and research. Proc AMIA Symp. 2002:792-5.

49. Aspden P, Corrigan JM, Wolcott J, Erickson SM, eds. Patient Safety: Achieving a New Standard for Care. Washington, DC: National Academy Press; 2003.

50. Rhodes H, Mon DT, Dougherty M. The drive for an EHR standard picks up speed. J Ahima. 2004;75:18-22.

51. Mon DT. Next steps for the EHR draft standard. J Ahima. 2004;75:50-1.

52. Mon DT. The EHR: life after the draft standard is approved. J Ahima. 2004;75:54.

53. Mon DT. Setting the right expectations for the EHR standard. J Ahima. 2004;75:52-4.

54. Leavitt M, Gallagher L. The EHR seal of approval: CCHIT introduces product certification to spur EHR adoption. J Ahima. 2006;77:26-30; quiz 33-24.

55. Metzger JB. EHR certification eliminates barriers. AHIP Cover. 2006;47:64,66,68.

56. Wang J, Gold JA. The DOQ-IT initiative: primary care physicians can get help implementing or expanding HIT. WMJ. 2005;104:77.

57. Columbus S. Small practice, big decision: selecting an EHR system for small physician practices. J Ahima. 2006;77:42-6.

58. Davis D. Does CME work? An analysis of the effect of educational activities on physician performance or health care outcomes. Int J Psychiatry Med. 1998;28:21-39.

59. Davis DA, Thomson MA, Oxman AD, Haynes RB. Changing physician performance. A systematic review of the effect of continuing medical education strategies. JAMA. 1995;274:700-5.

60. Kremsdorf R, Regan DW. Delivering first-class healthcare in today's environment means giving physicians easy access to computer-based patient information. Healthc Exec. Mar-1997;12:41-2.

61. Weiner M, Stump TE, Callahan CM, Lewis JN, McDonald CJ. Pursuing integration of performance measures into electronic medical records: beta-adrenergic receptor antagonist medications. Qual Saf Health Care. 2005;14:99-106.

62. O'Connor PJ, Pronk NP. Integrating population health concepts, clinical guidelines, and ambulatory medical systems to improve diabetes care. J Ambul Care Manage. 1998;21:67-73.

63. Honigman B, Lee J, Rothschild J, et al. Using computerized data to identify adverse drug events in outpatients. J Am Med Inform Assoc. 2001;8:254-66.

64. de Lusignan S, van Vlymen J, Hague N, Dhoul N. Using computers to identify non-compliant people at increased risk of osteoporotic fractures in general practice: a cross-sectional study. Osteoporos Int. Aug 24 2006.

65. Halvorson GC. Wiring health care. Healthcare cannot be reengineered without data. Health Aff (Millwood). 2005;24:1266-8.

66. Kumar S. Web-based tools aid Quality Improvement projects. Available at: http://www.psqh.com/julsep04/kumar.html. Accessed September 20, 2006.

67. Gill JM, Ewen E, Nsereko M. Impact of an electronic medical record on quality of care in a primary care office. Del Med J. 2001;73:187-94.

68. Mekhjian HS, Kumar RR, Kuehn L, et al. Immediate benefits realized following implementation of physician order entry at an academic medical center. J Am Med Inform Assoc. 2002;9:529-39.

69. Johnston D, Pan E, Walker J. The value of CPOE in ambulatory settings. J Healthc Inf Manag. 2004;18:5-8.

70. Wells BJ, Lobel KD, Dickerson LM. Using the electronic medical record to enhance the use of combination drugs. Am J Med Qual. 2003;18:147-49.

71. Benin AL, Vitkauskas G, Thornquist E, et al. Improving diagnostic testing and reducing overuse of antibiotics for children with pharyngitis: a useful role for the electronic medical record. Pediatr Infect Dis J. 2003;22:1043-7.

72. Katz SJ, Nissan N, Moyer CA. Crossing the digital divide: evaluating online communication between patients and their providers. Am J Manag Care. 2004;10:593-8.

73. Feldstein A, Elmer PJ, Smith DH, et al. Electronic medical record reminder improves osteoporosis management after a fracture: a randomized, controlled trial. J Am Geriatr Soc. 2006;54:450-7.

74. Gioia PC. Quality improvement in pediatric well care with an electronic record. Proc AMIA Symp. 2001:209-13.

75. Frank O, Litt J, Beilby J. Opportunistic electronic reminders. Improving performance of preventive care in general practice. Aust Fam Physician. 2004;33:87-90.

76. Gandhi TK, Sequist TD, Poon EG, et al. Primary care clinician attitudes towards electronic clinical reminders and clinical practice guidelines. AMIA Annu Symp Proc. 2003:848.

77. Tang PC, LaRosa MP, Newcomb C, Gorden SM. Measuring the effects of reminders for outpatient influenza immunizations at the point of clinical opportunity. J Am Med Inform Assoc. 1999;6:115-21.

78. Dexter PR, Perkins SM, Maharry KS, et al. Inpatient computer-based standing orders vs physician reminders to increase influenza and pneumococcal vaccination rates: a randomized trial. JAMA. 2004;292:2366-71.

79. Etzioni DA, Yano EM, Rubenstein LV, et al. Measuring the quality of colorectal cancer screening: the importance of follow-up. Dis Colon Rectum. 2006;49:1002-10.

80. Eysenbach G. What is e-health? J Med Internet Res. 2001;3:E20.

81. Tang PC, Ash JS, Bates DW, Overhage JM, Sands DZ. Personal health records: definitions, benefits, and strategies for overcoming barriers to adoption. J Am Med Inform Assoc. 2006;13:121-6.

82. Tang PC, Black W, Buchanan J, et al. PAMFOnline: integrating EHealth with an electronic medical record system. AMIA Annu Symp Proc. 2003:644-8.

83. Wang SJ, Middleton B, Prosser LA, et al. A cost-benefit analysis of electronic medical records in primary care. Am J Med. 2003;114:397-403.

84. Goodman C. Savings in electronic medical record systems? Do it for the quality. It is unrealistic to hold out widespread adoption of health information technology as a net cost saver. Health Aff (Millwood). 2005;24:1124-6.

85. Renner K. Cost-justifying electronic medical records. Healthc Financ Manage. 1996; 50:6364,66,68 passim.

86. Kian LA, Stewart MW, Bagby C, Robertson J. Justifying the cost of a computer-based patient record. Healthc Financ Manage. 1995;49:58-60,62,64-57.

87. McDonald CJ. The barriers to electronic medical record systems and how to overcome them. J Am Med Inform Assoc. 1997;4:213-21.

88. Menachemi N, Perkins RM, van Durme DJ, Brooks RG. Examining the adoption of electronic health records and personal digital assistants by family physicians in Florida. Inform Prim Care. 2006;14:1-9.

89. Kemper AR, Uren RL, Clark SJ. Adoption of electronic health records in primary care pediatric practices. Pediatrics. 2006;118:e20-24.

90. Lee J, Cain C, Young S, Chockley N, Burstin H. The adoption gap: health information technology in small physician practices. Understanding office workflow can help realize the promise of technology. Health Aff (Millwood). 2005;24:1364-6.

91. Burt CW, Sisk JE. Which physicians and practices are using electronic medical records? Survey data show limited use of these information tools. Health Aff (Millwood). 2005;24:1334-43.

92. Himmelstein DU, Woolhandler S. Hope and hype: predicting the impact of electronic medical records. RAND's vision of "gold in them than hills" owes more to Merlin than to metallurgy. Health Aff (Millwood). 2005;24:1121-3.

93. Bodenheimer T, Grumbach K. Electronic technology: a spark to revitalize primary care? JAMA. 2003;290:259-64.

94. Ford EW, Menachemi N, Phillips MT. Predicting the adoption of electronic health records by physicians: when will health care be paperless? J Am Med Inform Assoc. 2006;13:106-12.

95. Rosenfeld S, Bernasek C, Mendelson D. Medicare's next voyage: encouraging physicians to adopt health information technology. Policymakers seem to agree on the necessity of HIT in Medicare but need to commit the resources needed to effect change. Health Aff (Millwood). 2005;24:1138-46.

96. Crosson JC, Stroebel C, Scott JG, Stello B, Crabtree BF. Implementing an electronic medical record in a family medicine practice: communication, decision making, and conflict. Ann Fam Med. 2005;3:307-11.

97. Scott JT, Rundall TG, Vogt TM, Hsu J. Kaiser Permanente's experience of implementing an electronic medical record: a qualitative study. BMJ. 2005;331:1313-6.

98. Chaiken BP. Clinical ROI: not just costs versus benefits. J Healthc Inf Manag. 2003; 17:36-41.

99. Frisse ME. Comments on return on investment (ROI) as it applies to clinical systems. J Am Med Inform Assoc. 2006;13:365-7.

100. Kaushal R, Jha AK, Franz C, et al. Return on investment for a computerized physician order entry system. J Am Med Inform Assoc. 2006;13:261-6.

101. Shah NR, Seger AC, Seger DL, et al. Improving acceptance of computerized prescribing alerts in ambulatory care. J Am Med Inform Assoc. 2006;13:5-11.

102. Miller RH, Hillman JM, Given RS. Physician use of IT: results from the Deloitte Research Survey. J Healthc Inf Manag. 2004;18:72-80.

103. Edwards DB. Computer physician order entry. Ann Intern Med. 2004;140:669; author reply 669-70.

104. Nassberg BM. Computer physician order entry. Ann Intern Med. 2004;140:669; author reply 669-70.

105. Han YY, Carcillo JA, Venkataraman ST, et al. Unexpected increased mortality after implementation of a commercially sold computerized physician order entry system. Pediatrics. 2005;116:1506-12.

106. Scanlon M. Computer physician order entry and the real world: we're only humans. Jt Comm J Qual Saf. 2004;30:342-6.

107. de Lusignan S, Hague N, van Vlymen J, Kumarapeli P. Routinely-collected general practice data are complex, but with systematic processing can be used for QI and research. Inform Prim Care. 2006;14:59-66.

108. Gans D, Kralewski J, Hammons T, Dowd B. Medical groups' adoption of electronic health records and information systems. Practices are encountering greater-than-expected barriers to adopting an EHR system, but the adoption rate continues to rise. Health Aff (Millwood). 2005;24:1323-33.

109. Bates DW. Physicians and ambulatory electronic health records. U.S. Physicians are ready to make the transition to EHRs—which is clearly overdue, given the rest of the world's experience. Health Aff (Millwood). 2005;24:1180-9.

110. Ash JS, Sittig DF, Poon EG, et al. The Extent and Importance of Unintended Consequences Related to Computerized Provider Order Entry. J Am Med Inform Assoc. Apr 25 2007.

111. Ash JS, Sittig DF, Dykstra RH, et al. Categorizing the unintended sociotechnical consequences of computerized provider order entry. Int J Med Inform. 2007;76 (Suppl 1):21-7.

112. Weiner JP, Kfuri T, Chan K, Fowles JB. "e-Iatrogenesis": The Most Critical Unintended Consequence of CPOE and other HIT. J Am Med Inform Assoc. 2007;14:387-8.

113. Campbell EM, Sittig DF, Ash JS, Guappone KP, Dykstra RH. Types of unintended consequences related to computerized provider order entry. J Am Med Inform Assoc. 2006;13:547-56.

114. Hillestad R, Bigelow J, Bower A, et al. Can electronic medical record systems transform health care? Potential health benefits, savings, and costs. The adoption of interoperable EMR systems could produce efficiency and safety savings of $142-$371 billion. Health Aff (Millwood). 2005;24:1103-1117.

11

Physician Adoption Strategies

Lyle Berkowitz, MD

"*There are no benefits without adoption*". Remember this phrase, you may need to repeat it many times during your implementation and beyond.

There are many compelling reasons to believe that electronic health record (EHR) systems will become an integral part of improving our healthcare system in the future. They have the potential to improve the quality of care, increase efficiency, decrease costs, and strengthen relationships between hospitals, physicians, and patients. Additionally, data repositories created by their use will help create the framework by which we can improve disease management, preventive care, and quality improvement systems. However, these potential benefits will never be fully realized unless there is significant physician involvement and adoption of these systems. Instead, we will see feature-rich systems that fail because they are unable to achieve a critical mass of users and data.

As obvious as this concept appears, physician adoption has been the bane of many EHR projects. All too often, executives and leaders allow the creation of rigid and difficult-to-use EHR systems because they get caught up in the hype of trying to perfect quality and lose the proverbial forest for the trees. While it is important to keep long-term quality benefits in mind, they will only come to fruition by implementing a product, a workflow, and an atmosphere that encourages full adoption of an EHR system.

This chapter will discuss strategies and tactics to help healthcare leaders and organizations improve acceptance and use of an EHR system. Categories to be addressed include: Laying the Groundwork, Understanding Physicians, Physician Involvement, Supporting Physicians, Choosing the Right System, and the Science of Change Management.

Background

A variety of articles have been written on improving physician adoption of information technology (IT) systems (1-4) with key themes being the importance of understanding physician needs, keeping physicians educated and involved, and creating systems that solve physician workflows in an easy and fast manner. However, many promising attempts at computerizing the medical record have experienced trouble (and sometimes even revolt) because of poor physician adoption strategies (5,6). In fact, it is estimated that 20% to 30% of EHR systems are "de-installed" within a year, often due to physician dissatisfaction.

One group of authors superbly analyzed and described how their institution's computer-based patient record (CPR) system failed because it did not offer the advantage touted at the beginning of the process, but instead "resulted in information overload and standardization, clerical task load increase, work organization rigidity, and expert autonomy negation" (7). Furthermore, they noted that because a unilateral vision was chosen for the system, the project team could not benefit from the potential benefit of process innovation and instead made crucial design and implementation errors that resulted directly from the rigid vision that was used.

In another paper, the same authors recognized that the failure of their CPR project was also due to "profound misunderstandings, largely spread within the project team, that led to fatal decisions that resulted in the failure of the CPR experiment. These misunderstandings were of a dual nature: the true nature of the CPR on the one hand, and the reality of medical practice and informational needs of the experts on the other hand" (8).

It is important that we critically review both failures and triumphs so we can learn how to improve the likelihood of success in future systems. Further information on this topic can be found in an earlier chapter of this book ("Why do EHR Implementations Fail").

Important Trends

Information Technology and Electronic Health Record: Adoption Patterns

While a variety of studies have discussed the growing use of IT by physicians, the exact numbers remain difficult to decipher due to how questions were posed and how they may have been interpreted. For example, according to findings from the 2006 Community Tracking Study Physician Survey (9) (from the Center for Studying Health System Change), over 83% of physicians state they had access to IT applications in their practices. However, this number can be deceiving. First, IT applications could include things as simple as "obtaining information about treatment alternatives or recommended guidelines", presumably via the Internet or a CD-ROM. Access to more sophisticated applications like e-Prescribing was significantly lower at 21.9% of the physicians surveyed. In fact, the survey did not even ask about access to full-blown EHR functionality, which usually ranges from 5%-10% nationally. Second, because physicians were asked about IT availability in their practice but not whether they actually use the technology or the frequency or intensity of use, the authors noted that the "estimates presented here should be considered an upper bound on the proportion of physicians regularly using clinical IT in their practices."

Similarly, when one reads about EHR adoption at levels of 60%, a closer look usually reveals a report in which 60% of physicians have *the ability to look up some results or notes online*—hardly a full EHR adoption. So although we are certainly increasing IT and EHR adoption over time, it is important to be discerning about what you read or hear about in this quickly evolving space.

Revisions to Stark Law and Anti-Kickback Statute Emphasize EHR Sponsorship Models

The cost of purchasing, implementing, and maintaining EHR systems continues to prevent widespread use. While larger enterprises can more easily shoulder these costs, smaller practices cannot, creating a growing gap in implementation and use of ambulatory EHRs. In fact, a 2003 survey conducted by the New York-based Commonwealth Fund found that "the odds of a physician practicing in a high-tech environment are 7.7 times higher for physicians in large practices than if they are in a solo practice" (23).

Fortunately, this trend may have met its match in a business model based on strategic and financial logic that enables hospitals to function as "EHR sponsors" for smaller physician practices (10). Hospitals and similar health care systems are finding that their investment in enterprise EHRs can be successfully leveraged to create a high-value, low-cost system that can be offered to their affiliated physicians.

Examples of this type of centrally managed, remotely utilized model include PeaceHealth in Oregon, Evanston Northwestern Healthcare in Illinois, Blue Ox Medical Network in Delaware, and Sutter Health in California. And importantly, relaxations of both Stark Laws and the Anti-Kickback Statute safe harbors in 2006 will make this model increasingly common. Specifically, these new rulings will allow hospitals or health systems to significantly subsidize the expense of EHR software to physicians with whom they are affiliated. The result will likely be an increase in the number of EHR projects taking place across America.

Pay-for-Performance Initiatives

It is commonly known that America's healthcare system is not always aligned well, often rewarding volume over quality. However, with rising morbidity, mortality, and costs being associated with quality deficiencies, both employers and government agencies are creating new financial systems that reward improved quality along various metrics.

Employer coalitions such as the Leapfrog Group and Bridges to Excellence are creating quality standards that are then rewarded by local employers. Meanwhile, Medicare announced in 2006 that future payments will be tied in part to both hospital and physician quality metrics. And in 2007, Medicare hinted at the fact that future reimbursement cuts might only be reversed for physicians who were using at least ePrescribing components of an EHR.

Pay-for-performance initiative may therefore reward a range of activities, from using ePrescribing to measuring quality metrics to proving a high level of quality metrics. It is, however, clear that those using EHR systems will be at a distinct advantage in fulfilling these initiatives.

Laying the Groundwork: The Five Es

Enabling Infrastructure and Cultural Changes

A critical first step in establishing any clinical information system is to build a reliable computing infrastructure (hardware, software, and connectivity), which then starts both a cultural and technological shift towards IT-enhanced workflows. All physicians should become comfortable with using computers in their office well before an EHR system is installed. A physician should therefore have easy access to a computer with standard applications (e.g., email, word processing, Internet access), basic clinical software (e.g., patient education handouts, medical reference online), and an Intranet site that contains information such as hospital policies, web-based paging, physician and clinic directories, and local disease management guidelines. This computer network should be fast, reliable, and easy to use. If an information systems department can successfully roll out this infrastructure early on, they can gain significant credibility with the physicians they serve while laying the physical and cultural groundwork for future projects.

Extend to Practice Management Systems

An important strategy to consider is whether to optionally implement a new practice management system (PMS) either before or in conjunction with an EHR system. The obvious benefit is that with a single PMS in place, it is significantly easier to choose and install an EHR system since there will be more infrastructure in place and less interfaces required. Additionally, the experience an information services (IS) department receives will make them feel more comfortable working on large projects in an ambulatory setting. If moving ahead, it is most advisable to make a PMS choice in parallel with the EHR system to ensure good scalability and integration. However, the timing of the implementation may be staggered. For example, it may make sense to install the PMS initially, and then only implement the EHR system afterwards, perhaps starting before the PMS roll out is completed in every clinic.

On the other hand, many physicians are very committed to their current PMS and would not want to be told it has to change. So it is important to do thorough due diligence ahead of time to find out what physicians' perspectives are on their current PMS products, whether they understand the benefits of a tighter PMS-EHR integration, and how they feel about changing products. If the decision is to not roll out a single integrated PMS product, then large healthcare systems will need to accept the need for integration with multiple PMS vendors.

Executive Level Support

Physicians at any institution know that new programs and policies must be well supported by both the administrative and clinical executive level to achieve success. All members of the executive level must not only support the EHR project philosophically and financially, they must also vocalize that support to the medical staff. They should make it clear that they understand and accept that an EHR project may be a slow and costly process, but that it will eventually result in happier doctors, healthier patients, and a more financially fit enterprise. Other ways to show their support will be for executive level officers to become involved in both educational processes and committee meetings when appropriate. Lastly, the executive level will need to be willing to talk tough with their current vendors in order to ensure that there is support and integration with whichever EHR product is chosen.

Education

Formal education of physicians and their staff should address specific problems with the current paper-based system, potential benefits and risks of implementing an EHR system, and an explanation of the processes that will be involved in moving forward. A powerful strategic vision should clearly define the reasoning behind having an EHR system in a particular institution, and should include both immediate and long-range benefits. This vision should include the high-level goals or mission of the enterprise, as well as specific benefits for individual physicians. If possible, it additionally should describe the return on investment for both physicians and the enterprise.

A simple slogan or vision should be crafted and then repeated often at meetings, in newsletters, and during informal discussion so that everyone is on the same page. At Northwestern Memorial in Chicago, we used the mnemonic IMPACT for "Improving Patient Care Through Technology". At Boston's Children Hospital, they used CHAMPS for "Children's Hospital Applications Maximizing Patient Safety".

One of the difficulties in educating physicians on this topic is the amount of personal and public anecdotal stories that can bias their beliefs. While these stories can be beneficial to highlight a point, it is also important to detail the valid scientific literature on this topic. Previous chapters provide good references, but the following reports should be well known to your IT staff and clinicians:

◆ The Institute of Medicine's 1999 report "To Err is Human" (11), which many consider a call to arms. It describes how medical errors are the fourth leading cause of death in America.

◆ The Institute of Medicine's 2001 report "Crossing the Quality Chasm" (12), which many consider a call to action. This report describes multiple IT-based strategies to improve on their often quoted six key aims of quality ("Care should be safe, effective, patient-centered, timely, efficient, and equitable"). More specifically, the report describes ten rules for care delivery redesign as follows:

  1. Care should be based on continuous healing relationships.
  2. Customization should be based on patient needs and values.
  3. The patient is the source of control.
  4. Knowledge should be shared and there should be free flow of information.
  5. Evidence-based decision making is necessary.
  6. Safety is a system property.
  7. Transparency should be considered as necessary.
  8. Needs must be anticipated.
  9. Waste should be continuously decreased.
  10. There should be cooperation among clinicians.

◆ The Center for Information Technology Leadership's 2003 report (13) on the benefits of using electronic prescribing in the outpatient environment. Important findings included:

  1. The average outpatient physician using paper based prescribing has thirty-eight adverse drug effects (ADEs) per year, of which fourteen (about one-third) are preventable, and two are life-threatening.
  2. An electronic prescription system can stop 75% of preventable ADEs (eleven per year per physician, of which one may be life-threatening).
  3. Nationally, these statistics equate to eight million ADEs/year, 2.6 million of which are preventable, of which two million can be avoided with the use of electronic prescription systems, of which 130,000 are potentially life-threatening.

Finally, physicians should be educated about the problems with today's paper-based systems and be referred to studies that examine these problems (Table 11-1). In other words, let physicians know about problems and their inherent professionalism and desire to improve will help keep things moving forward.

Table 11-1

PROBLEMS WITH PAPER-BASED SYSTEMS IN CLINICAL PRACTICE

Problem	Reference Number/Study
Only 55% of adult patients receive recommended care.	14
Physicians greatly underestimate their informational needs (in one study, physicians found answers to only 30% of their questions).	15
Patient data is difficult to find (at least one piece of patient data missing in 81% of cases).	16
Access to historical data more difficult to find with paper-based systems.	17
Chart documentation may not always reflect the complete history.	18, 19
Chart documentation may not fully reflect a patient's medication list.	20, 21
Medication errors may be high (i.e., as high as 100 errors per 1000 cases) but often go unrecorded.	22
Drug-related illness due to inappropriate prescriptions.	23
Physicians do not always ensure that they receive the results of all ordered tests, that they report those results to patients, or that they document this notification.	24

Expectation Management

Some physicians believe that an EHR system can solve all of their problems, others believe an EHR can only bring despair, but most are in between these extremes. It will be important to identify these expectations early so they can be managed appropriately. Clarification of these expectations will come about by personal experiences, committee input, and workflow and need analysis studies.

Managing these expectations will involve both formal and informal education. Formal education may include newsletters, lectures, and other forms of correspondence, which focus on explaining the potential benefits and processes involved with an EHR system. Informal education relates to the inclusion of EHR strategies in other discussions that do not focus on the EHR itself. For example, a ground rounds lecture on the increasing problem of drug-to-drug interactions or hospital acquired infections might include a study that shows how an EHR system can help to significantly decrease those occurrences. Or a meeting with doctors about future incentive systems, such as "Pay for Performance", might include a review of how an EHR can both simplify reporting and improve clinical quality via decision support at the point of care.

One important caveat is to be very careful not to "oversell" the system. Healthcare leaders should try to provide realistic expectations for EHR systems, ideally enhanced with descriptions of case studies involving institutions who have gone through a similar process.

Understanding Physicians

To best understand how to improve physician adoption of an EHR system, it is important to understand how physicians work, think, and feel, and how computers can affect their lives. It is additionally useful to identify the bottlenecks in their information flow that cause them pressure and frustration. Equally important is identifying where individual physicians are on the IT Adoption Curve—how they feel about and respond to technology.

Define and Understand Goals

An important part of understanding physicians will be to understand their goals. While individuals in the administrative and executive level may have clear goals concerning quality and productivity, the goals of physicians may be somewhat different. And it will be crucial for all involved to fully understand that the organizational goals will best be met if the physicians' goals are satisfied as well.

An important method to understand these goals involves workflow and needs analysis studies, in which physicians describe what goals and benefits they expect, and why those would be important to them. These goals will likely focus on improving efficiency, decreasing "busy work" (e.g., filling out forms), and improving revenues.

Workflow and Needs Analyses

Workflow and needs analyses can help a healthcare system better understand how to identify and satisfy the true needs of physicians. The chances for successful adoption of an EHR system will therefore increase if the EHR can fulfill the specific needs that have been identified by the physicians themselves. For example, a needs analysis might reveal that physicians want to access clinic notes from home and, furthermore, that they want to review and document all results from home. The project team should thus ensure that the EHR can allow off-site access to physicians, and permits them to use an electronic attestation feature to confirm their viewing of any type of result.

Workflow Analysis

Workflow studies should define how physicians access, use, and document information. Specifically, they should identify current systems of information flow and clarify how physicians have adapted to it. For example, a workflow analysis can study how physicians currently retrieve and document a patient's lab results, how they exchange data with a colleague (e.g., phone, letters, fax, email), and how they document their visits (e.g. dictation, hand-written notes). Specific workflow questions to study include the following:

- **Documentation:** How is a patient visit documented. How is a telephone encounter documented. Describe the timing and modality, including free-form written notes, structured templates, and dictation.

- **Chart dynamics:** In how many physical locations can the chart potentially be found. For what circumstances is the chart pulled. Detail the physical flow of the chart in each of those circumstances.

- **Chart organization:** Describe how the chart is organized, including: demographics, problem list, allergy list, medication list, past history, flow sheets, visit notes, phone encounters, labs results, other test results, clinical correspondence (e.g., consult notes), administrative correspondence, other.

- **Chart utilization:** How do physicians use the chart when they see a patient or call them on the phone: do they look at a single summary sheet or problem list, or do they review their last note or leaf through multiple old notes, or other.

- **Ordering process:** Describe the ordering process for the following: lab tests, radiology reports, hospital-based studies, referrals, and billing. Include the timing and modality (e.g., paper-based, verbal, or electronic).

- **Result Process:** How are test and referral results obtained. Is there a process to ensure that all orders were done. Describe the process that ensures that a physician has seen the results and documents its review and any action taken.

- **Finding External Clinical Information:** How do physicians find useful clinical information external to the chart, such as drug dosages, formularies, and treatment options.

- **Finding administrative Information:** How do physicians find useful administrative information, such as specialist phone numbers and billing information.

- **Current Computer Use:** How are physicians currently using computers in their offices, the hospital, or at home. Describe both medical and non-medical applications.

- **Communication:** How do physicians communicate with their office staff, with each other in the same office, and with physicians in other offices.

- **Computer Space:** Where in the physician's office can a computer physically fit. Specifically, is there space in exam rooms for any type of computer system.

- **Typical Day Workflow:** Detail a typical day for a physician, from seeing patients, to returning phone calls, to filling out paperwork. Look for obvious inefficiencies and problems that can be automated or improved with a computerized system.

Needs Analysis

Needs analysis studies should further clarify what informational needs are most important to physicians and define how those needs can be best met. This is usually done by a survey or a face-to-face meeting. The following lists questions which would be helpful in a needs analysis study:

- Describe the most important pieces of information you would want to have about every patient. Rank the following in order of importance: demographics, problem list, allergy list, medication list, visit notes, phone encounter notes, labs results, other test results, and referral letters.

- How often do you believe the patient chart is not available when needed?

- How often do you believe certain test results are not in the patient chart when needed?

- Do you find it difficult to effectively communicate with your staff or other physicians?

- Describe other bottlenecks or sources of frustration in your daily workflow.

- How do you see using a computer system in your workflow in the next year? How about in the next five years?

- What are your expectations about computer systems with respect to size, speed, cost, and reliability?

- What are your expectations about EHR systems? Do you think an EHR can increase your efficiency, improve your quality of care, or increase your revenues?

- What are your expectations about the access and security issues involved with EHR systems? How do you feel about home access, assigned passwords, biometric authentication, hardware tokens, audit trails, and other authentication and security devices and strategies?

- How do you think your patients would react to having a computer in the exam room?

- How do you feel about electronic communications (e.g., email or a more secure messaging system)? Do you or your staff want to send messages to patients (e.g., summary of lab results)? Does your organization want to receive patient messages about appointments, administrative issues, and/or clinical issues?

♦ How do you feel about allowing a patient to view parts of their EHR online, such as allergies, medications, problems, lab results, past and pending appointment times, etc.?

♦ What are the "good things" done by the information systems department?

♦ What are the "bad things" done by the information systems department? How can this be improved?

The Four Types of Physicians: The Electronic Health Record User Continuum

Although physicians have a number of similar characteristics, they are a very heterogeneous group due in part to their high intellectual aptitude, their strong desire for independence, and their unrelenting quest for perfection. It is therefore important that an implementation team recognize that they are not dealing with a single type of individual. Not acknowledging this fact has meant the failure of many EHR projects because too much time and energy is wasted on trying to change physicians, when instead it is the strategies themselves that should be altered to fit the users.

With respect to EHR adoption strategies, an appropriate way to understand and work with physicians is to think of them as being in four different groups based upon their willingness to use computerized systems in the office setting. These groups can be called the "Four Physician Types", and have been described by at least two separate authors (14,18). Type 1 is a "Resistant User" or technophobe, who will not directly use a computer system. Type 2 is a "Variable User", who will only use a computer in specific situations (e.g., to use ePrescribing only, or just do a simple Medline search or print out a patient education handout). Type 3 is a "Consistent User", who will use an EHR system if it provides some reasonable benefits to their practice style. And Type 4 is a "Technophile User", who believes so passionately in the technology and "rightness" of these systems, that they are willing to use an EHR in their workflow, even if the benefits are not always clear.

Every health care system has an assortment of these different physician types. And while the two extremes (Type 1 and 4) may be the most vocal, the majority of physicians lie in between them. Many of the strategies described in this chapter can be used for all physicians, but there are also individualized strategies that can be used for each of the four types described. The general vision is to move the Type 1 and 2 physicians towards Type 3 status, while satisfying the Type 3 and 4 physicians at the same time. An example of one system that had success with this type of evolutionary approach found that by providing volunteers with basic information on computers, and gradually adding functionality over time, they were able to gain the support of the majority of physicians in their enterprise (15). The following sections will describe some of the strategies that can be used to move physicians along this information technology continuum.

Type 1 Physicians: Resistant Users

These doctors are a difficult group with which to work. In fact, it is usually best to not expend too many resources on these physicians initially, as they may just cause the project team to become frustrated. Instead, start a slow "cultural shift" towards computerization (as described previously). This will involve providing these physicians with computer resources, sharing some of the benefits of computerizing parts of the medical record, and letting them see how well their colleagues are doing with the EHR system.

Over time, there may be several opportunities to start changing the perceptions and actions of Type 1 physicians. These opportunities usually involve improved access to patient information through automation of their paper-based processes. One example is an application that automatically prints all of a patient's new test results in a physician's office, no matter the source of the data. This could cut down on waiting time and improve quality by consolidating multiple sources of data. Physicians might even start asking to see flow charts of the lab data or how to obtain other clinical reports, such as echocardiogram readings or discharge summaries. And they will hopefully come to the conclusion that they can best access and analyze those reports at their offices, in their hospitals or at home—if they are willing to use a computer.

At some point, there may come a time when these users need to either get on board the train or get left behind. Executive support is of utmost importance at these junctures, and it may need to be explained that physicians not willing to transfer to these systems will be let go for no longer practicing at the standard of care being delivered by a group or institution.

Type 2 Physicians: Variable Users

These physicians will also benefit from the process of a cultural and technological shift described previously. Fortunately, they are more willing to alter their workflow if they believe a system will help them improve their efficiency or quality. They may use a single EHR function with all patients (e.g., results reporting) or they may use the full EHR application for a selected group of patients (e.g., the chronically ill). The appropriate strategy is thus to support their current use of the system, while offering them an increasingly more sophisticated set of solutions.

For example, many physicians may just use the results reporting function of an EHR system. You should support and encourage this function by making sure as many pieces of data as possible are in the system. You can then try to introduce other high-value functions such as clinical messaging, patient education handouts, prescription writing, and problem list maintenance. As you begin to show physicians the vast possibilities of using computers in their workflow, you should then try to increase the demand for these products while carefully managing their expectations.

Type 3 Physicians: Consistent Users

These physicians want to use an EHR because they believe in its benefits, but they will not use a system if it slows them down significantly or makes their workflow too complex. The strategy for this group is thus to ensure that you provide a truly usable EHR system and support them well. Their success will be one of the major factors in advancing the Type 1 and 2 physicians along the curve. Additionally, there should be strong and frequent lines of communication between these physicians and the IS department. The requests made by them will be made by many others if they are not addressed quickly.

Because these physicians will use an EHR system with all of their patients, they can also be provided with special features that can only be utilized by consistent users. One of these features involves reporting capabilities that allow a physician to more easily identify high-risk patients. For example, they can be sent a report that lists all heart failure patients who are not on ACE inhibitors or they can be allowed to quickly create a mailing which reminds all appropriate individuals to get an annual flu vaccine. A more complicated report could attempt to predict which patients are sickest, thus allowing disease management protocols to be used more effectively. Another high-profile example of reporting involves how physicians deal with drug recalls such as Baycol and Vioxx. Non-computerized physicians will either have to look through their charts, take calls from upset patients, or simply wait for the patient to show up at their next visit. But the Type 3 physicians using an EHR can easily get a list of all patients on a recalled drug, and the computer can even print out a letter to be mailed to all of them. Ideally, these types of actions would cause the demand for an EHR system to increase quickly in the Type 1 and 2 groups.

Type 4 Physicians: Technophile Users

These doctors enthusiastically use computers and fully accept the vision of the EHR. The strategy for them is similar to that for the Type 3 users: provide a good EHR system, support them well, and listen closely to their advice and comments. These physicians are often on the cutting edge of how to use technology, and they should help to envision future plans for the use of information technology in their organization. But be careful of basing the results of a clinical computing project on the success of these physicians alone. While it is important that they use the EHR system, their success will not readily translate to the other physician types in the organization. Because they are so knowledgeable about computer systems in general, they will likely perform at a much higher level than any of the other physicians. Alternatively, they may have unrealistic expectations about what an EHR system can do, and they can even be disruptive to your project if they become too demanding. One expert who has dealt with this problem suggests that you assign these individuals to a special EHR development task force, where they can have an advanced forum to provide their input (16).

Physician Involvement: Definitions and Strategies

It is crucial to involve physicians and their staff throughout the process of choosing, implementing, and maintaining an EHR system. As noted in the previous paragraphs, education and expectation management are important first steps to involve the majority of stakeholders. However, a healthcare system should also plan to identify, provide incentives, and define roles for physician leaders in their organization. The level of physician involvement can range from a Chief Medical Information Officer (CMIO) or similar "Physician Champion" to a Physician EHR Committee or general communications with any physician who is part of the system. The following definitions and strategies will help to clarify the different characteristics and roles for the physicians most involved in the EHR process.

Physician Leaders

In small medical groups that have successfully implemented an EHR system, there is always at least one physician who leads the charge in getting the system in place. In larger systems, it is equally vital to have one or more physicians devoted to doing this job for the whole organization. Various titles may apply, such as Chief Medical Information Officer (CMIO), Medical Director of Information Systems, Clinical Informatics Director, VP of Quality and Efficiency, EHR Guru, or any combination, but it should be clear that it is someone who concentrates on the EHR and related projects. Depending on the size of the organization and the abilities of these individuals, the responsibilities might be split different ways, such as inpatient vs. outpatient, or quality vs. implementation.

This individual (or group) often is the driving force in a successful EHR implementation and therefore needs to be identified and utilized correctly. Hospitals or groups with an EHR project in place have usually created and funded full or part-time positions for these clinicians-IT hybrids. Ideally, this person will have a background and understanding of computers and medical informatics and at least five to ten years of clinical experience. Characteristics of these physicians usually include a person who can communicate well and bridge the gap between the technologists in the IS department, the administrators in the organization, and the physicians in the clinics.

This physician needs to be a leader who is "willing to learn about the nature of systems, how to control them, and how to improve them", and must also "look beyond their own professional or organizational identities and see themselves as part of the larger system" (17). In other words, they need to be able to analyze and improve the current clinical workflow, understand that the benefits from an EHR system will only result if the system is adequately used by the majority of physicians, and feel comfortable representing all of the various types of physicians found in the organization. Lastly, the physician needs to be committed because this role may take between 50% and 100% of their time and resources.

Beware of the "Techno-Geek" as Leader

A potential mistake is to choose a physician who is a highly charged "techno-geek" because they are often more enamored with the technology itself than widespread implementation. This person often has a very good understanding of computers but may be most interested in helping to write EHR software and set up the network architecture rather than shifting culture, optimizing established systems and providing higher level strategy. While these physicians can be helpful in other ways, it is unlikely they will perform well as the clinical leader of an EHR project.

The Anti-Champion

An important point about physician involvement is to realize that not everybody will be on board from the start. There will never be an EHR system that satisfies absolutely everyone from the very beginning. Physicians with negative viewpoints should certainly be heard, but it is advised to not get too involved trying to respond to a vocal minority, nor to force these negative physicians to use a system they do not like. This will not only fail with that one physician, but will very likely produce an angry user who may create negative feeling across the whole institution. Instead, listen to their opinions, identify their fears and needs, and realize that the success of the EHR system in their colleagues' offices should eventually win them over.

The Physician Electronic Health Record Committee

The physician champion attempts to represent most physicians in the organization, but other forms of physician involvement are crucial as well. A physician EHR committee should include a group of physicians who are well-respected, knowledgeable about the different types of clinicians and workflow in their organization, and are interested in the general concept of improving quality and efficiency. The mandate of this committee should be to represent the organization's physicians in choosing and using EHR systems, and to disseminate information to their colleagues about how and why the system can benefit them and their organization.

At the start of a project, this committee should try to meet every month, more often if there are many decisions to decide. However, caution must be used in fully respecting the physicians' time and workload. For example, all meetings should have a clear agenda and the committee should have the power to make appropriate decisions. It also may be important to provide incentives for these physicians. Depending on the organizational structure and the time of involvement, this may vary from a nice meal during meetings to a partial subsidy of their salaries.

Superusers

Superusers are usually defined as computer-literate physicians or clinical staff who are willing to become early adopters and high-volume users of the system. Their offices may be used as pilot sites, and their success often helps to break through barriers of resistance. Therefore, it is very important to identify these users and expend extra resources to make sure their use of the system is successful.

Office Staff

A physician's office staff can provide invaluable information and support to an EHR project. Make sure to include them in the evaluation, implementation, and continued management of any EHR system.

Supporting Physicians

Support Desk

An effective and efficient "Help Desk" is a critical piece of the physician adoption puzzle. Physicians feel that time is their most important commodity, so they will want to know they can call a single phone number to get immediate assistance with their projects. While this initially may be for basic computer applications, they will remember how the IS department handled these calls when they consider whether to use an EHR system controlled by the same department. It is thus crucial to acquire a great support staff that understands the technology and knows how to talk with clinicians. Ideally, set up a dedicated phone line and email contact (e.g., DOCS@hospital.org) for physicians only.

Clinical Liaisons

IS departments attempting an EHR project should ensure they have an appropriate number of clinical liaisons. These are usually nurses or other clinical staff who have a good understanding of information systems and an excellent ability to understand and communicate with physicians. This group will act as a vital link between the IS department and the physicians. Besides serving as the main educators and trainers, they will help to define problems, create solutions, overcome barriers, and serve on the front-line in improving physician use and acceptance of EHR systems. And to achieve the highest amount of acceptance, the majority of this interaction should ideally be done as one on one sessions with physicians.

Re-Training and Optimization

As with most any application, initial EHR training will leave physicians with only a limited amount of knowledge about the system. No matter how much is taught initially, users will only be able to absorb the key elements needed to survive their day. Additionally, new functionality will be added over time. Therefore, it is important to consider how to re-engage physicians in the learning process months and years after the initial implementation.

First, figure out where to focus. Standardized surveys can help to identify stronger and weaker EHR users, as well as functionality that is underutilized. Training projects can then be designed to focus on the weaker users and/or the underutilized functionality. Do not try to accomplish too much at once, but rather focus on a small set of users or a few functionalities every one to two months. Perhaps one month is focused on working with the 20% of weakest users, and another month is for making sure everyone understands a specific workflow that involves a feature not typically used.

Second, consider who or how you will train/re-train your users. An ideal situation would be for a clinical liaison to work one on one with each user. A more realistic situation would be for the clinical liaison to rotate for at least one day in all the groups and clinics once a month, to interact with as many physicians as possible during that time, and to hand off some information to the "Superusers" at that office. But besides working with pre-identified users or teaching a specific new workflow, the clinical liaisons should also answer any other question that comes up (or promise to get an answer), and ask for the kind of feedback that only happens in face-to-face situations. A report on these interactions should be prepared and then used in future meetings to help prioritize what functionality or user will be focused upon next.

However, many organizations do not have the manpower to send out as many trainers as desired. So an increasingly common technique is to transmit educational messages electronically, such as with emails or via screencasts. An email is certainly the easiest way to quickly educate users. But make sure it is relatively short and clinically oriented. A good model to use is the following:

♦ A short summary at the top, since some physicians will only read a few lines, they won't read a detailed email. For example, one could say "A new enhancement allows user to now pick a favorite pharmacy for patients upon which they prescribe- more details below".

◆ Following the summary, there should be a detailed "FAQ" section, in which questions are asked from the perspective of a "typical user" and should address anything from "How do I do this" to "Why should I do this" to "What if I have more questions".

A screencast is a newer communication tool that captures all activity on a computer screen and converts those images into movies that show users how to perform a specific action or workflow. Written and verbal instructions may accompany these movies. For example, a one-minute movie could show how to create an order for a medication and then save that order to a user's favorite folder. A narrator would describe the action as it unfolds on the screen. The medical group would then post this movie online so that their users could view it at any time. This can be a powerful addition to simple email descriptions because the visuals will make it much more clear. There are a variety of free or low-priced tools that capture these movies (e.g., CamStudio), as well as free web sites that allow users to post movie clips such as these (e.g. YouTube).

Electronic Health Record Assistants

One of the major problems with physician adoption has been the issue of data entry. In many cases, the process of entering data in a computerized system takes longer than traditional methods such as handwriting and dictation. So even if there are long-term benefits to entering this data, there are few immediate benefits, thus creating a large barrier to using the system. Physicians have been using "provider extenders" to help them with similar tasks in their daily workflow for years. These extenders range from medical assistants to nurses to physician assistants. So it is no surprise that there has been discussion about informatics assistants for many years. One author even discussed the creation of a new type of medical support personnel, which he called the "Physician's Information Assistant" or PIA (18).

These assistants would be responsible for using the EHR system to both retrieve and input information for the physician. Alternatively, there may be a middle ground, in which the typical physician extenders take on some of the responsibilities of retrieving or entering data for their physicians. Lastly, an increasingly attractive option will be for patients to input some of their own data online either before or during their visit. Several EHR vendors and independent companies are now offering secure messaging portals that are starting to allow for this type of data collection process.

Choosing the Right Electronic Health Record System

There is no perfect EHR system, but there may be some systems that are a better fit for your organization and physicians, and there are some you clearly want to avoid. The following section describes strategies and tools that focus on helping to ensure the choice of an EHR system that will be most successfully accepted and used by physicians. This section can be used in conjunction with an earlier section of this book ("EHR Selection") that reviews the whole EHR selection process.

The "FIRST" Principles

The following five principles are critical for the successful adoption of any EHR system. It should be noted that although there will continue to be a "commoditization" of EHRs as they each acquire the same checklist of features, the underlying tenets of these principles will differentiate the best EHRs from the not so best ones.

1. **Flexible:** Individual physicians need to be able to practice the way they feel is best. Therefore, an EHR system should allow for multiple methods to document a visit, including writing, typing, templates, and dictation (whether for voice recognition and/or transcription). Additionally, a flexible EHR should let physicians individualize screens and create their own order sets, but ideally in manner that preserves appropriate consistency across the enterprise.

2. **Intuitive:** The system should be so easy to use that only minimal training time is needed to get started (e.g., less than one hour). More in-depth training should also be offered for advanced features.

3. **Reliable:** The system needs to act the same way day after day and not have software failures or errors. This may seem obvious, but because EHR systems are quickly evolving pieces of software, it is advisable to get statistics and guarantees about this issue. Additionally, the system should have no down time during active hours and should thus be supported via hardware and software redundancy. Finally, there should be clear and easy backup plans in case a problem occurs.

4. **Speedy:** Screen changes should be less than one or two seconds, and signing in and out must be quick. Data entry should be kept to a minimum. Allow doctors to document by any means available, including writing notes, checking off templates, or dictating. Do whatever is needed to ensure that the system is at least time-neutral.

5. **Topical:** The system needs to speak to the physician's specific workflow and needs. For a physician to use an EHR system, they must see that there are clear benefits that personally mean something to them. For example, many physicians expect EHR systems to make them more efficient. It therefore makes sense to identify some particularly inefficient workflow patterns and determine whether the EHR system can immediately help with that. These small wins will help build up confidence and usage of the system.

Interfaces

Physicians will appropriately expect that the EHR system will be connected to all the other computerized systems in the organization. To help deal with this important expectation, real-time interfaces should be a crucial feature examined in all EHR systems. Specifically, physicians will be more likely to use an EHR system if it interfaces with their practice management system, their transcription service, their lab information system, and their hospital's clinical data repository (CDR). With these interfaces, they can retrieve demographics, schedules, dictated notes, lab results, and any other result held in the CDR. Additionally, they can order lab tests and perform billing electronically via the EHR system. These features help to quickly overcome the barrier that would be encountered by starting an EHR project with no information populating its database.

Site Visits

Before choosing an EHR vendor, it will be important to perform site visits to at least two or three institutions using the EHR in similar practices. It is equally important to involve physicians in these evaluations. Additionally, you should try to bring along anyone else who will be using the system, such as nurses, clinical assistants, front office staff, transcriptionists, and billing administrators.

Define Active Clinical Users

When vendors describe how many users they have at their "busy sites", be sure to clarify what that means. Some vendors will include every potential user (including physicians, clinical staff, and administrative staff), while others might just count the physicians. However, it is more important to define "active clinical users", and to further define exactly which functions are being used. An EHR system can have a "great feature", but there may be a problem if clinicians are not using that feature routinely. For example, if a vendor describes a formulary feature as a key component of their system, they should clarify how many physicians are using the EHR to electronically write prescriptions at the point of care and how many of those are actively using the formulary function. A feature is only beneficial if it gets used.

Site Visit Questions

At the sites themselves, physicians should have the opportunity to talk with their peers about the specific EHR system. It will be important for them to talk with a wide cross-section of physicians at the site, not simply the superusers that the vendor wants them to meet. Specifically, this means that they should talk to those physicians who use the system occasionally or only use parts of the system. And assuming physicians do use the system differently, it will be important to try to distinguish why that is the case.

High Impact and Quick Wins

While improved quality and research may be important drivers for an organization, they are often not the driving force to get most physicians to change their workflow. The paragraphs below describe some high value and immediate functionality that can be used to help satisfy the goals of physicians. It will be important to consider features such as these when evaluating and choosing an EHR system.

High Value Features

Certain EHR features, such as "Results Reporting", "Clinical Messaging", and "Orders", can offer high value functionality to physicians by addressing their needs for improved access to information and increased efficiency of their routine tasks. Results reporting functionality allows physicians to view labs and other reports and ideally be notified that tests they have ordered have finalized. Other relevant actions include electronic attestation, confirming a physician's review of results and automated letter writing to inform patients of results. Clinical messaging is a sophisticated email-like system that provides a secure and reliable way for physicians to communicate with their staff, colleagues, or even patients. Finally, order entry applications can increase efficiency by computerizing certain routine tasks (e.g., lab ordering, prescription writing, patient handouts, billing).

Cost-effectiveness and quality can be improved with all of these functions by capture of relevant patient data in a centralized repository and by providing decision support tools at the point of care (e.g., drug interaction checking, formulary and referral management, E&M Coding evaluation). Additionally, once physicians are using certain modules, there will be more inertia for their evolutionary movement towards use of the full EHR suite.

Another high value feature involves the use of EHR data for analysis and reports for individual physicians. An example would be a monthly clinical report automatically generated about a physician's diabetic patients. An internist or endocrinologist might be more apt to use a system if he knew he would receive a monthly report about the rate of opthamological referrals or glycohemoglobin tests in his diabetic patients, especially if there was the opportunity to easily send patients personalized reminders about those tests.

Immediate Benefits

An EHR function that can increase efficiency within the first few days of use will help to improve adoption and thus secure the long-term benefits that are of such great interest. To help define an immediate benefit, use information from physician advisors, as well as workflow and needs analyses, to identify "key functions" that the majority of doctors would use on a daily basis. An obvious source for these key functions will come from close examination of normal tasks that are long and repetitive. Examples might include results reporting, prescription refills, referral forms, or patient summaries.

A specific example of an immediate benefit involves prescription management. Even on the first day of use, a physician should be able to obtain some benefits with this function. For example, consider a scenario where a doctor documents a patient's new diagnosis of hypertension and the EHR system provides a list of potential anti-hypertensive medications based upon physician preference, formulary restrictions, and individual patient characteristics (i.e., age, sex, race, weight, and co-morbidities). After the doctor chooses the desired medication, an expert system could ensure that there are no drug interactions, the prescription could be printed (or sent to the patient's pharmacy), and the electronic chart documents it all. On return visits, the system can allow for easy drug refills.

The Science of Change Management

The preceding part of this chapter explained very specific strategies and tactics for improving physician adoption of EHRs. However, it should be noted that many other industries, such as banking and retail, have pushed IT adoption much farther along than in healthcare. While it is true that healthcare is a more complex business that has not funded IT as much as these other industries, there are many lessons learned from seeing how other organizations have succeeded with change management. A few effective books and techniques in this arena are described below.

Leading Change

In this book (19) and its various sequels, a professor of leadership at Harvard Business School explains that successful change management requires a strong leadership team that can push an organization through its usual corporate inertia. An eight-stage model for implementing change is described:

◆ **Stage 1. Establish a sense of urgency:** People need to be telling each other, "Let's go, we need to change things!"

◆ **Stage 2. Create the guiding coalition:** Build a powerful group that can guide change.

◆ **Stage 3. Develop a vision and strategy:** The guiding coalition needs to develop the right vision and strategy for the change effort.

◆ **Stage 4. Communicate the vision:** People should understand why change is needed and agree with the plan to change.

- **Stage 5. Empower action:** Encourage more people to act on the vision.
- **Stage 6. Create short-term wins:** Momentum builds as people try to fulfill the vision, and fewer people resist change.
- **Stage 7. Don't let up:** Continue making changes until the vision is fulfilled.
- **Stage 8. Make change stick:** Reinforce the winning behavior despite the pull of tradition or a change in leadership.

Crucial Conversations: Tools for Talking When Stakes Are High

This book describes seven well-studied techniques for resolving conflicts and influencing people (20). This quickly becomes a good skill set to have as a clinical or technical leader who often needs to communicate effectively with a variety of administrators, technical staff, and physicians.

- **Start with heart:** Figure out what you really want, and stay focused on that.
- **Learn to look:** Be aware of others and notice when safety is at risk.
- **Make it safe:** Create a discussion in which anyone can talk about almost anything.
- **Master your stories:** Practice stories that keep you focused on the important issues, and control your emotions by controlling your story.
- **State my path:** Speak persuasively, not abrasively.
- **Explore others' paths:** Make sure to listen when others blow up or clam up.
- **Move to action:** Turn these crucial conversations into actions and results.

Getting to Yes: Negotiating Agreement Without Giving In

This is another classic book that describes a straightforward five-step system for how to behave in negotiations with a goal of creating a win-win situation (21).

- Don't bargain over positions.
- Separate people from the problem.
- Focus on interests, not positions.
- Invent options for mutual gain.
- Insist on using objective criteria.

Crossing the Chasm: Marketing and Selling High-Tech Products to Mainstream Customers

This book can be used to help better understand the range of users and how to best relate to each one (22). Interestingly, it may actually be most appropriate for the vendor side of the equation, in which it discusses how to move a product used by selected visionary customers to a mainstream market that needs to satisfy more pragmatic users.

Conclusion

Electronic Health Record systems have the potential to help physicians, patients, and administrators practice healthcare with a higher quality and greater efficiency than ever before. Fortunately, physicians are becoming more accustomed to a variety of information technologies in their lives and financial barriers are falling as systems get cheaper, other entities are paying for them, and rewards are being planned for their use.

However, ensuring physician acceptance and use of EHR systems remains a complex and important issue. Common causes of low levels of acceptance include ingrained practice styles, inefficient systems, and difficulty in creating immediate value for physicians. The top ten tips for physician adoption are listed in Table 11-2. This chapter has provided advice on how to improve education, understanding, involvement and support of physicians while also optimizing the choice and implementation of the EHR so that it has the best chance to be initially accepted and used long-term in an organization.

Table 11-2

THE TOP TEN TIPS FOR PHYSICIAN ADOPTION OF EHR SYSTEMS

1. Create a cultural shift towards computerization.
2. Ensure there is strong strategic and financial support from the executive level.
3. Educate physicians and their staff about the reasoning and process of an EMR system.
4. Correctly define and manage both high and low expectations.
5. Use workflow and needs analyses to improve understanding of physicians.
6. Identify, provide incentives for, and define roles for physician leaders and participants.
7. Provide excellent support, including quick and personalized training.
8. Choose a system that is fast, flexible, easy to use, reliable, and physician-oriented.
9. Prioritize functions with immediate benefits for physicians.
10. Create an ongoing system of training to ensure that physicians know how to use the system most optimally.

Recommended Books

- The Physician-Computer Conundrum
- Crossing the Quality Chasm Series (Institute of Medicine)
- Leading Change
- The Heart of Change: Real-Life Stories of How People Change Their Organizations
- Crossing the Chasm: Marketing and Selling High-Tech Products to Mainstream Customers
- Crucial Conversations: Tools for Talking When Stakes are High
- Getting to Yes: Negotiating Agreement Without Giving In

References

1. Anderson JD. Increasing the acceptance of clinical information. MD Comp. 1999;16:62-5.
2. Berkowitz LL. Breaking down the barriers: improving physician buy in of CPR systems. Healthc Inform. 1997;14:73-6.
3. Bria WF, Berkowitz LL, Gaillour FR, Wald J. Physician Adoption Strategies for CPR Systems. 1999 HIMSS Proceedings. 1999; Volume 3: 11-20.
4. Weaver MJ. Improving Physician Participation and Satisfaction with Information Systems and Technology. 1999 HIMSS Proceedings. 1999; Volume 4: 39-48.
5. Dambro MR, Weiss BD, McClure CL, Vuturo AF. An unsuccessful experience with computerized medical records in an academic medical center. J Med Educ. 1988;63:617-23.
6. Massaro TA. Introducing physician order entry at a major medical center. I: Impact on organizational culture and behavior. Acad Med. 1993;68:20-5.
7. Sicotte C, Denis JL, Lehou P. The computer based patient record: A strategic issue in process innovation. J Med Systems. 1998;22:431-43.
8. Sicotte C, Denis JL, Lehou P, Champagne F. The computer based patient record: Challenges towards timeless and spaceless medical practice. J Med Systems. 1998; 22:237-56.
9. Reed M, Grossman J. Growing Availability of Clinical Information Technology in Physician Practices. Center for Studying Health System Change, Data Bulletin No. 31, June 2006.
10. Berkowitz LL. Hospital Sponsorship of Ambulatory EHR Systems. Most Wired Online. July 10, 2005.
11. Institute of Medicine. To Err Is Human: Building a Safer Health System. Kohn LT, Corrigan JM, and Donaldson MS, eds. Washington, D.C: National Academy Press. 2000.
12. Institute of Medicine. To Err Is Human: Building a Safer Health System. Hurtado MP, Swift EK, Corrigan JM, eds. Washington, D.C: National Academy Press. 2001.
13. Johnston D, Bates DW, Pan E, Middleton B. The Value of Computerized Provider Order Entry in Ambulatory Settings. HIMSS Publications. 2003. More information online: http://www.citl.org/research/ACPOE.htm.
14. Berkowitz LL. Diagnosing doctors. Four types of physicians require four approaches to promote clinical computing acceptance. Healthc Inform. 1998;15:93-6.
15. Dewey JB, Manning P, Brandt S. Acceptance of direct physician access to a computer-based patient record in a managed care setting. Proc Ann Symp Comput Appl Med Care. 1993:79-83.

16. Bria WF, Rydell RL. The Physician-Computer Connection. American Hospital Publishing; 1996:28.
17. Nolan TW. Understanding medical systems. Ann Int Med. 1998;128:293-8.
18. Sachs R. Ten predictions of the future of electronic medical records. 1999 HIMSS Proceedings. 1999;2:99-105.
19. Kotter J. Leading Change. Harvard Business School Press. 1996.
20. Patterson K, Grenny J, McMillan R, Switzler A. Crucial Conversations: Tools for Talking When Stakes are High. McGraw-Hill Publishing. 2002.
21. Fisher R, Ury WL, Patton B. Getting to Yes: Negotiating Agreement Without Giving In. Penguin Publishing. 1991.
22. Moore, GM. Crossing the Chasm: Marketing and Selling High Tech Products to Mainstream Customers. New York: HarperCollins Publishers. 2002.
23. Audet A, Doty M, Peugh J, et al. Information technologies: when will they make it into physicians' black bags? MedGenMed. 2004;6:2.

12

Legal Issues and Health Care Information

Terri Thompson Mallett

Traditionally, physicians have maintained medical information in paper charts and physically transmitted patient data. However, an increasing number of health care providers and provider networks, managed care organizations, and payors have switched to an electric method of patient information storage. Federal regulations lay a basis for the protection of electronic records.

An electronic health record (EHR) system has the ability to capture clinical information concerning each encounter that a patient has with practitioners who are geographically and often organizationally dispersed in a single longitudinal patient record. A patient-centered medical record makes possible improvements in the quality, continuity, and cost-effectiveness of health care that are not achievable if each provider treating a patient maintains a separate record. As providers continue to transition from a hospital-based organization model to an integrated health care delivery system ("IDS"), patient clinical information must travel throughout the system quickly and efficiently over increasing distances, particularly with the emergence of widely dispersed referral networks, and be available to practitioners along the continuum of care.

It is increasingly common for all providers within an IDS to have access to patient information (including medical records information) maintained by every other provider within the IDS. For example, master patient indexes are being established to identify each patient uniquely and to facilitate linking patient data across numerous care settings. In addition, clinical data repositories and other shared clinical databases permit participating providers to capture all of the clinical data recorded about a patient at any point of care within an IDS over time.

An electronic or fully computer-based medical record is created on a computer (i.e., optical, digital, or magnetic media), authenticated by computer (i.e., computer key or computer code) and stored on media readable and retrievable by computer. The fact that the law is trailing advances in health information technology means that there often is an uncomfortable fit between law developed in an era of paper records and the manner in which providers now share patient information electronically in integrated delivery environments. The utilization of an EHRS thus raises myriad legal issues not generally of concern in the context of paper-based medical records including regulatory compliance, identification of acceptable media to store patient records, the validity of electronic signatures, ensuring the accuracy and reliability of patient records, maintaining the confidentiality and security of patient records accessible by computer, ownership of patient data, and contracting with vendors. Indeed the Code of Medical Ethics of the American Medical Association contains extensive guidance on protecting computerized medical records.

Medical records not only supply physicians and other health care professionals with necessary patient information, including personal and historical dates, but also contain information on the course of treatment and treatment result (1). Medical records are one of the most important means of communication in health care and are necessary for health care providers to diagnose and treat patients (1).

Federal Law

The Privacy Act of 1974 (2) (the "Act"), which applies only to federal agencies and health care facilities and which expressly covers medical records, restricts disclosure of records by federal agencies, guarantees individuals access to records that concern them, and requires agencies to make annual discloses of the existence of identifiable, personal information in the Federal Register. The Act extends to health care facilities operated by the federal government as well as to medical records systems operated under contract to the federal government. The Act does not extend to private entities and therefore has no direct impact on the private health care industry.

The Health Insurance Portability and Accountability Act of 1996 (HIPAA) (3) requires the Department of Health and Human Services (HHS) to adopt standards for electronic medical transactions (4). These regulations were to be implemented to provide protections for individual health information (4). HHS developed a proposed privacy rule governing individually identifiable health information and released it for public comment on November 3, 1999. The final regulation, the Privacy Rule, was published December 28, 2000 (4). In March 2002, the Department proposed and released for public comment modifications to the Privacy Rule. The final modifications were published in final form on August 14, 2002 (5).

Sections 261 through 264 of HIPAA require the Secretary of HHS to publicize standards for the electronic exchange, privacy, and security of health information. Collectively these are known as the Administrative Simplification provisions. HIPAA's Administrative Simplification sections outline a process for protecting the privacy of health information (2). These sections address the necessary criteria for standardizing electronic transmission of health information by focusing on the need to protect security, integrity, and authenticity of health information (2,6,8). These sections also discuss whom the regulations are to cover, what information is to be covered, what types of transactions are to be covered, and what penalties should accrue for violations of HIPAA (7).

The Privacy Rule (8), as well as all the Administrative Simplification rules, applies to health plans, health care clearinghouses, and to any health care provider who transmits health information in electronic form in connection with transactions for which the Secretary of HHS has adopted standards under HIPAA (the "covered entities") (8,9).

HIPAA states "covered entities are required to protect the confidentiality or integrity of medical information stored in electronic records and integrated information systems against 'reasonably anticipated threats'" (10). Under HIPAA, covered entities must implement safeguards that include regularly reviewing records that track patient information system activity, identifying and responding to security violations, and applying appropriate sanctions against employees who do not comply with a covered entity's security procedures and policies (8,10). Addressable safeguards include, but are not limited to: 1) implementation of procedures for the termination of access to electronic health records when employment ends; 2) implementation of procedures to determine whether or not the access of an employee is appropriate; 3) implementation of electronic procedures that would terminate an electronic session once a predetermined time has expired; and 4) implementation of electronic mechanisms that would corroborate whether electronic medical information has or has not been destroyed or altered (8,10).

In deciding which security measures to use, a covered entity must consider several factors, including: the size, complexity, and capabilities of the covered entities; the covered entity's technical infrastructure and hardware and software security capabilities; the cost of security measures; and the probability and criticality of potential risk to electronic protected health information (12). However, a covered entity generally has much flexibility in deciding what security measures to use in accordance with these factors because entities "differ not only in the nature and scope of their businesses, but also in the degree of sophistication of their information systems and information needs" (4,13).

Although HIPAA mandates efficiency and security in an electronic system, it fails to sufficiently protect private information by allowing an entity to determine how it will protect sensitive information. This is problematic because HIPAA serves the public interest in health care but does not adequately safeguard the personal interest in privacy. Privacy concerns and social goals are not absolutes (13). Achieving one and not the other is insufficient. The implementation of these safeguards should b stricter, monitored more closely, and enforced with sanctions for covered entities that fail to comply.

The Standards for Privacy of Individually Identifiable Health Information (the Standards) "protect the privacy of individually identifiable health information in prescribed settings" (4,5), and their general purpose s to "improve the efficiency and effectiveness of public and private health programs and health care services by providing enhanced protections for individually identifiable health information" (4,5). The Privacy Rule standards address the use and disclosure of individuals' health information (called "protected health information" by organizations subject to the Privacy Rule) called "covered entities," as well as standards for individuals' privacy rights to understand and control how their health information is used (4,5). In addition, public concern for the breakdown of the privacy surrounding individually identifiable health information maintained by health care providers was recognized regarding electronic technology in the health care industry (4,5).

A major goal of the Privacy Rule is to ensure that individuals' health information is properly protected while allowing the flow of health information needed to provide and promote high-quality health care and to protect the public's health and well being. The Rule strikes a balance that permits important uses of information, while protecting the privacy of people who seek care and healing. Given that the health care marketplace is diverse, the Rule is designed to be flexible and comprehensive to cover the variety of uses and disclosures that need to be addressed.

The Privacy Rule protects all "individually identifiable health information" held or transmitted by a covered entity or its business associate, in any form or media, whether electronic, paper, or oral. The Privacy Rule calls this information "protected health information (PHI)" (14). The Privacy Rule excludes from PHI employment records that a covered entity maintains its capacity as an employer and education and certain other records subject to, or defined in, the Family Educational Rights and Privacy Act (15).

The Standards seek a balance between the needs of patients and needs of society and create a "framework of protection" that sets rules that can be strengthened by both the federal government and the states as health information systems continue to evolve (15).

The responsibility for enforcing the Standards has been delegated to the HHS's Office for Civil Rights (OCR) (15). The OCR s responsible for working with covered entities to secure voluntary compliance through the provision of technical assistance; responding to questions regarding the regulations and providing interpretations and guidance; responding to state requests for exception determinations investigating complaints and conducting compliance reviews; and, where voluntary compliance cannot be achieved, seeking civil monetary penalties and making referrals for criminal prosecution (15). The Standards promulgated by the HHS are seemingly protective, and the OCR's enforcement activities encompass a great deal. However, these provisions may not be enough to secure patient privacy in an increasingly electronic health care system.

Federal officials say electric records can make hospitals more efficient, reduce medical errors, and lower health care costs (16). However, confidentiality and privacy, if unaddressed, are in jeopardy in an electronic system. In addition, judicial precedent protects the right to privacy but also promotes overriding public policy.

"A right to privacy in personal information has historically found expression in American law." (4). Individual rights traditionally have been placed at the forefront of democracy (4,5). Several rights in the Constitution attempt to protect individual privacy "while balancing it against the larger social purposes of the nation" (4,5). The courts, however, have struggled with the balancing of new technological advancements against a constitutional "right to privacy."

Covered Entities

Health Plans

Individual and group plans that provide or pay the cost of medical are covered entities (14,17). Health plans include health, dental, vision, and prescription drug users, health maintenance organizations, Medicare, Medicaid, Medicare supplement insurers, and long-term care insurers (excluding nursing home fixed-indemnity policies). A group health plan with fewer than 50 participants that is administered solely by the employer that established and maintains the plan is not a covered entity. Two types of government-funded programs are not health plans: 1) those whose principal purpose is not providing or paying the cost of health care, such as food stamp programs; and 2) those programs whose principal activity is directly providing health care, such as a community health center, or the making of grants to fund the direct provision of health care (2,8). Even if an entity, such as a community health center, does not meet the definition of a health plan, it may meet the definition of a health care provider, and, if it transmits health information in electronic form in connection with the transactions for which the Secretary of HHS has adopted standards under HIPAA, may still be a covered entity. Certain types of insurance entities are also not health plans, including entities providing only workers' compensation, automobile insurance, and property and casualty insurance (2,8).

Health Care Providers

Every health care provider, regardless of size, who electronically transmits health information in connection with certain transactions, is a covered entity. These transactions include claims, benefit eligibility inquiries, referral authorization requests, or other transactions for which HHS has established standards under the HIPAA Transaction Rule (14,17). Using electronic technology, such as email, does not mean a health care provider is a covered entity; the transmission must be in connection with a standard transaction. The Privacy Rule covers a health care provider whether it electronically transmits these transactions directly or uses a billing service or other third party to do so on its behalf. Health care providers include all "providers of services" and "providers of medical or health services" as defined by Medicare, and any other person or organization that furnishes, bills, or is paid for health care (2,8).

Health Care Clearinghouse

Health care clearinghouses are entities that process nonstandard information they receive from another entity into standard, or vice versa (14). In most instances, health care clearinghouse will receive individually identifiable health information only when they are providing these processing services to a health plan or health care provider as a business associate. Health care clearinghouses include billing services, re-pricing companies, community health management information systems, and value-added networks and switches if these entities perform clearing house functions.

Business Associates

In general, a business associate is a person or organization, other than a member of a covered entity's workforce, that performs certain functions or activities on behalf of, or provides certain services to, a covered entity that involve the use or disclosure of individually identifiable health information. Business associate services to a covered entity are limited to legal, actuarial, accounting, consulting, data aggregation, management, administration, accreditation, or financial services. Business associate functions or activities on behalf of a covered entity include claims processing, data analysis, utilization review, and billing (14).

When a covered entity uses a contractor or other non-workforce member to perform "business associate" services or activities, the Rule requires that the covered entity include certain protections for the information in a business associate agreement. In the business associate contract, a covered entity must impose specified written safeguards on the individually identifiable health information used or disclosed by its business associates (20), and a covered entity may not contractually authorize its business associate to make any use or disclosure of protected health information that would violate the Rule (8,21).

Protected Information

The Privacy Rule protects all individually identifiable health information held or transmitted by a covered entity or its business associate, in any form or media, whether electronic, paper, or oral. Individually identifiable health information is information, including demographic, data that relates to:

♦ the past, present, or future physical or mental heath or condition of an individual,

♦ the provision of health care to the individual, or

♦ the past, present, or future payment for the provision of health care to the individual

and that identifies the individual or for which there is a reasonable basis to believe it can be used to identify the individual (14). The Privacy Rule excludes from protected health information employment records that a covered entity maintains in its capacity as an employer and education and certain other records subject to, or defined in, the Family Educational Rights and Privacy Act (23).

Health information can be de-identified in one of two ways: 1) a formal determination by a qualified statistician; or 2) the removal of specified identifiers of the individual and of the individual's relatives, household members, and employers is required, and is adequate only if the covered entity has no actual knowledge that the remaining information could be used to identify the individual (23).

Uses and Disclosures

A major purpose of the Privacy Rule is to define and limit the circumstances in which an individual's protected health information may be used or disclosed by covered entities. A covered entity may not use or disclose protected health information, except either 1) as the Privacy Rule permits or requires or 2) as the individual who is the subject of the information (or the individual's personal representative) authorized in writing (24).

A covered entity must disclose protected health information in only two situations: 1) to individuals (or their personal representatives) specifically when they request access to, or an accounting of disclosures of, their protected health information and 1) to HHS when it is undertaking a compliance investigation or review or enforcement action (24).

A covered entity is permitted, but not required, to use and disclose protected health information, without an individual's authorization, for the following purposes or situations:

1. to the individual (unless required for access or accounting disclosures),

2. treatment, payment, and health care operations,

3. opportunity to agree or object,

4. incident to an otherwise permitted use and disclosure (24),

5. public interest and benefit activities, and

6. limited data set for the purposes of research, public health or health care operations (24).

Covered entities may rely on professional ethics and best judgments in deciding which of these permissive uses and disclosures to make.

A covered entity may disclose protected health information for the treatment activities of any health care provider, the payment activities of another covered entity involving either quality or competency assurance activities or fraud and abuse detection and compliance activities, if both covered entities have or had a relationship with the individual and the protected health information pertains to the relationship.

- **Treatment (25)** is the provision, coordination, or management of health care and related services for an individual by one or more health care providers, including consultation between providers regarding a patient and referral of a patient by one provider to another.

- **Payment (25)** encompasses activities of a health plan to obtain premiums, determine or fulfill responsibilities for coverage and provision of benefits, and furnish or obtain reimbursement for health care delivered to an individual and activities of a health care provider to obtain payment or be reimbursed for the provision of health care to an individual.

- **Health care operations (25)** are any of the following activities:
  1. quality assessment and improvement activities,
  2. competency assurance activities, including provider or health plan performance evaluation, credentialing, and accreditation,
  3. conducting or arranging for medical reviews, audits, or legal services,
  4. specified insurance functions,
  5. business planning, development, management, and administration, and
  6. business management and general administrative activities of the entity.

Most uses and disclosures of psychotherapy notes for treatment, payment, and health care operations purposes require an authorization (26).

Obtaining written permission from individuals to use and disclose their protected health information for treatment, payment, and health care operations is optional under the Privacy Rule for all covered entities (27). The content of a consent form, and the process for obtaining consent, are at the discretion of the covered entity electing to seek consent.

Informal permission may be obtained by asking the individual outright, or by circumstances that clearly give the individual the opportunity to agree, acquiesce, or object. Where the individual is incapacitated, in an emergency situation, or not available, covered entities may make such uses and disclosures if in the exercise of their professional judgment the use or disclosure is determined to be in the best interest of the individual. A covered health care provider may rely on an individual's informal permission to list their name, general condition, and location in the facility in its directory (28). The provider may then disclose the individual's condition and location in the facility to anyone asking for the individual by name. Religious affiliation may also be disclosed to members of the clergy.

A covered entity also may rely on an individual's information permission to disclose to family, relatives, or friends or to other persons whom the individual identifies, protected health information directly relevant to that person's involvement in the individual's care or payment for care (29). This provision, for example, allows a pharmacist to dispense filled prescriptions to a person acting on behalf of the patient.

The Privacy Rule also permits use and disclosure of protected health information, without authorization or permission, for 12 national priority purposes (30). Specific conditions or limitations apply to each public interest purpose, striking the balance between the individual privacy interest and the public interest need for this information. Such priority purposes include the following:

1. Covered entities may use and disclose protected health information without authorization as **required by law** (30-32);

2. Covered entities may disclose protected health information to accomplish **public health activities** (30);

3. In certain circumstances, covered entities may disclose protected health information to appropriate government authorities regarding **victims of abuse, neglect, or domestic violence** (30);

4. Covered entities may disclose protected health information to health oversight agencies for purposes of legally authorized **oversight activities**, such as audits and investigations necessary for oversight of the health care system and government benefit programs (30);

5. Covered entities may disclose protected health information in a **judicial or administrative proceeding** if the request for the information is through an order from a court or administrative tribunal or in response to a subpoena or other lawful process (30,33,34);

6. Covered entities may disclose protected health information to law enforcement officials for **law enforcement purposes** under specific circumstances and subject to specified conditions (27,30);

7. Covered entities may disclose protected health information to funeral directors, as needed, and to coroners and medical examiners

to identify a deceased person, determine the cause of death, and perform other functions authorized by law (30);

8. Covered entities may use or disclose protected health information to facilitate the **donation and transplantation of cadaveric organs, eyes, and tissue** (30);

9. The Privacy Rule permits a covered entity to use and disclose protected health information for **research** purposes, without authorization, provided the covered entity obtains 1) documentation that an alteration or waiver of authorization for the use or disclosure of protected health information about them for research purposes has been approved by an Institutional Review Board or Privacy Board; 2) representations from the researcher that the use or disclosure of the protected health information is solely to prepare a research protocol, that the researcher will not remove any protected health information from the covered entity and that protected health information for which access is sought is necessary for the research; or, 3) representations from the researcher that the use or disclosure sought is solely for research on the protected health information of decedents, that the protected health information sought is necessary for the research, and, at the request of the covered entity, documentation of the death of the individuals about whom information is sought (25). A covered entity also may use or disclose a limited data set of protected health information for research purposes without authorization (23);

10. Covered entities may disclose protected health information that they believe is necessary to prevent or lessen a **serious or imminent threat to the health or safety** a person or the public, when such disclosure is made to someone they believe can prevent or lessen the threat (30);

11. An authorization is not required to use or disclose protected health information for certain essential government functions. Such functions include: assuring proper execution of a military mission, conducting intelligence and national security activities that are authorized by law, providing protective services to the President, making medical suitability determinations for U.S. State Department employees, protecting the health and safety of inmates or employees in a correctional institution, and determining eligibility for or conducting enrollment in certain government benefit programs (30); and,

12. Covered entities may disclose protected health information as authorized by, and to comply with, workers' compensation laws and other similar programs providing benefits for work-related injuries or illnesses (30).

A limited data set is protected health information from which certain specified direct identifiers of individuals and their relatives, household members, and employers have been removed (23). It may be used and disclosed for research, health care operations, and public health purposes, provided the recipient enters into a data use agreement promising specified safeguards for the protected health information within the limited data set.

Authorized Uses and Disclosures

A covered entity must obtain written authorization for any use or disclosure of protected health information that is not for treatment, payment, or health care operations or otherwise permitted or required by the Privacy Rule (26). A covered entity may not condition treatment, payment, enrollment, or benefits eligibility on an individual granting an authorization, except in limited circumstances. A covered entity, however, may condition the provision of health care solely to generate protected health information for disclosure to a third party on the individual giving authorization to disclose the information to the third party (26).

All authorizations must be in plain language and contain specific information regarding the information to be disclosed or used, the person(s) disclosing and receiving the information, expiration, right to revoke in writing, and other data.

A covered entity must obtain authorization to use or disclose psychotherapy notes (25), except that the covered entity who originated the notes may use them for treatment and a covered entity may use or disclose the psychotherapy notes for its own training and to defend itself in legal proceedings brought by the individual without authorization.

A covered entity must obtain an authorization to use or disclose protected health information for marketing, except for face-to-face marketing communications between a covered entity and an individual, and for the provision of promotional gifts of nominal value by a covered entity (24,26). No authorization is needed, however, to make a communication that falls within one of the exceptions to the marketing definition (8).

Limiting Uses and Disclosures

A covered entity must make reasonable efforts to use, disclose, and request only the minimum amount of protected health information needed to accomplish the intended purpose of the use, disclosure, or request (4). When the minimum necessary standard applies to a use or disclosure, a covered entity may not use, disclose, or request the entire medical record for a particular purpose, unless it can specifically justify the whole record as the amount reasonably needed for the purpose.

A covered entity must develop and implement policies and procedures that restrict access and uses of protected health information based on the specific roles of the members of their workforce. These policies and procedures must identify the persons, or classes of persons, in the workforce who need access to protected health information to carry out their duties, the categories of protected health information to which access is needed, and any conditions under which they need the information to do their jobs.

The policies and procedures must also address routine, recurring disclosures, or requests for disclosures, that limit the protected health information disclosed to that which is the minimum amount reasonably necessary to achieve the purpose of the disclosure. Individual review of each disclosure in not required. For non-routine, non-recurring disclosures, or requests for disclosures that it makes, covered entities must develop criteria designed to limit disclosures to the information reasonably necessary to accomplish the purpose of the disclosure and review each of these requests individually in accordance with the established criteria.

If another covered entity makes a request for protected health information, a covered entity may rely, if reasonable under the circumstances, on the request as complying with this minimum necessary standard. Similarly, a covered entity may rely upon requests as being the minimum necessary protected health information from 1) a public official, 2) a professional who is a business associate of the covered entity seeking the information to provide services to or for the covered entity, or 3) a researcher who provides the documentation or representation required by the Privacy Rule for research.

Individual Rights

A covered health care provider with a direct treatment relationship with individuals has been required to deliver a privacy practice notice to patients since April 14, 2003 (35).

- Not later than the first service encounter by personal delivery, by automatic and contemporaneous electronic response, and by prompt mailing;
- By posting the notice at each service delivery site in a clear and prominent place where people seeking service may reasonably be expected to be able to read the notice; and
- In emergency treatment situations, the provider must furnish its notice as soon as practicable after the emergency abates.

The Privacy Rule requires that the notice contain certain elements (8), which include:

1. The notice must describe the ways in which the covered entity may use and disclose protected health information;

2. The notice must state the duties of the covered entity to protect privacy, provide a notice of privacy practices and abide by the terms of the current notice;

3. The notice must describe individuals' rights, including the right to complain to HHS and to the covered entity if they believe their privacy rights have been violated (36-40);

4. The notice must include a point of contact for further information and for making complaints to the covered entity.

Covered entities must act in accordance with their notices. The Rule also contains specific distribution requirements for direct treatment providers, all other health care providers, and health plans.

Covered entities, whether direct treatment providers or indirect treatment providers, such as laboratories, or health plans must supply notice to anyone on request (35). A covered entity must also make its notice electronically available on any web site it maintains for customer service or benefits information.

The covered entities in an organized health care arrangement may use a joint privacy practices notice, as long as each agrees to abide by the notice content with respect to the protected health information created or received in connection with participation in the arrangement (35). Distribution of a joint notice by any covered entity participating in the organized health care arrangement at the first point that an OHCA member has an obligation to provide notice satisfies the distribution obligation of the other participants in the organized health care arrangement.

A health plan must distribute its privacy practices notice to each of its enrollees by its Privacy Rule compliance date. Thereafter, the health plan must give its notice to each new enrollee at enrollment, and send a reminder upon request. A health plan satisfies its distribution obligation by furnishing the notice to the "named insured" (the subscriber for coverage that also applies to spouses and dependents).

A covered health care provider with a direct treatment relationship with individuals must make a good faith effort to obtain written acknowledgement from patients of receipt of the privacy practice notice unless in an emergency treatment situation (35). The Privacy Rule does not prescribe any particular content for the acknowledgement. However, the provider must document the reason for any failure to obtain the patient's written acknowledgement.

Administrative Requirements

HHS recognizes that covered entities range from the smallest provider to the largest, multi-state health plan. Thus, flexibility and scalability of the Rule are intended to allow covered entities to analyze their own needs and implement solutions appropriate for their own environment. To ensure compliance with the Rule, a covered entity must:

♦ Develop and implement written privacy policies and procedures that are consistent with the Privacy Rule.

♦ Designate a privacy official responsible for developing and implementing its privacy policies and procedures, and a contact person or contact office responsible for receiving complaints and providing individuals with information on the covered entity's privacy practices.

♦ Train all workforce members on its privacy policies and procedures, as necessary and appropriate for them to carry out their functions (14). A covered entity must have and apply appropriate sanctions against workforce members who violate its privacy policies and procedures or the Privacy Rule.

♦ Mitigate, to the extent practicable, any harmful effect it learns was caused by use or disclosure of protected health information by its workforce or its business associates in violation of its privacy policies and procedures or the Privacy Rule.

♦ Maintain reasonable and appropriate administrative, technical and physical safeguards to prevent intentional or unintentional use or disclosure of protected health information in violation of the Privacy Rule and to limit its incidental use and disclosure pursuant to otherwise permitted or required use or disclosure.

♦ Establish procedures for individuals to complain about its compliance with its privacy policies and procedures and the Privacy Rule. The covered entity must explain those procedures in its privacy practices notice (35).

♦ Maintain, until six (6) years after the later of the date of their creation or last effective date, its privacy policies and procedures, its privacy practices notices, disposition of complaints, and other actions, activities and designations that the Privacy Rule requires to be documented (41).

A covered entity may not retaliate against a person for exercising rights provided by the Privacy Rule, for assisting in an investigation by HHS or another appropriate authority, or for opposing an act or practice that the person believes in good faith violates the Privacy Rule (4). A covered entity may not require an individual to waive any right under the Privacy Rule as a condition for obtaining treatment, payment, and enrollment or benefits eligibility (41).

The only administrative obligations with which a fully insured group health plan that has no more than enrollment data and summary health information is required to comply are the 1) ban on retaliatory acts and waiver of individual rights and 2) documentation requirements with respect to plan documents if such documents are amended to provide for the disclosure of protected health information to the plan sponsor by a health insurance issuer or HMO that services the group health plan (41).

Enforcement and Penalties for Noncompliance

All covered entities, including small health plans, were required to be compliant with the Privacy Rule by April 14, 2004 (14,42). Consistent with the principles for achieving compliance provided in the Rule, HHS will seek the cooperation of covered entities and may provide technical assistance to help them voluntarily comply with the Rule (43). The Rule provides processes for persons to file complains with HHS, describes the responsibilities of covered entities to provide records and compliance reports and to cooperate with, and permit access to information for, investigations and compliance reviews.

HHS may impose civil money penalties on a covered entity of $100 per failure to comply with a Privacy Rule requirement (44). That penalty may not exceed $25,000 per year for multiple violations of the identical Privacy Rule requirement in a calendar year. Additionally, HHS may not impose a civil money penalty under specific circumstances, such as when a violation is due to reasonable cause and did not involve willful neglect and the covered entity corrected the violation within 30 days of when it knew or should have known of the violation.

A person who knowingly obtains or discloses individually identifiable health information in violation of HIPAA faces a fine of $50,000 and up to one year imprisonment (45). The criminal penalties increase to $100,000 and up to five years imprisonment if the wrongful conduct involves false pretenses, and to $250,000 and up to ten years imprisonment if the wrongful conduct involves the intent to sell, transfer or use individually identifiable health information for commercial advantage, personal gain, or malicious harm. Criminal sanctions will be enforced by the Department of Justice.

State Law

Several states have laws that contemplate the use of EHR services (46-51). These statutes and/or regulations reinforce the importance of safeguarding the authenticity, security, and confidentiality of computerized medical records. In some states that lack any meaningful statutory or regulatory guidance on the use of EHRS, such as Wisconsin, case law authority has begun to define what state legislatures and health departments have not. In these states, hospitals should determine whether, and to what extent, the state courts have interpreted existing statutory or regulatory law to apply to EHR services. For hospitals in other states, it may be prudent to look for guidance to the standards set forth in New York's current medical records amendments. Since there are a number of ways for a hospital to customize such a system, each hospital should consider designing its own system with the proper safeguards for authenticity, security, and confidentiality.

In states lacking statutes and regulations that directly relate to the use of EHR services, hospitals may need to determine whether existing law has been interpreted by the courts to apply to electronic systems. In Wisconsin, for example, a court recently ruled that the existing statute requiring written prescription orders be signed by the prescribing physician, could be interpreted to allow the use of computer-transmitted prescriptions (52). Recognizing that the existing statute did not contemplate the use of computers to transmit prescriptions electronically from physician to pharmacy, the Wisconsin Court of Appeals held that such transmissions were similar to prescriptions transmitted orally by telephone, which the statute expressly allowed to be filled without being signed by the physician.

Missouri and Kansas have implemented provisions for hospital records. States also have confidentiality requirements for other types of health care providers. "The patient's medical records shall be maintained to safeguard against loss, defacement, and tampering and to prevent damage from fire and water. Medical records shall be preserved in a permanent file in the original, on microfilm, or within other electronic media." (50) "Each medical record shall be treated as confidential. Only persons authorized by the governing body shall have access to the records.... Medical records shall be the property of the hospital and shall not be removed from the hospital premises except as authorized by the governing body of the hospital or for purposes of litigation when specifically authorized by Kansas law or appropriate court order" (51).

Case Law

In United States v. Westinghouse Electric Corp. (52), the Court of Appeals for the Third Circuit attempted "to reconcile the privacy interests of employees in their medical records with the significant public interest in research designed to improve occupational safety and health" by determining whether the National Institute for Occupational Safety and Health (NIOSH) could direct an employer to produce documents under the Occupational Safety and Health Act of 1970 (52).

In 1978, NIOSH received a complaint from a workers' union at Westinghouse Electric Corporation's plant, alleging that workers were suffering allergic reactions. In response, NIOSH initiated an investigation and visited the site and requested access to company medical records of potentially affected employees (52). Westinghouse supplied a list of employees then in the area affected, but denied information regarding present employees no longer working in the affected area and denied access to all medical records. Thereafter, NIOSH issued a subpoena duces tecum requiring Westinghouse to produce the medical records. Westinghouse refused, and the district court granted NIOSH's petition and ordered full enforcement of the subpoena.

On appeal, the circuit court found

> proliferation in the collection, recording and dissemination of individual information has made the public, Congress and the judiciary increasingly alert to the threat such activity can pose to one of the most fundamental and cherished rights of American citizenship, falling within the right characterized by Justice Brandeis as "the right to be let alone." (52,54)

The court went on: "Information about one's body and state of health is a matter which the individual is ordinarily entitled to retain within the 'private enclave where he may lead a private life'" (52,53). To weigh the competing interests of privacy and public interest, the court said it must consider several factors, including the type of record requested, the adequacy of safeguards to prevent unauthorized disclosure, and whether there is an express statutory mandate, articulated public policy, or other recognizable public interest militating toward access. Other factors considered by the court include "the information (a requested record) does or might contain, the potential for harm in any subsequent nonconsensual disclosure, the injury from disclosure to the relationship in which the record was generated" and "the degree of need for access."

In light of these considerations, the court held "the most appropriate procedure is to require NIOSH to give prior notice to the employees whose medical records it seeks to examine and to permit the employees to raise a personal claim of privacy, if they desire" (52). However, once medical records are integrated into the electronic world, courts may not be able to protect how they are used, in what way they are used, and for which purposes they are used.

In Whalen v. Roe (60), the United States Supreme Court addressed the issue of whether a state may record, in a centralized computer file, the names and addresses of persons who have obtained a prescription for certain drugs for which there is both a lawful and unlawful market. In response to concerns that drugs with both legitimate and illegitimate uses were being diverted into unlawful channels, the New York state legislature created a special commission to evaluate the state's drug-control laws. The resulting statute classified potentially harmful drugs in five schedules, of which Schedule II contained the most dangerous drugs used for legitimate purposes and were required all Schedule II prescriptions to be forwarded to the New York State Department of Health and to be sorted, coded, logged, and recorded for processing by a computer.

Before the statute was to take effect, a group of patients regularly receiving Schedule II prescriptions, physicians who prescribe such drugs, and two associations of physicians filed suit, alleging that such a recording violated their constitutionally protected right to privacy. The court held, by recording private prescription information in a centralized database, the state had not invaded any right or liberty of its citizens protected by the Fourteenth Amendment (60).

References

1. Briggs W. Andrews, Medical Records Liability, 6 HEALTH LAW 11, 11 (Summer 1992).
2. 5 U.S.C. §552a. Available at: www.usdoj.gov/oip/privstat.htm.
3. Public Law 104-191 (codified at 42 U.S.C.A. §§1320 et seq.). Available at: aspe.hhs.gov/admnsimp/pl104191.htm.
4. Standards for Privacy of Individually Identifiable Health Information, 45 C.F.R. Parts 160 and 164. Available at: www.hhs.gov/ocr/hipaa/finalmaster.html.
5. Standards for Privacy of Individually Identifiable Health Information, 67 FR 53182 (August 14, 2002).
6. Veling W. Tsai, Cheaper and Better: The Congressional Administrative Simplification Mandate Facilitates the Transition to Electronic Medical Records, 19 J. LEGAL MD. 549, 51 (1998).
7. S.C. Med. Ass'n v. Thompson, 327 F.3d 346 (4th Cir. 2003).
8. http://www.hhs.gov/ocr/hipaa.
9. http://cs.hhs.gov/hipaa/hipaa2/support/tools/decisionsupport/default.asp.
10. Michelle C. Pierre, Note, New Technology, Old Issues: The All-Digital Hospital and Medical Information, Privacy, 56 RUTGERS L. REV. 541 550 (2004).
11. 45 C.F.R. §164.308(a).
12. 45 C.F.R. §164.306(b)(2).
13. Melissa Steward, Electronic Medical Records: Privacy, Confidentiality, Liability, The Journal of Legal Medicine 26: 461-506 (2005).
14. 4 CFR §160.103.
15. 20 U.S.C. §1232g.
16. Associated Press, Hospitals Move toward "Paperless" Age, Aug. 4, 2004. Available at http://msnbc.msn.com/id/5592501.
17. 45 CFR §§160.102.
18. Social Security Act, §1172(a)(3).
19. 42 U.S.C. §1320d-1(a)(3).
20. 45 CFR §§164.502(e), 164.50(c).
21. http://www.hhs.gov/ocr/hipaa/contractprov.html
22. The Family Educational Rights and Privacy Act is found at 20 USC §1323g.
23. 45 CFR §164.514(b).
24. 45 CFS §164.502(a).
25. 45 CFR §164.501.
26. 45 CFR §164.508(a)(2).
27. 45 CFR §164.506(b).
28. 45 CFR §164.510(a).
29. 45 CFR §164.510(b).
30. 45 CFR §164.512.
31. Ohio Legal Rights Service v. Buckeye Ranch, Inc., 365 F.Supp.2d 877, 886 (S.D. Ohio 2005) (Subsection (1) is an exception that stands on its own, allowing a covered entity to make a disclosure otherwise prohibited by HIPAA if that disclosure is required by another law.).
32. Protection & Advocacy System, Inc. v. Freudenthal, 412 F. Supp. 2d 1211, 1218 (D. Wyo. 2006) (The Privacy Rule was intended to develop a procedure for handling protected health information and not to create or change substantive law).

33. Crenshaw v. Mony Life Insurance Co., 318 F. Supp. 2d 1015, 1029 (D. Cal. 2004).
34. Hutton v. City of Martinez, 219 F.R.D. 164, 167 (D. Cal. 2003).
35. 45 CFR §164.520.
36. Johnson v. Quander, 370 F. Supp. 2d 79, 100 (D.D.C. 2005).
37. O'Donnell v. Blue Cross Blue Shield of Wyo., 173 F. Supp. 2d 1176 (D. Wyo. 2001).
38. Brock v. Provident Am. Ins. Co., 144 F. Supp. 2d 652 (N.D. Tex. 2001).
39. Means v. Indep. Life and Accident Ins. Co., 963 F. Supp. 1131 (M.D. Ala. 1997).
40. Wright v. Combined Ins. Co. of Am., 959 F. Supp. 356 (M.D. Miss. 1997).
41. 45 CFR §164.530.
42. 45 CFR §164.534.
43. 45 CFR §160.304.
44. Pub. L. 104-191; 42 USC §1320d-5.
45. 42 USC §1320d-6.
46. Alaska Stat. § 18.23.100 (2007); KRS § 205.566 (2006)
47. Miss. Code Ann. § 41-9-64 (2007).
48. N.C. Gen. Stat. § 90-412 (2006).
49. R.I. Gen. Laws § 23-77-1 (2007); 18 V.S.A. § 9417 (2007).
50. Mo. Code Regs. Ann. Tit. 19, 30-20.021(3)(D)(15)(1996).
51. Kan. Admin. Regs. 28-34-9a (d)(1997).
52. Walgreen Co. v. Wisconsin Pharmacy Examining Board, No. 97-1513, 217 Wis.2d 290, 577 N.W.2d 387, 1998 WL 65551 at 4 (Wis. App. Feb. 19, 1998) Eich, J.
53. Westinghouse Electric Corp., 638 F.2d 570 (3d Cir. 1980).
54. United States v. Grunewald, 233 F. 2d 556, 581-82 (2d Cir. 1956).
55. Olmstead v. United States, 277 U.S. 438, 478 (1928) (declaring the right to be let alone "the most comprehensive rights and the right most valued by civilized men") (Brandeis, J., dissenting).
56. 429 U.S. 589 (1977).
57. Mo. Code Regs. Ann. tit. 19, 30-20.021(3)(D)(15)(1996).
58. Kan. Admin. Regs. 28-34-9a (d)(1997).
59. 638 F.2d 570 (3d Cir. 1980).
60. Whalen v. Roe, 429 U.S. 589 (1977).

13

Privacy and Security of Health Information

Merida L. Johns, PhD

D uring the past three decades phenomenal changes have occurred in the collection and use of health information. Environmental forces coupled with technological advances have played primary roles in these changes. As a result we are experiencing an unparalleled growth in the depth and breadth of the collection and use of personal health information. The extent of primary and secondary uses of health information has grown tremendously. Primary uses of patient-specific information have traditionally included patient care delivery, support, and management as well as billing and reimbursement. This information is usually collected and maintained by the provider in the course of delivering health care services to the patient. However, there are other secondary users not directly involved with the care of the patient, who collect and maintain health care information. Among these are educational institutions, civil and criminal justice systems, pharmaceutical companies, health and life insurers, credit agencies, banking centers, and medical and social researchers (1). In addition some secondary users and other private companies have "begun to act on the commercial incentive to collect health care data" (2) gathering and selling aggregate data without the patient's knowledge.

The patient medical record includes some of the most sensitive, private, and intimate information about an individual's life. It is also the primary source of information to health care providers in the delivery of direct patient care. The Institute of Medicine's report, The Computer-Based Patient Record: An Essential Technology for Health Care, envisioned that computerization of health information would play an increasingly important role in the health care environment, providing opportunities for improving quality of care, reducing administrative costs, and capturing relevant data necessary for provider and consumer education, technology assessment, and health services and outcomes research (3). More than a decade later in 2004, President Bush outlined a plan for adoption of health information technology and the implementation of electronic health records within ten years to address longstanding problems of preventable errors, uneven quality, and rising costs in the nation's health care system (4). Computerization of health information has the potential, if appropriately implemented, to provide support for streamlining and improving the health care delivery system. However, it also heightens concerns surrounding the protection of individual privacy and the provision of adequate data security. The implementation of technology solutions for the capture, storage, and use of health information must be coupled with strong institutional data security programs and legislative initiatives that protect privacy interests.

Privacy, Confidentiality, and Security of Health Care Information

The importance of privacy and confidentiality has been acknowledged for over 2000 years, having its roots in the Hippocratic Oath, which compels physicians to keep confidential any information obtained during the attendance of the sick. Other health-related professions have acknowledged the confidential nature of information obtained during the course of health-care delivery and have adopted similar oaths (5). In 1994, the Computer-Based Patient Record Institute (CPRI) prepared a position paper on "Access to Patient Data," which advocated the establishment of a national regulatory framework to protect patients' informational privacy (6). Several governmental reports over the years have recommended that an environment must be maintained in which the patient, who discloses personal information in the course of health care delivery, is free from fear of improper re-disclosure of this information (1,7).

Frequently the terms "privacy", "confidentiality", and "security" are misunderstood, resulting in their misuse. Privacy, in the health care context, is usually understood to mean the right of individuals to limit access to information about their person; this is also called "informational privacy" (8). Informational privacy includes the right of individuals to determine at what time, in what way, and to what extent information about them is shared with others. Confidentiality, on the other hand, refers to the expectation that information shared by an individual with a health care provider during the course of care will be used only for its intended purpose. Disclosure of information beyond its intended purpose would not be accomplished without the patient's knowledge and consent.

The Center for Democracy and Technology has defined the terms "personal information", "information privacy", "data confidentiality", and "security" in an attempt to clarify the terminology associated with privacy and security issues in health information (9). The CPRI also published a glossary of terms related to information security (10). Personal information is health information that contains data that identifies or can reasonably identify an individual. Examples of such data include name, social security number, and date of birth. Personally identifiable information may also include data that together contain a sufficient number of variables to allow identification of an individual.

Privacy as defined by the CPRI is "the right of individuals to keep information about themselves from being disclosed to anyone" (11). The Center for Democracy and Technology elaborates on information privacy by saying that it encompasses the individual's right to control the collection, use, and disclosure of personal information.

As opposed to privacy, the CPRI defined confidentiality as the act of limiting disclosure of private matters. Ball and Collen (12) further explain that confidentiality is a status accorded to information that indicates that it is sensitive. By conferring a confidential status on data, there is an assumption that specific controls will be established to ensure against its theft, improper use, or inappropriate disclosure.

Security provides the protection measures and tools for safeguarding information and information systems. The National Research Council (13) has defined security as the protection of information systems against unauthorized access to or modification of information, denial of service to authorized users, and provision of service to unauthorized users. The American Society for Testing and Materials (ASTM) has divided security into two concepts: data security and system security (14). **Data security** encompasses protection measures that safeguard data and computer programs from undesired occurrences and exposures. This includes measures that would safeguard data against: 1) accidental or intentional disclosure of information to unauthorized users; 2) accidental or intentional alteration of data; 3) unauthorized copying; and 4) theft of data or loss of data through hardware or software failures. **System security,** as defined by the ASTM, includes the totality of security safeguards associated with hardware, software, personnel, and enterprise-wide institutional policies. Table 13-1 provides a comparison among CPRI, Center for Democracy and Technology, and ASTM of definitions of these various terms.

Uses and Users of Health Information

With the fundamental restructuring of the U.S. health care delivery system, there has been a parallel increase in the collection and use of patient-related data. Certainly development of integrated delivery systems, managed care programs such as health maintenance organizations, and general concerns over the rising cost of health care services has stimulated the demand for more and more information. The availability of information technologies has provided the conduit for data sharing within and across organizational boundaries. Estimates for expenditures on health information technology are cited between $11 billion and $15 billion a year in 1997

Table 13-1

COMPARISON OF DEFINITIONS OF SECURITY TERMS

Terms	CPRI	ASTM	Center for Technology & Democracy
Information Privacy	The right of individuals to keep information about themselves from being disclosed to anyone.	A state or condition of controlled access to personal information; the ability of an individual to control the use and dissemination of information that relates to himself or herself; the individual's ability to control what information is available to various users and to limit re-disclosures of information.	Specific right of an individual to control the collection, use, and disclosure of personal information
Confidentiality	The act of limiting disclosure of private matters	Status accorded to data or information indicating that they are sensitive for some reason and therefore need to be protected against theft, disclosure, and improper use.	Tool for protecting privacy
Security	Means to control access and protect information from accidental or intentional disclosure to unauthorized persons and from alteration, destruction, or loss.	Totality of safeguards including hardware, software, personnel policies, information practice policies, disaster preparedness, and oversight of these components.	Encompasses all the safeguards in an information system.

to $17 billion and $42 billion in 2004 and are expected to grow over the next few years (15).

There are various accounts of the number of individuals who have access to an individual's health information. Estimates range from 150 to as many as 400 individuals who may see the sensitive data that are collected in a patient's medical record (16,17). Individuals having access to health care data fall within two categories: those classified as health care providers and those classified as non-health care providers.

To support a patient care encounter, many functions must be performed that require internal data sharing. For example, registration and admission functions, direct patient care functions, case management and utilization review, and discharge planning all require internal data sharing. Ancillary departments whose functions support the delivery of patient care require data from the patient care areas in order to carry out their activities. Such departments include dietary, laboratory, pharmacy, social services, physical therapy, and respiratory therapy. Internally, an organization also shares data to support disease registries, risk management, outcomes and quality management, and infection control. Information to support research and education is also abundantly shared internally.

Data distribution also occurs to external entities such as county and state health departments, state disease registries, state data commissions, and contract outcomes management databases. Reports to third-party payers contain patient-specific data and determine a patient's initial and continued eligibility for coverage. While third-party payer organizations may vary in their activities, many do have data sharing relationships, which are either direct or indirect, with employers, third-party benefits managers, marketers and database developers, and life insurers. The American Health Information Management Association has developed a situation analysis and position paper on the Confidentiality of Medical Records that presents a schema for health information and how it is used (18). The Health Privacy Project illustrates how personal medical data flows to downstream users such as drug marketers, law enforcement agencies, public assistance programs, and information brokers (19).

The National Research Council identified new entrants to the information sharing market (13). The new users of health information are typically those who provide products and services to the health care industry and have significant business interests in the collection of individually identifiable health information. Examples of such companies include medical and surgical suppliers, pharmaceutical companies, reference laboratories, and companies that provide information technology services. Table 13-2 provides a listing of typical individuals and organizations that could receive personal health information related to one clinical encounter.

Breaches in the protection of confidential data have become widespread as a consequence of the pressures for more information, the technology capacity to deliver such data, and the potential commercial advantage to collecting health care information. In some instances these breaches occur within the parameters of present law, while others have been illegal. Prior to implementation of the Health Insurance Portability and Accountability Act (HIPAA), pharmacies in some states could legally sell individual prescription records to pharmaceutical companies for use in marketing, and mailing list brokers could sell the names of individuals suffering from specific conditions to those marketing specific products or services (18). More recently in 2003, The Privacy Rights Clearinghouse (PRC), a San Diego–based nonprofit consumer information and advocacy organization, filed a lawsuit in California Superior Court charging Albertsons and its affiliated companies with violating the privacy rights of thousands of its customers by illegally selling their confidential prescription information to drug companies (19).

Table 13-2

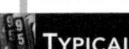

TYPICAL USERS OF HEALTH INFORMATION*

Patient

Primary care physician

Health insurance company

Clinical laboratory

Local retail pharmacy

Pharmacy benefits manager

Consulting physician

Local hospital

State bureau of vital statistics

Accrediting organization

Employer

Life insurance company

Medical Information Bureau

Managed care company

Attorney

State public health and family physician

State agency collecting hospital discharge data

Medical researcher

*National Academy of Sciences. Washington, DC. For the Record: Protecting Electronic Health Information by Committe on Maintaining Privacy and Security in Health Care Applications of the National Information Infrastructure, Commission on Physical Sciences, Mathematics, and Applications, National Research Council. Copyright 1997 by National Academies Press. Reproduced with permission of National Academies Press in the format Other book via Copyright Clearance Center.

Illegal breaches in the protection of confidential data run the gamut of re-leasing personal medical information of politicians during campaigns, leak-ing names of HIV-positive patients to newspapers to selling patient records to lawyers soliciting malpractice plaintiffs (17). Specific privacy violations cited in the Center for Democracy and Technology report include (9):

♦ During the 1992 campaign of a congresswoman from New York, confidential medical records were faxed to a local newspaper. The Congresswoman won her seat in the House only after overcoming the fallout from the unauthorized disclosure of her medical history.

♦ In December 1994 six pages of detailed data on the HIV status and drug abuse history of volunteers in an AIDS-prevention unit were faxed to an organization.

♦ An HMO plan recently admitted to maintaining detailed notes of psychotherapy sessions in computer records that were accessible by all clinical employees.

♦ In Maryland, eight Medicaid clerks were prosecuted for selling computerized record printouts of recipients' financial resources and dependents to sales representatives of managed care companies.

The PRC maintains a chronology of healthcare and other data breaches (20). A few of the health information data breaches listed in the chronology include:

♦ A stolen computer in November 2006 from Electronic Registry Systems that manages a cancer patient registry database for Geisinger Healthcare. Patient data included names, addresses, birthdates, medical record numbers, and social security numbers, dating back to 1980, and included records of 25,000 patients.

♦ Two stolen computers from an Indian state health department contractor containing the names, addresses, birth dates, social security numbers, and medical and billing information for more than 7500 women. The data were collected as part of the state's Breast and Cervical Cancer Program.

♦ Stolen names, birth dates, and social security numbers from 1100 patients who were hospitalized or had day-surgeries from June 22 to Sept 21 by an employee at Swedish health system. The employee used three patients' information to open multiple credit accounts.

The corresponding social consequences of breaches in safeguarding confidential information have far-reaching results. The aftermath of inappropriate information disclosure includes the denial of employment, insurance, healthcare, and housing. As more information is collected at even greater levels of granularity than in the past, the inappropriate dissemination of information may potentially be more devastating. This is particularly the case with genetic information. A recent article in the *Journal of the American Medical Association* notes that:

> Participants in genetic testing should be informed that the genetic testing for cancer susceptibility may limit their ability to obtain health, life, or disability insurance; may lead to limitations in health insurance coverage; or may result in higher premiums for insurance products. Participants also should be informed that genetic testing might pose a risk to their present or future employment (21).

Growth and Impact of Information Technologies

The threat to informational privacy due to technology advance and capacity continues to be a challenge today. Computer and network security is one of the most difficult issues facing the computer technology industry today. Experts in 1985 estimated that the real cost of computer/network crime was in the area of $15 billion annually (23). Today, companies in the United States could be losing hundreds of billions annually to information thieves. The 2005 Computer Security and Crime Survey conducted jointly by the

Computer Security Institute (CSI) and the Federal Bureau of Investigation (FBI) found virus attacks were the most common computer breach, followed by unauthorized access, theft of proprietary information, and denial of service attacks. The survey also found that breaches by insiders within an organization were as likely as external attacks (24).

It is true that the application of security measures can greatly reduce the threat to informational privacy, to the extent, some believe, that protections in the computerized environment offer more security opportunities than in the paper world (25). Nonetheless, these opportunities can only be realized when security systems are properly designed and implemented, monitored, and managed through an appropriate security organizational infrastructure.

Several technology advances have allowed greater depth and breadth of data collection, storage, and dissemination. Certainly the computer network revolution and the development and refinement of distributed processing technology have provided greater opportunities for data access and dissemination. Such systems are remarkably complex and heterogeneous and pose some of the most confounding security concerns to ever face the information systems environment. Threats to information security are particularly heightened when networks go beyond the physical boundaries of the enterprise campus. Computer and network security have been cited as two of the largest problems in the computer technology industry today.

Maturing of information technologies that allow for the development of data repositories and warehouses also has a great impact on data access, dissemination, and potential for security breaches. Older technology allowed for the infamous "silos" of information. While this approach hindered data access and integrity and encouraged data redundancy, it did provide some intrinsic security by separating data. Today, however, the very nature of aggregating data in one virtual space causes a breakdown of physical boundaries between records and data and those who may want to access them. In addition to greater access opportunities, the aggregation of data provides a broader range and depth for information access. While this is useful to the organization for clinical and management decision support, it also provides more opportunity for intrusion into sensitive information.

The application of technologies such as data mining, neural networks, and artificial intelligence to large data stores also poses new and potentially ominous security threats. As defined above, personally identifiable information includes data that together contain a sufficient number of variables to allow identification of an individual. With the combined application of sophisticated statistical techniques, data visualization, pattern recognition, and machine learning, individuals can be uniquely identified given a set of variables that may not necessarily by themselves contain personally identifiable information.

The explosion of the Internet brings immense security and law enforcement challenges. Reports indicate the growing vulnerability of information systems connected to public infrastructures such as the Internet, which have allowed interlopers a frequently easy avenue for intrusion (7). Interstate and international consumer fraud have been made significantly easier in a number of respects as a result of the Internet, and jurisdiction and identification issues have also complicated the prosecution of Internet crime (26). The exponential growth of electronic mail, a result of the Internet, also brings with it its own security problems. Electronic mail can be intercepted and read or even altered during transit by unauthorized intermediaries. Even the authenticity of an email sender cannot be ensured because email headers can be easily altered or faked. The Internet and explosion of the use of electronic mail provide avenues for any individual to intrude into private health information.

The Imperative for Health Information Security

The imperative for health information security is greater today than ever before. Technological advances and increases in information systems capacity bring opportunities to streamline health care delivery, reduce costs, and improve quality. These advances, however, when associated with increased collection and storage of personal information also create greater vulnerabilities in safeguarding and protecting privacy. The traditional paper environment inherently provided some protection of privacy (9). Information on a given individual was more difficult to aggregate, to access and to analyze.

In today's sophisticated electronic environment the collection and storage of aggregate data on an individual is much easier. The granularity of data is greater; the number of users of health data has exploded; and database technology and networks have opened up an entirely new world for information aggregation, sharing, and access. Data mining and other analytical techniques cannot only invade patient privacy but provider privacy as well. Information about corporate activities is just as vulnerable in today's world as patient-specific data.

No private practice, institution, organization, or enterprise is free from cyber-intrusion by people either inside or outside the corporate walls. The scope of the problem must be recognized and dealt with through the development of a systematic and encompassing security program. Such a program must be directed toward protecting information from insider attacks from current and former employees, onsite contractors, consultants, partners, and suppliers. The security program must also safeguard information from outsiders who may attempt to steal or corrupt information through electronic break-ins, employing surveillance technologies, or engaging in competitive intelligence. As reports cited previously indicate the stakes and costs are just too large to ignore. Protecting patient's right to privacy and respect for the confidentiality of health information has been an important underpinning in the provision of health care for over two thousand years. To continue to safeguard personal health information will require a concerted effort on the part of health care providers, health care organizations, health policy developers, the information technology industry, and the government.

Security Threats to Healthcare Information

Security of healthcare information encompasses three basic concepts. The first of these is **protection of the information.** Specifically this includes the defense or safeguard of information against attack through either intentional or unintentional acts. This concept encompasses informational privacy concerns. The second concept involves **data integrity.** This includes assurance that quality characteristics are maintained and that data are relevant, comprehensive, appropriate, timely, current, and consistent. The third concept involves **reliability.** This means the dependability of a system to perform exactly as expected and without error. Thus, given these principles, the major goals of any security program are to provide for information privacy, integrity, and availability.

Threats to healthcare information can be identified in terms of threats to informational privacy, data integrity, and information availability. Table 13-3 presents a matrix of common threats that can interfere with achievement of security program goals.

Threats to Informational Privacy

The following are common threats to informational privacy:

- **Insider accidental disclosures/errors:** This is probably the most common threat to informational privacy. In this case the employee, due to lack of knowledge of organization policy or some other reason, releases private information to unauthorized individuals.

- **Abuse by insiders of their access privileges:** In this case individuals who have authorized access to target data violate the trust associated

Table 13-3

COMMON THREATS TO HEALTHCARE INFORMATION SECURITY GOALS/THREATS

Goals/Threats Information Privacy	Information Integrity	Information Reliability
Insider accidental disclosure	Insider accidental errors	Natural hazards
Insider abuse of access privileges	Insider malicious attack	Equipment failure
	Intruder accidental or malicious attack	Software failure
Insider unauthorized access		Human error
Outsider intruders	Equipment failure	Theft
	Software failure	Malice
	Strategic attacks (e.g., virus)	Strategic attack

with that access. For example, an employee who reviews the medical information of a colleague, family member, or friend for non-healthcare delivery purposes.

- **Insider unauthorized access:** This includes those cases where an employee may have access to the information system but targets access to unauthorized information through exploitation of system vulnerability or through other means. Frequently this type of action will be for spite or profit.

- **Outside intruders:** Individuals who do not have authorized access to the system but gain such access through exploitation of system vulnerabilities or other means to explore information stores or mount attacks to damage systems or disrupt operations.

Threats to Information Integrity

Several of the threats to informational privacy also apply to those related to information integrity.

- **Insider accidental error:** In this case the employee inputs incorrect values or collects data inappropriately. This may be due to a lack of knowledge or to poor system constraints.

- **Insider malicious attack:** In this case the employee purposefully corrupts data for which there may be authorized or unauthorized access.

- **Intruder attack:** In this case an intruder gains access to the system by exploitation of system vulnerability or other means and either accidentally or purposefully corrupts or destroys data.

- **Software failure:** Failure of application or system software due to performance, inadequate code, or other reason fails to adequately protect data integrity.

- **Strategic attack:** Includes purposeful attack, such launching of a computer virus that corrupts or destroys data.

Threats to Information Reliability

Threats to information reliability involve a wide spectrum of incidents ranging from natural disasters to human error. Among these are:

- **Natural hazards:** This includes such things as earthquakes, tornadoes, ice storms, fires, floods, electrical storms, and so on.

- **Equipment and software failures:** This includes hardware breakdowns and software failures that cause unexpected systems suspension or shutdown.

- **Human error:** This includes any human error that would cause hardware or software to improperly function, causing unexpected system disruption or shutdown.

◆ **Theft, malice, or strategic attack:** Includes purposeful theft or attack on any component of the information system with the intent of causing system disruption or shutdown.

Governmental and Legislative Protections

Until 2003, there were no uniform federal privacy protections for health information. The fragmented, state-by-state approach to that time yielded little uniformity to protect the confidentiality of health information and provided no consistent or comprehensive privacy protection for health information. The range of medical privacy law did not address the practice of compiling medical information about patients, with or without their consent, or the identification of personal information for sale to business with a financial interest in the data (1). State statutes also varied in regard to allowing patients a right to access their own information. Furthermore, most statutes did not address redisclsoure of health information and lack penalties for misuse or misappropriation (27).

On the federal level, only the Privacy Act of 1974 provided protection of confidential information, and this was limited only to the disclosure by the government of individual health records maintained by government agencies. In its report, the Office of Technology Assessment concluded that:

> This patchwork of State and Federal laws addressing the question of privacy in personal medical data is inadequate to guide the health care industry with respect to obligations to protect the privacy of medical information in a computerized environment. It fails to confront the reality that, in a computerized system, information will regularly cross State lines, and will therefore be subject to inconsistent legal standards with respect to privacy. The law allows development of private sector businesses dealing in computer databases and data exchanges of patient information without regulation, statutory guidance, or recourse for persons who believe they have been wronged by abuse of data. These laws do not address the questions presented by new demands for data prompted by computerization, and the obligations of secondary users in accessing and maintaining data. Lack of legislation in this area will leave the health care industry with an uneven sense of their responsibilities for maintaining privacy (1, p. 15).

Legislative Initiatives

Beginning in 1980 Congress attempted to pass health privacy legislation. During the 1990s several bills were introduced to address privacy protection of healthcare information that provided varying degrees of protection. Among these were:

◆ The Fair Health Information Practices Act of 1997 (HR52)

◆ The Medical Privacy in the Age of New Technologies Act of 1997 (HR 1815)

◆ The Consumer Health and Research and Technology Protection Act (HR 3900)

- The Medical Information Privacy and Security Act (S1368)
- The Healthcare Personal Information Nondisclosure Act (S 1921)
- The Medical Information Protection Act of 1998 (S 2609)
- The Medical Information Privacy and Security Act (S 573)
- The Health Care Personal Information Nondisclosure Act (S 578)
- Medical Information Protection Act (S 881).

None of the above bills were considered for legislative action prior to the end of their legislative sessions. Several issues, however, arose during hearings held on the above bills. Some groups felt that many of the bills did not go far enough to safeguard confidential information. Other groups were concerned about how healthcare information is used outside the care setting, especially in areas of law enforcement and employment. Still other groups had concerns about the restrictive nature of some federal legislation, particularly in the area of healthcare information use in research, evaluation of utilization of services, and outcomes of care research. Federal preemption of state statutes has also been a major issue, even among groups that support federal legislation.

In 1996 Congress took up the issue of health privacy legislation within the context of the Health Insurance Portability and Accountability Act (HIPAA). The Administrative Simplification provisions of HIPAA were designed to encourage the development of electronically based health information exchange. An important component in developing such a system was to ensure privacy protections for health information. Congress set itself a three-year deadline for enacting comprehensive health privacy legislation. If Congress failed to act within that time, the Department of Health and Human Services (HHS) was directed to write and issue health privacy regulations. Congress was unable to pass comprehensive health privacy legislation within the three-year period. Accordingly, HHS then developed federal health privacy protections. The Privacy and Security Rules are minimum federal standards, providing a "floor" of protection, and do not supercede state laws affording higher protections.

While the HIPAA provides protections to health information that is collected and exchanged between "covered entities" such as healthcare providers, health plans, and insurance companies, no uniform national standard, currently exists that protects the confidentiality of all personally identifiable health information. There are many loopholes in HIPPA, and information that might be provided, for example, to an online e-mail list or to a health fair or free medical screening is not likely covered by HIPAA protections.

HIPAA Privacy Protections

The Privacy Rule is included in the Administrative Simplification provision of Title II of the Health Insurance Portability and Accountability Act along with the HIPAA security standards and the transaction and code set standardization requirements. The following discussion provides a high level overview of the HIPAA Privacy Rule. Additional information can be found in the Code of Federal Regulations (28).

The HIPAA privacy standards apply to covered entities that are health care providers (i.e., hospitals, long-term care facilities, physicians, pharmacies, clinics), health plan, or healthcare clearing houses that transmit any healthcare information in electronic form in connection with a transaction covered by the regulations. Some examples of electronic transactions include health claims and encounter information, health plan enrollment and disenrollment transactions, healthcare payment and remittance advice, health plan premium payments, health claim status, referral certification, and coordination of benefits.

HIPAA privacy standards apply to all protected health information (PHI). PHI is defined as individually identifiable health information that is transmitted by electronic media, maintained in any electronic medium or maintained in any other form or medium (i.e., paper or oral forms). Information is considered to be individually identifiable if it either identifies the person or there is a reasonable basis to believe that a person could be identified from the information given.

Guiding Principles

HIPAA privacy protections are based upon several guiding principles. These include:

◆ Setting boundaries for the use of health information and imposing a legal duty of confidentiality on those who provide and pay for health care and on other entities that receive health information from them

◆ Requiring measures for protection of health information

◆ Providing consumer control over individual information

◆ Establishing sanctions for the misuse of information

◆ Balancing individual rights with the public good

Individual Rights

The HIPAA Privacy Rule provides patients with specific rights for control over their own information. These rights allow individuals the right of access to inspect and obtain a copy their own PHI that is included in a designated record set, such as a health record. However, there are exceptions to what PHI may be accessed in specific circumstances. For example, information compiled in reasonable anticipation of a civil, criminal, or administrative action is an exception.

The Privacy Rule also provides for the right of an individual to request that a covered entity amend PHI or a record about an individual in a designated record set. The request for amendment can by denied by the covered entity in specific situations. For example, when the information is determined to be accurate or complete as it appears or if the information was not created by the covered entity.

The Privacy Rule contains a specific standard requiring the monitoring and tracking of disclosures of PHI. Individuals have the right to receive an accounting of certain disclosures made by a covered entity within six years prior to the date on which the accounting is requested. However, the type of disclosures included in this record keeping is limited. For example, disclosures made to carry out treatment, payment and health care operations and those pursuant to an authorization are exceptions.

Individuals are afforded additional rights to control their PHI. Among these is the opportunity to request confidential communication of their PHI by a covered to an alternative location (i.e., to an alternative address). For example, if an individual did not want their PHI sent to their home address, but provided an alternative location.

Uses and Disclosures

The Privacy standards include permitted uses and disclosures of PHI with and without patient authorization. For example, patient authorization is not required for treatment, payment and operations; disclosures required by law, public health activities; healthcare oversight activities; judicial and administrative proceedings; and some law enforcement purposes. Individuals must be provided an opportunity to agree or object to their information being included in a patient directory or to notification of relatives and friends of their treatment, if they are otherwise able to make healthcare decisions. Except for the purposes and circumstances specifically mentioned in the Privacy Rule that do not require an authorization for uses or disclosures, all other uses and disclosures require an individual's authorization.

Administrative Requirements

The Privacy Rule contains several standards that apply to administrative requirements. Among these are the designation by each covered entity of a privacy officer who is responsible for developing and implementing privacy policies and procedures for the organization. In addition to a privacy officer, covered entities are required to designate a person or office as the responsible party for receiving privacy-related complaints.

Every member of a covered entity's workforce must be trained in privacy policy and procedures. New employees must receive training within a reasonable period of time after joining the workforce. Whenever privacy policies or procedures are changed or there is a change in privacy law, workforce members must receive updated training. Covered entities are required to maintain documentation showing that privacy training has taken place.

The Privacy Rule requires covered entities to implement policies and procedures to ensure that it is in compliance with all HIPPA privacy standards, implementation specifications, and other requirements of the Privacy Rule. This includes conducting ongoing review of privacy policy to ensure appropriateness and maintaining all required documentation as specified in the Privacy Rule.

Privacy Rule Documents

The Privacy Rule requires that covered entities develop two key documents that serve to inform individuals of their privacy rights and provide them a measure of control over their PHI. These documents include the notice of privacy practices and authorization for use and disclosure of information are required.

The notice of privacy practices explains how an individual's PHI is used and disclosed. The notice explains the patient's rights and the covered entity's responsibilities and legal duties with respect to the individual's PHI. The notice of privacy practices must be provided to an individual at the first contact with the covered entity, for example at a first clinic visit or first hospitalization. The Rule outlines specific requirements for the privacy notice content.

Except for the purposes and circumstances specifically identified in the Privacy Rule that do not require an authorization for use and disclosure of PHI (i.e., for treatment, payment, and healthcare operations), a signed authorization form is required for use and disclosure of PHI in all other circumstances. The authorization must be written in plain language and contain at least the following elements:

♦ Description of the information to be used or disclosed

♦ Name or other specific identification of the person(s) or class of persons authorized to make the requested use or disclosure

♦ The name or other specific identification of the persons(s) to whom the covered entity may make the requested use or disclosure

♦ An expiration date or event that relates to the individual or the purpose of the use or disclosure

♦ A statement of the individual's right to revoke the authorization in writing and the exceptions to the right to revoke, together with a description of how the individual may revoke it

♦ A statement that information used or disclosed pursuant to the authorization may be subject to redisclosure by the recipient and no longer protected the Privacy Rule

♦ Signature of the individual and date of authorization

♦ When the authorization is signed by a personal representative of the individual, there must be a description of the representative's authority to act for the individual

Safeguarding Healthcare Information Security

To protect informational privacy, specific measures must be in place for safeguarding information and information systems. Security can be defined as the protection measures and tools for safeguarding information and information systems. The NCR defines security as (29):

♦ The protection of information systems against unauthorized access to, or modification of, information

♦ The denial of service to unauthorized users

♦ The provision of service to authorized users

Various security strategies and countermeasures can be employed to help ensure information security. To be successful, however, these must be embedded within an overall enterprise-wide security program. A piecemeal approach to implementation of countermeasures, techniques, and safeguards will not ensure a robust security program that will protect the interests of the enterprise or public.

Security Program Components

Several security strategies make up the components of a strong security program. Among these are development of a formal security organization; development and implementation of administrative, physical, and technical controls such as the establishment of a risk analysis program and development of a business continuity plan.

Development of the Security Organization

The most fundamental security strategy is the establishment of a formal security organizational structure. Frequently in health care institutions security functions have been placed under the direct control of the information systems department or delegated to those who operate departmental information systems. A security program, however, because of its multifaceted purposes, is multidisciplinary, and no one person or department will likely have the knowledge and skills to staff the security function adequately (5). Thus, the security organization should include the appropriate mix of personnel with skills to carry out the security function and also include a variety of individuals who function in an oversight or matrix organizational structure.

In order for the security function to be successful, it must have the support of executive management. Security programs require resources and delegation of appropriate authority and responsibility to individuals to carry out security management functions. The support of top management signals clear support for the security initiative and indicates that responsibility and associated accountability has been delegated.

Various organizational structures can be used to support the security function. Most importantly, though, the security function should be positioned within an organization so that it has significant authority to successfully carry out the functions of a security program. Furthermore, the security organization should be independent of those organizational units that are subject to security measures. In other words, the security function should not report to the information systems department or internal audit department. Frequently institutions will designate a chief security officer (CSO) or information security officer (ISO) with overall responsibility for the security function. The CSO may report directly to the Chief Information Officer or report to another top executive officer of the organization. The CSO will normally be responsible for the design, implementation, and evaluation of the total security program encompassing information protection, integrity, and availability. Typical functions of a CSO are listed in Table 13-4. In addition to the CSO, the formal security organization should be staffed by individuals who have both technical and managerial expertise in the area of systems security. Depending on the organization, this may include individuals with special expertise in personal computing, local area networking, access control administration, contingency planning and training and awareness development.

In addition to staffing, the security organization must also define resource requirements, develop and manage a budget, establish job descriptions, develop mission, goals, and strategies for the security initiative, and develop and foster interdepartmental relationships. Additionally, a formal information security management committee should be established that is multidiscipli-

Table 13-4

TYPICAL FUNCTIONS OF THE CHIEF SECURITY OFFICER

Security strategic planning

Development of enterprise-wide security policy for safeguarding the access, integrity, and availability of information and information systems

Development of enterprise-wide procedures and standards for security policy implementation

Coordinate the administration of security software

Manage confidentiality agreements for employees and contractors

Coordinate security procedures

Coordinate employee security training

Monitor audit trails to identify security violations

Conduct risk assessment of enterprise information systems

Develop business continuity plan

nary and composed of departments that represent major computer users and those that have a significant responsibility for information security.

Administrative Controls

Administrative controls consist of management constraints, operational procedures, accountability procedures, and supplemental controls that provide an acceptable level of protection for computing resources. One of the best preventive controls is employee education and training. Security awareness training helps employees understand the importance of security practices and includes heightening awareness of general overall policies as well as training in fundamental technical techniques. For example, awareness of the destructiveness of a computer virus can help employees understand why external software or files should not be loaded on individual workstations. Understanding procedures for backing up files can save the company and the employee enormous amounts of time and cost should there be a software or equipment failure. Frequently, simple preventive measures will result in major cost and timesavings.

Every organization should have appropriate recruitment and termination procedures. While this preventative measure seems simplistic, it is surprising to note how many organizations do not do an adequate job of screening individuals prior to hiring or employ appropriate computer security procedures at the time of termination. Regardless of the conditions of termination, all access rights should be immediately discontinued upon cessation of employment. In cases of involuntary termination, the employee should be asked to leave the premises immediately; computer rights should be discontinued; all badges, keys or other devices should be confiscated; and all locks to computer resource areas should be changed.

Security policies and procedures should be established that are enterprise-wide. These include policies and procedures that cover the use and control of computing resources such as equipment, files, and software; access to and use of organization information; protection of confidential information; security incident reporting; and potential consequences of employee noncompliance with security policy or procedures. All employees, volunteers, contractors, students, consultants, or others who may use computer resources or have access to organizational information should sign a confidentiality statement or agreement at time of employment, and the statement should be updated on a yearly basis. Samples of such agreements can be obtained from the The American Health Information Management Association (30).

Another type of administrative control is a security review or audit. Such reviews should be periodically scheduled to ensure those policies and procedures are being followed. For example, periodic review or audit of local workstation drives may reveal the presence of unauthorized software or application programs, inappropriate use of local passwords, or other violations of security policy.

Physical Controls

Physical controls fall into two categories: preventive and detective. The use of locks, badges, and alarms helps to control access to physical computing resources. Physical controls can also provide protection to the computing resource from theft and destruction or damage from accident, fire, or natural disasters.

Some very simple and inexpensive measures can provide a wide umbrella of protection of computing resources. A fundamental strategy is storage of backup files and documentation off-site so that one incident will not destroy both active data files and software and back-up copies. Back-up copies should be afforded the same security as active data files and stored in a secure location with appropriate environmental safeguards. Backup power supply should be used to ensure that computing resources are available should there be a power outage. Backup power should be minimally available to allow for an appropriate period of time to safely shutdown the computer systems so that files and/or software are not damaged during a power outage of long duration.

Badge systems, locks, and keys should be used at all entrances to restrict access to computing resource areas. Closed-circuit television monitors may also be employed to monitor access to computing rooms and equipment. Various sensors and alarms should be used to detect dangerous changes in air or cooling systems or to detect fire or smoke.

Technical Controls

A wide variety of technical controls should be used to protect the information resource. Access control software is a fundamental technique for security protection and is used to limit access of computer data files to approved users. This type of software verifies computer users and limits their privileges to view, copy, delete, or otherwise alter files. Frequently this type of software is used in conjunction with the categorization of the degree of confidentiality, class or security of information. For example, military organizations give access rights to classified, confidential, secret, or top secret information according the corresponding security clearance level of the user.

Associated with access control software is the use of fixed and dynamic password protections. Passwords are used to verify that the user of identification is the owner of the identification. To be effective, **fixed passwords** must be difficult to guess and should not be composed of meaningful words or something that is associated with the user (i.e., pet's name, user birthdate, etc.). Ideally, fixed passwords should contain both alphabetic and numeric characters and be at least six characters in length. Fixed passwords should be changed on a regular basis and ideally no less than every 90 days.

Dynamic passwords are created by a token that is programmed to generate passwords randomly. Tokens are tamper-resistant plastic cards that contain a microprocessor chip that contain a stored password that automatically and frequently changes. When a token is used to access a computer, the computer reads the token's password, reads another password entered by the user, and matches these two to an identical token password generated by the computer and user's password. Tokens are expected to be reinforced by biometric identification such as unique personal characteristics such as fingerprints, retinal patterns, skin oils, voice variations, and keyboard-typing rhythms (31).

Encryption is another technical security control and is a method by which data is made unintelligible to those who do not have appropriate access. Usually encryption is used with network transmissions. Essentially with encryption, information is changed from readable text to ciphertext or unreadable data. This is accomplished by scrambling data using mathematical equations and secret codes called keys. Two keys are usually used, one used by the sender to change the data into ciphertext and one used by the receiver of a message to decode the data. Encryption is considered to be the only sure way of protecting data during network transmission (32) (see Chapter 5 for more information on encryption.)

In addition to the above methods, **detection and intrusion systems** can be used to protect data. The most commonly used detective method is the audit trail. The audit trail or log is a record of system activities. The log captures various types of data. These data include a record of logins and logouts; specific events that have been taken against data such as reading, writing, modification, or creation; date and time of events and identification of the user associated with the event; and success or failure of the event. Violation reports can be automatically generated that can indicate potential significant security violations. However, audit trails and logs are not effective unless there is a procedure in place for regular and frequent review of their results. Furthermore, procedures need to be activated whereby possible security violations are investigated.

Intrusion detection systems use artificial intelligence methods to identify possible security breaches. Such systems track users while they are using the computer system and, based upon a unique user profile, determine whether or not the users' actions are consistent with their personal profile or an established norm. A user profile can be composed of various elements including usual CPU, input/out usage, command, compiler, or editor use. Such profiles often contain information about what files the user usually accesses, what programs are usually executed, types of errors frequently made, and usual hours and days of use.

Computer networks pose an enormous security threat to any organization. Protection of data within a computer network is very complex and involves the application of a number of **security services.** Among these are integrity services, authentication services, access control services, confidentiality services, and nonrepudiation services. All of these services must be well organized, interfaced, and managed by skilled professionals. In addition to these services, networks are also protected from outside intruders through the use of firewalls and security gateways. Essentially these methods filter access to the network while still allowing users access to the outside world. Firewalls limit the types of information that can be passed to or from computers located on the internal network.

To be effective technical controls must be implemented in a deliberate and organized manner into a system of controls. Application of control techniques must be based on a systematic plan that identifies potential risk of exposure (risk analysis), levels of information security, and the degree of consequence to the organization should data become altered, destroyed, or unavailable (risk assessment).

Risk Analysis and Assessment

A critical part of any security program is the management of risk. Risk management encompasses the identification, management, and control of untoward events. Conducting a risk analysis includes: 1) identifying threats or risks to security; 2) determining how likely it is that any given threat may occur; and 3) estimation of the impact of an untoward event. Among the threats to security are human error, such as a data entry mistake, unauthorized physical access to data, sabotage, power failures, and malfunction of software or hardware.

In addition to identifying risks, their likelihood of occurring, and their impact, informational assets must also be identified. Not all information is equal in importance or criticality to the operation of the organization. Determining the value of information is based on several factors. For example, what impact would a security breach have on quality of care, revenue, service, or organizational image?

Several different methodologies, ranging in complexity and computation, can be used to carry out a risk analysis. Calculation of risks based on unintentional occurrences such as power failures or data entry error are usually based on the probability of the specific event occurring. Calculation of risk for intentional risk such as fraud or theft are usually based on such factors as the attractiveness of a system to a perpetrator and the degree of vulnerability of the system.

Business Continuity Planning

A frequently overlooked security measure is the business continuity plan. The purpose of the business continuity plan (BCP) is to ensure that an organization is able to deliver its goods and services without interruption. Frequently the BCP is referred to as the disaster plan. However, BCP goes far beyond the response to a disaster. The goals of a BCP are to:

◆ Identify potential disasters and their effects
◆ Taking preventative measures to minimize the likelihood of disasters occurring

◆ Develop an organized response should a disaster strike

◆ Ensure that business processes continue during the disaster recovery period

The BCP is based on the information gathered during the risk assessment and analysis. Using this information, the BCP is developed based on the following steps: 1) identification of minimum allowable time for system disruption; 2) identification of alternatives for system continuation; 3) evaluation of cost and feasibility of each alternative; and 4) development of procedures required to activate the plan. The typical contents of a BCP include:

◆ **Responsibility for development and implementation of the plan:** security management team, emergency operation team, damage assessment team, and coordination and implementation

◆ **Disaster identification:** definition of disaster and its identification, notification procedures; identification of disaster cause; and communication procedures

◆ **Recovery plan:** organization and staffing; vendor contracts; backup plans, recovery plans, and alternate-site contacts

◆ **Plan testing:** method and frequency of testing the plan

Status of Data Security

Protection of computerized information must be a top priority for health care enterprises. As previously cited, cost of security breaches reach into the billions of dollars each year for American industry in general. For the health care industry, costs of security breaches must also measured in relation to the degree to which informational privacy is jeopardized and the extent to which quality of patient care is threatened.

The protection of electronic information results when a combination of administrative, technical, and physical controls are developed and implemented within a framework of a total security program. Each of these controls is equally important in providing a safety net surrounding information and information systems. The National Research Council's Report indicated that "health care organizations will have to work individually, collectively, and with relevant government entities to address the broad scope of concerns regarding privacy and security (7, p. ES-4). The Council also made five overriding recommendations for improving the privacy and security of electronic health information at the level of both individual organizations and the health care system as a whole that are still relevant today (7, p. ES5-12). Among these were:

1. All organizations that handle patient-identifiable health care information, regardless of size, should adopt the set of technical and organizational policies, practices, and procedures as outlined in their report.

2. Government and health care industry should take action to create the infrastructure necessary to support the privacy and security of electronic health information.

3. The federal government should work with industry to promote and encourage an informed public debate to determine an appropriate balance between the privacy concerns of patients and the information needs of various users of health information.

4. Any effort to develop a universal patient identifier should weigh the presumed advantages of such an identifier against potential privacy concerns.

5. The federal government should take steps to improve information security technologies for health care applications.

HIPAA Security Provisions

As part of the Administrative Simplification provisions of HIPAA, security standards for the safeguarding of health information were established. These standards support and work in conjunction with the HIPAA Privacy standards.

All healthcare providers, healthcare clearing houses, and health plans that electronically maintain or transmit patient health information must comply with these standards. The HIPAA security standards evolved directly from the first and third recommendations set forth in the NRC report cited above. Thus, HIPAA security standards represent an attempt to establish best practices for health information security. The HIPAA data security provisions are divided into the following:

◆ General rules

◆ Administrative safeguards

◆ Physical safeguards

◆ Organizational requirements and policies

◆ Procedures and documentation requirements.

The content of each section closely parallels the strategies for minimizing security threats discussed earlier. Basically, the HIPAA security provisions follow what has already been established in the information systems field as best practices for the development and implementation of good security policy.

The following discussion of HIPAA Security is based upon the Security Standards Final Rule (33) and adapted from HIPAA Security: Computer Based Training Modules (34).

General Rules

The General Rules provide the objective and scope for the HIPAA security rule as a whole. They specify that covered entities must develop a security program that includes a range of security safeguards that protect individually identifiable health information maintained or transmitted in electronic form. Examples of requirements that all covered entities must follow include:

◆ Ensuring the confidentiality, integrity, and availability of all electronic protected health information (ePHI) that is created, received, maintained, or transmitted by the covered entity

◆ Protecting PHI against any reasonably anticipated threats or hazards to the security or integrity of PHI

◆ Protecting PHI against any reasonably or anticipated uses or disclosure that are not permitted under the HIPAA Privacy Rule

◆ Ensuring compliance with HIPAA security rules by workforce members

Administrative Provisions

Administrative provisions are documented, formal practices for management of data security strategies throughout the organization. They require the facility to establish a security management process similar to the concepts discussed earlier in this chapter. Written policies and procedures are required. A formal policy manual should be developed and the organization should issue a statement of its philosophy on data security. An organizational chart outlining data security authority and responsibilities throughout the organization also should be developed.

The administrative provisions include the following nine standards that must be implemented by covered entities:

◆ **Security management process:** An organization must have a defined security management process. This means that there is a process in place for creating, maintaining, and overseeing the development of security policies and procedures and conducting risk analysis, risk management, development of a sanction policy, and review of information system activity.

◆ **Assigned security responsibility:** Each covered entity must identify a security official who is assigned security responsibility for the development and implementation of the policies and procedures required by the HIPAA Security Rule. Frequently, this individual is given the title of chief security officer (CSO).

◆ **Workforce security:** The covered entity must ensure appropriate access to individually identifiable information to workforce members who need to use electronic PHI to perform their job duties. Likewise, covered entities must prevent access to information to those who do not need it.

◆ **Information access management:** The fourth standard requires covered entities to implement a program of information access management. This includes specific policies and procedures to determine who should have access to what information.

- **Workforce security awareness and training:** Employees and other workforce members have formal training in proper data security handling.

- **Security incident procedures:** Organizations must establish security incident procedures so that management and employees know what to do in the event of a security breach.

- **Contingency plan:** A contingency plan be developed and tested. This is to ensure that procedures are in place to handle an emergency response in the event of an untoward event such as a power outage.

- **Evaluation:** A periodic technical and nontechnical evaluation must be performed in response to environmental or operational changes affecting the security of electronic PHI.

- **Business associate agreement:** A business associate agreement is required whenever electronic PHI is handled or exchanged through a third party who is not a covered entity. This is a written contract whereby the business associate agrees to handle data in a secure manner that meets HIPAA stipulations.

Physical Safeguards

Physical safeguards include the protection of computer systems from natural and environmental hazards and intrusion. This provision consists of the following (34):

- **Facility access controls:** Safeguards to prohibit the physical hardware and computer system itself from unauthorized access while ensuring that proper authorized access is allowed.

- **Workstation use:** Require that policies and procedures be in place that document the proper functions to be performed on workstations.

- **Workstation security:** Physical safeguards must be implemented to ensure workstation security. There must be safeguards in place to protect any workstations that access PHI from unauthorized access. Automatic logoffs are an example.

- **Devices and media:** Devices and media on which data are stored must be protected. Policies and procedures that ensure that disks, tapes, and videos are physically protected from harm or intrusion must be developed. Examples include controls for tracking the access, removal, and disposal of hardware and software such as sign-out logs. Organizations must have procedures to follow for data backup as well as for the disposal of disks and other media, including paper reports and records.

Technical Safeguards

The technical safeguard provisions consist of five broad categories. The provisions include those things that can be implemented from a technical standpoint using computer software. These provisions include:

- **Access controls:** Requires implementation of technical procedures to control access to health information, executed through some type of software program. This requirement ensures that individuals are given access to only the data they need to perform their jobs. The regulations state that access should be determined by one of three techniques: context-based, role-based, and user-based access schemes.

- **Audit controls:** Requires that audit controls be established so that system activities can be monitored through documented logs of system access and access attempts. Audit trails are an example of an audit control.

- **Data integrity:** Requires policies and procedures to protect electronic PHI from improper alteration or destruction.

- **Person or entity authentication:** Requires procedures that verify that a person or entity seeking access to electronic PHI is the one claimed. For example, an entity can be a human user of a system or another machine that has access to or transmits electronic PHI. Assignment of a unique identifier (such as a password) to workforce members is an example of person authentication.

- **Transmission security:** The controls applicable in transmission security are similar to those discussed already. HIPAA requires organizations to have integrity and access controls in place as well as entity authentication and audit trails.

In addition, the standard requires the use of encryption, when deemed appropriate, for data transmitted over public networks or communication systems.

Organizational Requirements

These requirements include just two standards: one addresses requirements for business associates and the other addresses requirements for group health plans.

- **Business associate contracts:** Covered entities must obtain a written contract with business associates who handle electronic PHI. The written contract must stipulate that the business associate will implement administrative, physical, and technical safeguards that reasonably and appropriately safeguard the confidentiality, integrity, and availability of the electronic PHI that it creates, receives, maintains, or transmits on behalf of the covered entity. The contract must ensure that any agent, including a subcontractor, agrees to implement reasonable and appropriate safeguards. Specifically, HIPAA requires a business associate to report to the covered entity any security incident of which it becomes aware. The covered entity must authorize termination of the contract if it determines that the business associate has violated a material term of the contract.

- **Group health plans:** Requirements for group health plans specify that plan sponsors must reasonably and appropriately safeguard electronic

PHI that they create, receive, maintain, or transmit. The Privacy Rule limits the health information that health plans, health insurance companies, and HMOS can disclose to plan sponsors. For example, this information is limited to summary health information for the purposes of obtaining premium bids from health plans for health insurance coverage or modifying, amending, or terminating the plan or for providing information on whether or not an individual is participating, enrolled, or disenrolled in the plan.

Health plan documents must include requirements for a plan sponsor to:

- Implement the same security measures required by the HIPAA Privacy Standard for information it creates, receives, maintains, or transmits on behalf of the health plan

- Ensure that the sponsor's employees' duties are adequately separated to ensure that PHI is not being used for employment or other employee-benefit decisions

- Require agents of the sponsor to provide reasonable and appropriate protection of health information provided to them by the plan sponsor

- Report any security incident of which it becomes aware to the health plan

Policies and Procedures and Documentation Requirements

Covered entities must have security policies and procedures documented in written format. Other information about any actions, assessments, or activities associated with the HIPAA Security Rule also must be in a written format. Documentation must be retained for six years from the date of its creation or the date when it last was in effect, whichever is later. It must be made available to those individuals responsible for implementing security procedures. Further, it must be reviewed periodically and updated, as needed, in response to environmental or organizational changes that affect the security of electronic PHI.

Summary

Privacy and security of health information are integral to the successful adoption of electronic technologies for electronic health records. Every healthcare organization must make the protection of healthcare information a top priority. The cost of privacy and security breaches reaches into the billions of dollars every year for American industry in general, not to mention the human costs associated with such breaches.

Health information can be protected through a total security program that combines administrative, technical, and physical controls and is associated with a privacy program. The Health Insurance Portability and Accountability Act contains provisions that have become the basis for national privacy and security standards. Each of the controls for privacy and security is equally important in providing a safety net for information. When any one control is lacking, the security program is vulnerable to many potential threats from both within and outside the healthcare organization.

References

1. U.S. Congress, Office of Technology Assessment, Protecting Privacy in Computerized Medical Information, OTA-TCT-576 (Washington, DC: U.S. Government Printing Office, September 1993).
2. U.S. Congress, Office of Technology Assessment, Protecting Privacy in Computerized Medical Information, OTA-TCT-576 (Washington, DC: U.S. Government Printing Office, September 1993). Page 11.
3. Institute of Medicine, The Computer-Based Patient Record: An Essential Technology for Health Care, Richard S. Dick and Elaine B. Steen, eds. Washington, DC: National Academy Press, 1991.
4. Department of Health and Human Services, Office of the National Coordinator of Health Information Technology (ONCHIT), The Decade of Health Information Technology: Delivering Consumer-centric and Information-rich Health Care Framework for Strategic Action. July 21. 2004. Available at: http://www.hhs.gov/healthit/documents/hitframework.pdf
5. Johns, M. L. Information Management for Health Professionals. Albany: Delmar, 1997.
6. Computer-Based Patient Record Intitute, Inc. Position Paper: Access to patient data. Chicago, Il. April 1994.
7. National Academy of Sciences, For the Record Protecting Electronic Health Information. National Research Council, Computer Science and Telecommunications Board, Committee on Maintaining Privacy and Security in Health Care Applications of the National Information Infrastructure, Computer Science and Telecommunications Board, Commissionn onPhysical Sciences, Mathematics, and Applications. Washington, DC: National Academy Press, 1997.
8. Gostin LO, Turek-Brezina J, Powers M, Kozloff R. Privacy and security of health information in the emerging health system. Health Matrix. Journal of Law-Medicine. Winter, 1995;8.
9. The Center for Democracy and Technology, Prviacy and Health Information Systems: A Guide to Protecting Patient Confidentiality. Seattle: Foundation for Health Care Quality.
10. Computer-based Patient Record Institute, Glossary of Terms Related to Information Security. Schaumburg, Il: CPRI, 1996.
11. Computer-based Patient Record Institute, Glossary of Terms Related to Information Security. Schaumburg, Il: CPRI, 1996;10.
12. Ball MJ, Collen MF, eds. Aspects of the Computer-based Patient Record. New York: Springer-Verlag, 1992.
13. National Research Council, Computers at Risk:Safe Computing in the Information Age. System Security Study Committee, Computer Science and Telecommunications Goard, Commission on Physical Sciences, Mathematics, and Applications. Washington, DC: National Academy Press.
14. American Society for Testing and Mateials. E1869-97 Confidentiality, Privacy, Access, and Data Security Principles for Health Information Including Comper-Based Patient Records. West Conshohocken, PA: American Society for Testing and Materials, 1997.
15. Office of the National Director of Health Information Technology (ONCHIT), Health Information Technology Leadership Panel Final Report. March 2005. Page 26. Available at: http://www.hhs.gov/healthit/HITFinalReport.pdf

16. Goldman, J, .and Hudson, Z. Exposed: A Health Privacy Primer for Consumers. Health Privacy Project. 1999. Available at: http://www.healthprivacy.org/usr_doc/34775.pdf

17. "Who's Looking at Your files," Gorman, Time, May 6, 1996, p. 60, et.seq.

18. Ganzer, Donna, Community Concers on Information Security, Presentation delivered at the 1996 Annuyal Meeting of the Healthcare Open Systems & Trials, March 21, 1996. Cited in Privacy and Health Information Systems: A Guide to Protecting Patient Confidentiality. Center for Democracy and Technology. Seattle WA: Foundation for Health Care Quality, 1996.

19. Privacy Rights Clearinghouse (PRC). Superior Court of the State of California, County of San Diego. Complaint filed by Utility Consumers Action Network on behalf of the Privacy Rights Cleraninghouse v. ALBERTSONS, INC.; SAV-ON-DRUG STORES, INC.; OSCO DRUG, INC.; JEWEL OSCO, INC.; and DOES 1 through 50, inclusive. Available at: http://www.privacyrights.org/ar/PharmComplaint.htm.

20. Privacy Rights Clearinghouse (PRC). Chronology of Data Breaches website.http://www.privacyrights.org/ar/ChronDataBreaches.htm.

21. American Health Information Management Association, Confidenitality of Medical Records Situation Analysis and AHIMA's Position. Chicago, IL: American Health Information Management Association.

22. Galler et al. Genetic testing for cancer. JAMA. May 14, 1997.

23. Shaffer SL, Simon AR. Network Security. Boston: Harcourt Brace & Company, 1994.

24. Federal Bureau of Investigation and Computer Crime and Security Institute.2005 CSI/FBI Computer Security Survey. Available at: http://www.fbi.gov/page2/july05/cyber072505.htm.

25. Computer-based Patient Record Institute, Security Features for Computer-based Patient Record Systems. Schaumburg, Il: CPRI, 1996.

26. Statement of Robert S. Litt, Deputy Assistant Attorney General, Criminal Division, United States Department of Justice before The Subcommitee on Technology, Terrorism, and Government Information. United States Senate, March 19, 1997.

27. Frawley, K.A. Federal Legislation on Confidentiality: Possibility or Insurmountable Challenge? Journal of the American Health Information Management Association. 1999;70:19-22.

28. Standards for Privacy of Individually Identifiable Health Information.2003. April 17. Code of Federal Regulations 45 CRF 160 and 164.

29. National Research Council, System Security Study Committee, Comuter Science and Telecommunications Board, Commission on Physical Sciences, Mathematics, and Applications. 2000. Computers at Risk: Safe Computing in the Information Age. Washington, DC: National Academy Press.

30. American Health Information Management Association, Chicago, IL http://www.AHIMA.org.

31. Parker, Donn B. Computer Security, Microsoft Encarta Encyclopedia. Http://encarta.msn.com/encarta.

32. Ruthberg, A., Tipton, H (eds) Handbook of Information Security Management Boston: Auerbach, 1993.

33. Department of Health and Human Services. 2003.45 CRF Parts 160, 162, and 164. Federal Register. Vol 68, Now. 34. February 20, 2003.

34. Johns, M.L. HIPAA Security: Computer Based Training Modules. Chicago: Holistic Training Solutions, 2003.

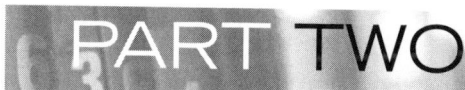

PART TWO

Electronic Health Records
Selection and Implementation:
Workbook

Workbook Introduction

The first 3 sections of this text provide the background information required to understand EHR-related technologies and concepts. Sections IV and V are intended to act as a "workbook" to help the reader apply the information learned in earlier sections. Since those engaged in EHR implementations run the gamut from solo practices to hospitals and large multi-specialty groups, we have endeavored to adapt these chapters to reflect these varied backgrounds. These chapters reflect the insights and the experiences of the authors and were written with an eye to providing practical advice. Particular attention has been given to the needs of ambulatory practices since they often cannot afford expert advice in areas such as change management, project management and security and frequently have more difficulty preparing for an implementation.

Sample forms for EHR product evaluation and RFP creation appear as appendices to chapters 17 and 19 respectively. A vendor evaluation form appears in Chapter 18. Appendix B offers a list of useful resources.

14

Starting the Electronic Health Record Selection Process

Jerome H. Carter, MD

The fact that you are reading this chapter indicates that you are seriously interested in implementing an electronic health record (EHR) system. A survey conducted in solo and small group practices revealed an estimated initial cost of up to $44,000 per fulltime FTE and with on-going costs of about $8500 per year for a typical installation (1). Aside from the dollar cost, there is a price to be paid in lost income, low morale, and simple frustration when an implementation goes sour. Getting your EHR system successfully implemented requires planning and attention to detail. This chapter offers an easy to follow plan and a few words of advice.

Take Your Time and Study Your Practice

There is no rush. You do not have to worry about being the last on your block to have an EHR. Prudence dictates that you assess your short- and long-term practice goals, current economic situation, employee skills and attitudes, and your ability to deal with fear, uncertainty, and doubt. Talk to your accountant in order to determine how much you can afford to spend and what overall economic benefit you may expect from your EHR. Increased productivity does not necessarily mean fewer staff FTEs. Along the same lines, how will you manage the slow-down that frequently occurs after a new system is installed? How do your employees feel about an EHR? Will their fears of being replaced lead to destabilizing resignations? Finally, do you have the patience to see this through to the end? Addressing these issues takes time and thought. Don't rush.

What Worked in a Friend's Practice Will Not Automatically Work in Yours

EHRs are not "one size fits all". Your practice environment (patient mix, employee skills, and specialty) will play a substantial role in determining the type of EHR product that best meets your needs. What works for surgeons may not work for family physicians, and what works for a solo practitioner may not work for a large multi-specialty group. Remember, when viewing demonstrations or conducting site visits, "your mileage may vary". Keep this in mind. When comparing your practice to another, always match as many practice variables as possible to ensure that the respective practices are similar. Your colleague is a touch typist; are you?

On the Surface Most Products Are Similar

EHR products have come a long way over the last five years. Most are the products of professional developers, are technically sound and offer similar features. However, the way that features are implemented may lead to significant differences in ease-of-use or utility. Consider a feature as basic as automatic drug interaction checking. Most EHRs offer this feature. However, all do not allow you to turn off the feature easily, adjust the number or type of interactions which are flagged, or check for food-drug interactions. You would be surprised to find how much the ability to adjust any of these features affects your comfort in using a product. Also, you may find that accomplishing the same task such as writing a prescription takes more steps in one product as compared to another.

The Vendor Is as Important as the Product

Quality, service, and continued existence count whether you are buying an EHR or an automobile. New vendors may have great products, but will they be around next year? Vendors may tout the fact that they have been in business for 10 years, but how often have they updated their products? Does the vendor offer interfaces to other important types of software found in medical offices (i.e., practice management systems, outside labs). How do they handle upgrades? Do they have a local office? Can they provide service during all hours that your practice site operates?

Another key issue is market focus. Few vendors have a service model that allows them to handle solo practices and large multi-specialty groups with equal aplomb. The same is true of specialty practices. Unfortunately, many vendors will sell to anyone who wishes to buy their product even when they know the practice is not typical for their customer base. The result of these mismatches is usually bad service from the vendor if the practice is too far removed from their usual customer base. Always check the market focus; you really don't want to be the five-person group that buys an EHR from a vendor that sells mostly to hospitals.

Do Not Confuse Quality with Price

When you research products you will notice a significant variability in price. This should not be used to determine the quality of the product. Quality should be determined by independent reviews, speaking to current users, length of time the product has been on the market, de-installation rate (removal of the EHR from the practice), and other factors. Quality and price are not synonymous.

After pondering the above points, if you still feel that you are ready to plunge ahead, then the next step is to draw up a plan for selecting and implementing a system. Success depends upon your willingness create a plan and stick to it. Please take planning seriously.

Developing Your Plan

Your EHR project will occur in two major phases: product selection and implementation. Each phase should be conducted using a formal plan. Product selection should begin with a focus on practice issues: goals, budget constraints, information needs (reporting and querying), employee skills, and process analysis (understanding the key tasks that must be performed in your practice). This will lead quite naturally to an RFP that truly reflects practice needs. Once a product has been selected the implementation phase begins. Here attention must be directed to fitting the practice to the EHR product. This entails workflow analysis (how each task is performed by each staff member) and reengineering (refitting the practice to achieve identified goals and to complement the EHR's features and functions). Table 14-1 presents an EHR project plan outline with suggested steps. The suggested completion times assume a practice at a single site with three or four physicians. It also assumes that an "EHR Team" (Chapter 21) consisting of key practice staff has been formed. Solo practices will have much shorter timelines.

Notice the time allotted for setting goals/objectives and for practice analysis steps. These steps, which are dedicated to understanding the fine points of how your practice operates, are the most important of the group. It is in these steps that you develop the vision and define the outcomes that, once realized, will result in the practice improvements that initially led to you consider implementing an EHR. The remainder of this book is dedicated to helping you to both understand and carry out each step of your plan.

Table 14-1

EHR Implementation Plan Outline

Product Selection	Suggested Time for Completion
Set Goals and Objectives (be specific)	1 month
Practice Analysis:	
◆ Process Identification	1 month
◆ Process Analysis	2-3 months
Requirements Specification	1 month
Product Evaluation	1-2 months
Vendor Analysis	1 month
Create and submit Request For Proposal (RFP)	1-2 months
Contract Negotiation	1 month or less
Implementation	
Workflow Analysis and matching to EHR	1-2 months
Re-engineering	1-2 months
Hardware/Software Installation & Testing	1 month or less
Training	1 week
Go-live until normal patient flow returns	2-3 months

Goals and Objectives

What problems are you trying to solve? Frame your answers in the most concrete terms possible. Are you hoping to increase productivity, reduce staff FTEs, improve access to patient data, improve safety, participate in pay-for-performance programs, or improve quality? These are a few of the reasons most often given for investigating EHR systems. Unfortunately, the next step is frequently a call to an EHR vendor. The more appropriate action would be to look at each problem more closely and determine what exactly would be required to address it. A good way to start is with staff interviews. Have each person create a list of common problems that they regularly encounter or how they would like to see the practice improve and then group them by type (goals, problems, wish list, etc.). Typical goals/objectives and problems are discussed below.

"We would like to increase productivity"

Productivity is a fairly vague concept in many practice situations. If increased productivity is the goal, it would be very helpful to know what is currently impeding an increase in productivity. If you wish to increase productivity, you must first define it in terms of what happens on a daily basis in your practice. Let us assume that in your practice productivity is defined as the number of patients seen per day. The obvious next step is to determine why more patients cannot be seen each day.

If a good deal of time is spent looking for charts or if needed information is frequently unavailable when seeing patients, then you have identified a common cause of decreased productivity. Assuming that locating charts during patient visits is an issue, it would be helpful to categorize this as a chart access problem.

Once chart access issues are on the table, try to determine if there are other chart access problems. Remote access to patient data, especially while on-call, is a well recognized access issue. Similarly, concurrent access (multiple users at the same time) may be an issue in large practices where more than one provider may need access to the paper chart at the same time. Finally the simple, but very common, problem of temporarily misplaced charts is one that many practices deal with daily.

Once you are satisfied that you have a fairly complete issue list, turn your attention to understanding why they exist. At this point you are trying to determine which issues may be addressed by changes in administrative policy and procedures as opposed to those that can only be solved by an EHR. Consider the example of an office where there is a thirty-minute lag-time between patient sign-in and placement in an examining room. If the delay is due to problems locating the patient's chart, then an EHR might help. However, if the delay is due to poorly trained staff, an EHR may actually result in a decrease in productivity. Table 14-2 contains a list of causes of low productivity that an EHR will *not* improve. Make sure that none are present in your practice before purchasing an EHR. No amount of technology will resolve these issues; sound administrative policies are required.

"We would like to implement quality improvement, safety, and pay-for-performance programs"

Quality improvement starts with the implementation of best practices for common ailments. The key is ensuring that all patients receive the proper interventions at the proper times. EHRs support quality improvement by

Table 14-2

COMMON ISSUES THAT AFFECT PRODUCTIVITY

Poor staff training

Poorly defined staff duties

Lack of formal administrative policy

Ineffective process for handling telephone calls

Ineffective process for managing charts

Ineffective process for managing information flow into the practice (labs, x-rays, referrals, etc.)

Poor resource scheduling (e.g., procedure suites)

making it much easier to identify patients who have specific diagnoses and to ensure that they receive the required interventions. This is often difficult to do with paper charts because of the time required for case finding and follow up.

Not harming patients while providing care is at the heart of patient safety. The medication features of EHRs provide the most obvious example of patient safety features. Drug-drug interactions checking and automatic allergy checks during prescription writing are good examples. Creating a legible prescription contributes to patient safety in a less "high-tech" way.

In addition to quality and safety issues, EHRs also help with other types of "outcomes" studies. Provider profiles, patient satisfaction, and simple performance studies are well within the capabilities of the average practice. Each may be done manually, but an EHR will certainly make things much easier. Of course, proper administrative policies must be in place to ensure that data are collected and entered in a systematic manner.

Pay-for-performance is another side of the quality/safety coin having the same basic requirements for the use of standardized protocols. Participating in these programs requires submission of patient data. Therefore, one important feature required of an EHR for pay-for-performance is the ability to create and export data sets using common informatics standards (Chapter 6).

Review your practice with an eye toward standardizing as many common activities as possible. You may, for example, reduce the number of laboratory service providers utilized. This will decrease the number of lab order forms that staff must use and remove the need for remembering multiple names for various combinations of common lab tests (e.g.; chem-7 vs. electrolyte panel). Do you have a process for ensuring that all diabetic patients receive yearly eye exams? Do you conduct chart reviews to determine if all required documentation is present? How are common interventions such as flu shots recorded? Do you have a special form or flow sheet for interventions or are these items included only in the provider's note? Table 14-3 list suggestions for preparing your practice for quality, safety and pay-for-performance programs

Table 14-3

STEPS FOR PREPARING FOR QUALITY, SAFETY, AND PAY-FOR-PERFORMANCE

Implement standard preventive health measures

Implement standard protocols for accepted clinical practices (ACE inhibitors for CHF, inhaled steroids for asthma, etc.)

Standardize documentation (templates) for common procedures and interventions

"We need to get a better handle on costs"

Cost control is a major issue for many practices, especially for those with significant numbers of capitated patients. An EHR can help in this area. However, an EHR alone is not enough; your practice management system is important as well. When dealing with capitation the costs generated from a patient encounter are derived from three main sources: diagnostic interventions (labs, x-rays, procedures), referrals, and therapeutic interventions (depending upon the amount of risk taken on by the practice). Begin your analysis by reviewing use of medications and diagnostic studies by diagnosis. For example, in managing patients with headaches, how often do you order CT scans or refer to neurologists? How often do providers order electrolyte studies for patients taking diuretics? Many common prescribing habits may confer little real benefit to the patient. An excellent example of this is the widespread use of antibiotics for common upper respiratory infections. Another cost saving measure that is also good medicine is the use of prophylactic medications for patient who suffer from migraine headaches. Effective prophylaxis may result in less use of expensive pain medications and fewer emergency room visits. Table 14-4 offers suggestions for reviewing practice patient care related costs.

"We need better access to patient information"

Timely access to information is a cornerstone of good patient care. Large practices and those with multiple sites are most likely to have problems with chart access. Remote access, while on call or simply away from the office, provides an additional example of the need for easy and rapid access to patient data. This is perhaps one of the clearest benefits of EHR technology.

Table 14-4

COMMON ISSUES THAT AFFECT PRODUCTIVITY

Review use of disposable supplies for unnecessary use/overuse

Review practice guidelines for common diseases for suggestions for best use of diagnostic studies and interventions

Look at antibiotic prescribing habits for over use

Look at outside referral patterns for common procedures/diagnoses

Review emergency room visits with particular emphasis patients with the following diagnoses: asthma, chest pain, headache, URI, UTI, abdominal pain

Review use of patient educational materials/walk-out instructions

Access to patient data for internal care processes or for sharing with other providers is not a function of EHR technology alone. Data quality is important and has to be managed carefully. As with many other things in a practice, high quality data requires well-defined administrative policies that are adequately enforced. Proper respect for the importance of properly managing patient information for legal and regulatory reasons must be emphasized and reflected in practice policies .

Take time to sit down with your medical records staff and review any issues they may have regarding current policies. Ask for suggestions for new policies or changes to current ones. Standardize forms placed on charts, look for redundant forms and practices, and optimize those procedures deemed worth keeping. Obviously, staff training is a major component of sound patient information management activities. Keep in mind that your EHR will become your legal record and must be treated accordingly. You must be able to demonstrate that the contents of your EHR are tamper-proof and that all signatures are valid and cannot be forged.

This is also a good time to look at communications with outside clinical consultants or facilities. Can paper-based reports be transmitted in electronic form? Would consulting providers be willing to send reports via disk, e-mail, or fax? Try polling consultants/groups with whom your practice has frequent interactions to determine if better ways of moving patient information can be agreed upon. Finally, when evaluating EHRs, look for systems that permit easy import of outside data and allow for remote access with good security protocols.

Parting Advice

You are about to start on a journey that will never really end. New technologies will appear, new reporting requirements will be mandated, your needs will evolve. Therefore, it is very important that you keep your goals firmly in mind. Monitor and evaluate your practice on a regular basis, look for inefficiencies and opportunities to improve. Remember, successful implementation of an EHR is very much dependent on your ability to identify and analyze your information needs. The remaining chapters of Section IV EHR Selection (Chapters 15-20) and Section V, EHR Implementation (21-25) will help you through each step.

References

1. Miller RH, West C, Brown TM, et al. The value of electronic health records in solo or small group practices. Health Aff (Millwood). 2005;24:1127-37.

15

How to Use Consultants Effectively

Erica L. Drazen, ScD, BS

Planning for, selecting, and implementing an electronic health record (EHR) is something a practice will do once every decade, so most practices do not have a lot of expertise or tools to make the process efficient and to ensure that the right decisions are made. There are hundreds of product options on the market, so even creating a short list of products to look at is a daunting task. Implementation of an EHR is not only expensive, it also requires a huge change in operations—you need to get it right on the first try! Because of these challenges, many organizations use experienced consultants to help select and implement EHR systems.

There are four basic reasons businesses hire information technology consultants:

1. **To access skills that are needed on a one-time or intermittent basis:** Electronic record system selection and implementation is a process that a practice will do no more than once every five years. It is impractical to acquire staff that is skilled in the facets of information systems planning, selection, or implementation for what amounts to episodic needs. Consultants present a reasonable solution, offering ready expertise in a timely and cost-efficient manner.

2. **To supply in-depth knowledge that is not resident in the organization:** Along with their technical expertise, consultants bring an insider's knowledge of key vendors, products, and services. The EHR vendor world changes frequently. Technology is continually evolving and products evolve at very different rates. New vendors enter the market and others close their doors, and the existing vendors' business fundamentals may change through market success, partnerships, mergers, or acquisitions. In the absence of a dominant EHR vendor, market shifts affect all players in the market.

Keeping up to date on the status of available products and vendors requires an on-going data collection process. Interpreting changes requires an understanding of the history of the market and the market participants.

3. **To provide an independent viewpoint:** In a market with so many vendors and so little long-term experience, vendors offering "solutions" can deluge physicians and physician office staff. This frequently causes more confusion than clarification. It is also not unusual for different participants in the decision process to have very different priorities and viewpoints. A physician with a hospital-based practice may be partial to a product offered by the hospital's vendor. Another physician may prefer to purchase a system she has used in a prior institution; if anyone has already purchased a system that meets their needs, they will want that to be the official solution. It is very helpful to be able to offload some of the tough political calls to someone whose only interest is doing what is best for the practice overall and who can leave at the end of the project.

4. **To provide supplementary resources for a short period of time:** The final reason to hire a consultant is for an "extra set of hands." Selection and implementation of a new EHR system will require a significant investment of time. Your staff knows the practice better than any consultant, and their expertise is essential to optimize processes in the automated environment. However, your staff cannot possibly supply all the resources needed to implement a system; they need to be supplemented with outside resources. These resources should be familiar with ambulatory care and the EHR system you have selected.

A Glimpse into the Consulting Business

To understand how to select and use a consultant effectively, it is helpful to understand the economics of consulting. Consulting firms hire skilled professionals and make major investments to ensure that those professionals expand their skills and build their knowledge base. The "product" that the consulting firm sells is time. Since "time" has no shelf life, a successful consulting firm must maximize the time available staff are working on client projects. This results in lower costs for the consulting firm and, hence, lower rates for consulting services.

One challenge in providing services to the physician practice market is that the time to sell a project is almost as long and involves a similar effort to selling to a large health plan or IDN, yet the revenue will be smaller. Also, small projects offer less flexibility to reallocate staff time among tasks if there are delays in scheduling meetings, waiting for decisions, etc. An effective collaboration between a consultant and a physician practice needs to recognize the realities of each other's business drivers.

An "ideal client" understands what they want from a consulting project, designs an efficient approach to selecting the consultant, recognizes the need to plan for using the consultant's time, and commits to minimize the changes to that plan.

Finding a Consultant

One could go to a consulting directory, wander the trade show at meetings, or look for advertising in trade magazines. However, the most common, and probably the best, way to select a consultant is through a personal referral. Who do you know that recently made a similar EHR decision? What consultant did they use? What consultant does the hospital or health plan use for IT planning or selections: do they have experts in EHR systems?

Some professional organizations and state medical societies maintain lists of recommended consultants; a few actually offer consulting services. Another approach is to look for consultants who are active in the Center for Certification of Healthcare Technology (CCHIT), relevant standards organizations, or groups such as AMIA or AHIMA. Consultants who have served as judges for the Davies EHR award also have demonstrated their commitment and knowledge of the field.

KLAS (www.healthcomputing.com) ranks consultants based on ratings submitted by customers. Their Top 20 Year-End Best In KLAS Report for 2006 listed Hayes Management, FCG, and IBM as the top three vendors for planning and assessment and IBM, FCG, and McKesson as the top three vendors for clinical systems implementation. The ratings include work for more hospitals than practices, but it could provide a useful starting point.

Before implementing any of these approaches, you need to decide:

1. Why you need a consultant

2. What you want the consultant to do

3. Your selection criteria for choosing your consultant

At a minimum, items one and two should be shared with consulting teams you are considering.

Selecting a Consultant

There are four elements that are essential to selecting the right consultant: skills, knowledge, fit, and aligned interests. The optimal balance of these elements depends on the role you want the consultant to play. The elements are attributes of both the individual consultants you will be working with and attributes of the consulting firm. Except when dealing with individual consultants, the firm and the individuals both need to be evaluated to select the ideal consultant.

If you expect a consulting firm to assist you in planning, selection, and implementation of your EHR system, it is important to evaluate whether a consulting firm selected for an earlier task (e.g., planning) has skills in selection and implementation also. Selecting one firm that can provide all the services you need decreases your investment in bringing outsiders "up the learning curve." Also consultants who have implemented EHR systems have a detailed knowledge of what makes these systems work; this knowledge can be invaluable in the early stages of planning and selection.

When you are looking for a consultant to help in an EHR project, you want more than generic skills. You want someone who is knowledgeable about your business and the EHR industry. You should be in a good position to judge the knowledge of your business. You can also ask, "What are the challenges you have seen in similar projects for similar organizations?" "How have your dealt with them?" "What value should we expect from this project?" "How can it be measured?" Any consultant you are considering should be able to answer the question: "Across the industry, what do you feel are the top five vendors and why?" They should also have an opinion on "up and coming" vendors. If the answers to these questions ring true and the consultants demonstrate operational knowledge, in similar settings, you can feel comfortable. Another (useful but dreaded) test is the pop quiz. Twenty-four to forty-eight hours before interviewing the consultant, you present a real-life issue you have faced or are currently facing and ask for advice during the interview.

You expect an EHR to provide benefits to your organization. To make sure you achieve this goal, you need to have realistic expectations, select an EHR system that provides the right support, and be willing to redesign processes to use the system effectively. Any consultant should be able to provide information on what goals have been achieved in other sites and what features and redesign are essential to attain the benefits.

At the current pace of change in industry players, products, and technology, it is impossible for any person to have complete and current knowledge of all industry products in memory. You certainly do not want to pay for a comprehensive inventory of vendors to be compiled. Therefore, any consultant should have a database of vendors available to be used to match your needs to possible solutions. You will want to check out:

◆ The size of the database (number of vendors)

◆ The topics covered (at a minimum, it should cover product features, technology, business metrics, and implementation experience)

◆ The sources of information (hopefully not solely from the vendor themselves)

◆ The currency of information and the updating process

Any vendor who does not track more than a dozen EHR vendors regularly probably is not ideally suited to consult on EHR issues.

Fit is the match between the consultant's style and knowledge and your needs. One aspect of "fit" is "chemistry": whether you feel comfortable with the consultant, the consultant's interaction with staff at all levels is appropriate, you think you could work with these people. This can be tested only with a face-to-face interaction with the principals who will be working with you. In some cases you may want to select a consultant because they would not fit your culture. If you tend to have difficulty making efficient business decisions, you might want to pick a consultant who does not. If you tend to get mired in detail, you might want a consultant who has a bias toward the strategic level, etc. In general you want a consultant who will challenge you, but who will not make unnecessary waves in your organization and you definitely want someone you can work with for several months. For the reasons discussed earlier, no firm can commit a team to a project until a start date is established; however, you should be able to meet the person who will have lead responsibility. You may also want to reserve the right to interview and approve any member of the team who will be working on site.

When considering the potential biases a consultant might bring to the relationship, the real question is "Does this consultant have a reason to alter their advice to you because of other financial interests?" The most obvious bias is involvement with a vendor. Clearly you run a risk if you ask a potential supplier of your EHR to be your consultant or your implementation partner, but this does happen. Less visible biases you need to worry about include whether the consultant has any direct financial interest in an EHR vendor or has an exclusive implementation agreement with a vendor. There are also potential biases if the consultant has other business relationships with you. Your law firm, or your accounting firm, may be inclined not to "rock the boat" and could shy away from giving advice that they think you are not ready to hear.

Many consultants have implementation agreements with vendors: they are certified to install the vendor's product and may sell these services either directly or through the vendor. Implementation experience is very valuable in your consultant because a consultant with implementation experience must have an in-depth knowledge of the product, and they have a better understanding of the total cost of ownership of the products that you may be considering. Rather than excluding any consultant who has implementation agreements with potential vendors, it could be helpful to select a consultant who has non-exclusive agreements with a large number of EHR vendors. Consultants should be willing to disclose any vendor relationships so you can assess whether you have confidence you will be getting independent advice.

Most processes of selecting a consultant include checking references. However, any consultant certainly can give you three or four great references.

Unless you know the references personally, the loyalty of the references to the consultant may be stronger than their relationship to you. On the other hand, it is unrealistic to ask the consultant to give you a list of all their clients and just randomly call whomever you want. You would not want to be the recipient of a large number of such calls. A good compromise is to ask the consultant for a list of current clients (for the last six months, a year, etc.) and review the list to find references you know personally or you think are similar to you. Select a few (two or three should be sufficient) and then provide the consultant with the opportunity to make a courtesy call to let the reference know you will be calling.

The Partnership

There is much talk about "partnerships" today. Every vendor and consultant wants to be your "partner." Clearly, what they really want is for you to be their customer. In many cases "partnership" is no more than "buzzword." What makes a partnership work is aligned incentives. Any established consulting firm that is dedicated to the healthcare industry has a built-in incentive for a project to be successful. This is a small industry and consultants know that they must maintain a reputation for the quality of the work and for successful outcomes.

One technique that is talked about is putting the fees or part of the fees at risk to be paid only if a certain level of performance is achieved. The two questions are: "Is there a measurable outcome?" and "Is the outcome within the consultant's control?" If the answer to these questions is "yes" then performance guarantees can be effective. For instance, a part of an implementation consultant's fee could be dependent on a successful "go live" by a specified time frame. It is also reasonable to hold a software developer accountable for on-time delivery of working code.

Contract negotiations are the time to really test the partnership. Is the consultant willing to share information on project costs by task? Can you have a productive discussion of where the approach could be changed to lower costs? Is the consultant willing to name staff who will be assigned? Two questions that are useful to ask are: "What activities are likely to provide marginal value? And, "If we had more money, what activities would you suggest we add to the project?"

Although it will be tempting, beware of consultants who are willing to cut the price of an engagement without changing the scope of work. They may have padded the original bid, cut corners, or ask for additional money later, when you really are in no position to say "no." Small discounts, or discounts for prompt start or prompt pay, are sometimes offered and may be advantageous for both sides.

Custom crafting of contract language is rarely needed and is costly for both sides. Typically, the consultant has a standard contract: if you have one too, you can just compare and negotiate differences. You also might want to review your employee agreement and add any items that are relevant, including, for instance, provisions to protect confidential patient information. If you get to the point where you have to pull out a contract to reach agreement, the relationship is over anyway.

Obviously, selecting a consultant is only the first step in building a successful relationship. As part of the final selection process you should agree on a schedule for the work, roles and responsibilities, and work products that will be delivered. The most important part of the scheduling is arranging for interviews and group meetings, especially any that will require scheduling physician's time.

Most consultants prefer to work with you rather than independently. However, the "collaboration" can vary from review at check points to a joint team. If there is valuable knowledge that you can gain from the consultant and apply in the future, you will want to have a joint team. An extreme example would be teaming on the initial implementation of a system that will be installed in multiple clinics. As the implementation progressed, the consultant staff numbers could decrease and your staff complement increase. However, typically you do not have the staff available to be a full-time part of the consultant's team. Even in that case, it is vital to have a project manager on your side that does have time available to stay in contact with the consulting team, monitor progress, and provide direction. It also makes sense for your staff to take responsibility for tasks that you can do much more quickly and efficiently than the consultant. This might include scheduling interviews (your staff knows how each office works), digging out financial data, or creating an inventory of existing systems.

Finally, it is important to keep channels of communication open. If the project seems to be getting off track, raise the issue early, have an open discussion, and agree on changes to be made. The decision you are making is an important and expensive one. You need to make sure you are getting the best help and advice available.

16

From Process Analysis To Product Evaluation

Jerome H. Carter, MD

Work in a medical practice consists of many common clinical and administrative activities such as writing a prescription, scheduling a referral, ordering labs, and registering a new patient, all of which occur on a daily basis as a series of "steps" carried out by one or more members of the staff. Each activity, along with the steps required to complete it, is referred to as a "process". The "work" that is accomplished as processes move from step to step is referred to as the workflow (1). Since processes form the basis for all work that occurs in a practice, we naturally want to analyze them to determine if they are efficient, effective, invariant, and properly documented (Table 16-1). In anticipation of an electronic health record implementation, process analysis also helps to determine which product will best support the needs of the practice. Electronic health record (EHR) features and functions are designed to support the individual steps of common processes, and therefore selecting the best EHR for your practice necessitates understanding what your most important processes are and the steps involved in completing them. That, in a nutshell, is process analysis and why it is important.

The list of EHR features and functions generated based on the process analysis we refer to as a requirements document (RD). The requirements document, along with practice profile (Chapter 14) and vendor qualification (Chapter 18), comprise the core components of the request for proposal (RFP) (Chapter 19) that is sent to prospective vendors. If process analysis is done with the proper attention to detail, you will find that determining which EHR product is best for your practice is not only much easier, but also that the overall EHR selection process becomes much more rational. There is no one "correct" way to do process analysis, and the approach taken varies from organization to organization. The approach to process analysis outlined in this chapter has EHR evaluation and selection as its main goals and has been used

Table 16-1

ANALYSIS CRITERIA

Criteria	Definition
Efficient	Process is completed with fewest possible steps
Effective	Always results in the desired outcome
Properly Documented	Process is documented in a manner that meets all billing, legal, and regulatory requirements
Invariant	There is only one accepted way of completing the process

by the author for a number of projects. This method of using process analysis to guide product selection may be adapted to any size practice. There are six steps: 1) process identification, 2) process analysis, 3) reengineering, 4) matching EHR features to processes, 5) creation of the request for proposal document, and 6) product evaluation.

Step 1: Identifying Processes for Analysis

When attempting process analysis for the first time, it is easy to be intimidated by the apparent scope of the task. However, keep in mind that analyzing every single process in your practice is not important. Instead, the focus should be on the most common processes and those that are specific to your practice or specialty. Remember, the focus of process analysis at this stage is to help you select the EHR that has the features and functions that you require.

Table 16-2 has a list of common processes for the average practice. Within any process there are specialty-specific variations. For example, pediatricians use growth charts during regular visits and oncologists have very specialized requirements for calculating medication doses that other specialties do not require. A good way to generate the best list of processes for your practice is to have everyone (or a representative group) participate in a brainstorming session. Have everyone list the things they do every day and then group and compare them to those in the table. Brainstorming is a great way to identify processes because it also provides a mechanism for staff to begin to discuss what is broken and what works well.

Step 2: Starting Your Analysis

Once you have a list of processes to analyze, the next step is to determine how well things are working currently. Take the list and create a matrix similar to Table 16-3. Then for each process on your list discuss each of the four global process traits as listed in Table 16-1. Be sure to get as many

Table 16-2

COMMON PRACTICE PROCESSES

Administrative

Patient registration

Appointment

Make outside referral

Create Bill

Telephone triage

Schedule procedure

Clinical

Order test

Review lab results

Start new medication

Prescription renewal

Document encounter

Patient education

New patient visit

Nurse only visit

Document Procedure

Preventive care/quality assessment

Hospital admission

members of the staff involved as possible in order to ensure a good flow of ideas. For each issue or problem identified, record potential solutions and work-arounds. Once initiated, these "practice improvement" sessions will become an integral part of EHR implementation planning. If the practice does not have a formal polices and procedure manual, this is the time to start to write one. (Start with the most common processes and those that are shared by the most job positions.)

Efficiency

Inefficient processes waste staff time and money. Review each step in the process and determine if it is necessary. If forms are involved in the process, look for duplication between data elements of the forms. For example, if two forms are involved in the same process and each requires the patient's name, address, and medical record number, it may be possible to combine both forms into one with two sections, cutting down on paper cost and the bulk of the chart. Also make sure that all staff members conduct the process with the same number of steps and with the same forms. Even in small practices it is surprising how much variation can exist and how different staff members complete the same task in different ways.

Table 16-3

GLOBAL PROCESS TRAITS

Process	Efficiency	Effectiveness	Documentation	Variations
ADMINISTRATIVE				
Patient registration				
Patient appointment				
Make outside referral				
Create Bill				
Telephone triage				
Scheduled procedure				
CLINICAL				
Order test				
Review lab results				
Start new medication				
Prescription renewal				
Document encounter				
Patient education				
New patient visit				
Nurse only visit				
Document Procedure				
Preventive care/quality assessment				
Hospital admission				

Effectiveness

Effective processes always produce the intended outcome. If the process is "making an appointment", then patients always receive the intended appointment with the appropriate provider. If the process is writing a prescription, then it always results in the proper medication and proper dose for the correct patient. Ineffective processes result in frustration for the patients as well as practice staff. Examples of ineffective processes are: failure to notify patients of lab results, prescription refill never called to pharmacy, requested appointment was never made. Every busy practice has plenty of examples of processes that are broken or ineffective.

Proper Documentation

Proper documentation is required to meet billing, legal, and regulatory needs. Many patient-related tasks often are poorly documented due to time pressures and hassle involved in pulling charts. Telephone calls are a good example. When a patient calls the practice to discuss an issue related to their medical care, the content and outcome of that conversation should be properly recorded.

Another common and poorly documented process is follow-up of abnormal lab results. Appropriate documentation should include signing of the report, note of the intended plan of action, and what was discussed with the patient. Many practices attempt to improve documentation for practice activities by using forms. This approach only works to the extent that staff are willing to follow the required procedures. More often than not, adding more forms tends to make documentation even more problematic because the forms are not used consistently.

Variation

Process variation is usually the result of physician work habits, poor staff training, absence of formal policies and procedures, or lack of administrative oversight. Every process should have, as a matter of policy, a specific set of steps that are required to produce the expected result. Any deviation (adding, altering, or deleting steps) creates variation that represents an unauthorized pathway. For example, say that as a matter of policy new patients must have insurance eligibility reviewed and approved prior to receiving an appointment. Any patient who receives an appointment without an insurance review represents an alternative (variant) appointment pathway. Variation is best addressed by proper training of staff, attentive administrative oversight, and clearly written policies and procedures.

Physician work habits are more difficult to address because they are so personal. They are also the greatest single source of implementation problems. Each EHR product is designed to carry out tasks in a specific manner. Using an EHR means one has adapt to its way of doing things. This requires that every provider adopt a standard way of accomplishing every task. Changing long-held practice habits in order to adopt to an EHR system is always a source of frustration (at least temporarily) and occasionally leads to a complete rejection of the EHR system. Standardization across all providers of common clinical tasks such as preventive care intervetions, abnormal results management, and clinical documentation should be a major focus of all process analysis and reengineering activities.

Identifying Steps

Concurrent with the discussion of global traits, create a flowchart (Figure 16-1) that illustrates process steps in the order of occurrence. Collect all forms that are used in the process and note in your flowchart where the forms appear. Be sure that all steps are represented and in the proper order. Figure 16-1 shows the steps for a typical "Review Lab Results" process. At this point it is not necessary to delve into the specifics of how each step is carried out, simply focus on accounting for all steps.

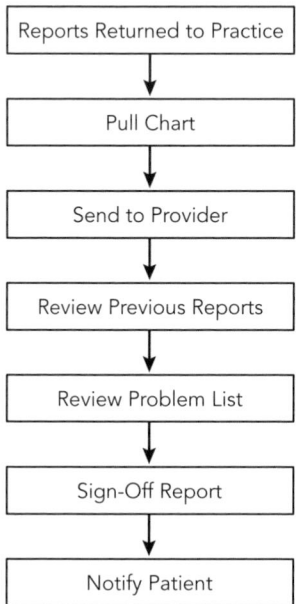

Figure 16-1   Review of Labs Process Steps

Step 3: Begin Optimizing Processes

When processes are found that require improvement, make the necessary changes, test the new version of the process, and then reevaluate. Since an EHR implementation is planned, focus on improvements to manual processes that affect are critical areas or that are badly flawed (e.g. frequent billing errors, poor follow-up for abnormal results, poor preventive care procedures). Although every practice is different, there are a few general measures that can be used to guide reengineering initiatives. Review Table 16-4 and see if any apply to your situation. If done conscientiously, process analysis can yield significant practice improvements even if no EHR implementation occurs. For a 3-5 provider practice allot two to four months for an analysis.

Level of analysis

One danger in doing process analysis is becoming too detailed early on. This is especially true when the ultimate goal is EHR implementation. Until a specific product has been selected it is not possible to decide how all key tasks will be performed. Therefore, initially process analysis should focus on major process steps and obvious problems. Once a specific product has been selected and the final stages of implementation planning has be-

Table 16-4

GENERAL PRACTICE IMPROVEMENT MEASURES

◆ Combine forms with many common elements into single form with multiple sections.

◆ Create an official version of each key process and use this for training and auditing purposes.

◆ Create a policy and procedure manual. The P&P manual is where the official version of how the practice operates is recorded. It will help with employee training and future improvement efforts.

◆ Institute regular process audits. Audits can begin with paper and continue with the EHR.

◆ Assign information gathering responsibilities exclusively to specific job roles. For example, allow only front office staff to gather and update patient demographic information.

◆ Create a formal employee orientation and training program. This will assure that everyone learns the "official" way of doing things.

◆ Create a permanent practice improvement committee.

gun then the level of analysis moves lower and becomes more detailed. At this point work processes are identified that must be adapted to utilize the functions and features of the EHR. The focus of analysis then moves to how each individual will interact with the EHR to accomplish their "work" as well as how work will move from person to person in the practice. (This is often referred to as "workflow analysis"). This is the final phase of process optimization.

Step 4: Matching Processes to Electronic Medical Records Features

Once major processes have been identified and rendered as flowcharts, it is time to work on the requirements specification. Start by creating a form or spreadsheet similar to that in Table 16-5. List each step of the targeted process in the left column and list the EHR feature required to support that step in the right column. To complete this step you will need familiarity with common EHR features and functions. Chapter 17 provides a review of the major features and functions of EHR products grouped by subject area (medications, labs, clinical encounter, etc.). Read the descriptions of the various features until you have a good understanding of what they are and why they are useful. After reading Chapter 17 you may wish to visit the website for the Certification Commission for Health Information Technology (CCHIT, www.cchit.org) and review the criteria used by the commission to certify electronic health record products (this is also a list of features and functions).

Table 16-5

MATCHING PROCESS STEPS TO EHR FEATURES/FUNCTIONS

Review of Labs Process Step	Supporting EHR Feature/Function
Reports return to practice	External Lab interface with automatic lab download
Pull chart	Search patients by name, SSN, MRN or other identifier
Send to Provider	Provider "Inbox", Task list or message alert
Review previous reports	Lab Result screen view, lab results report generation, flowsheet view, ability to display one or more results as a graph
Review problem List	Problem List view, display problems by type (acute, chronic, active, resolved)
Sign-off report	Electronic signature, role-based security
Notify patient	Automatic creation of patient letters when results are normal. Add report to provider "task list" or "desktop" if abnormal. Allow electronic messages to be sent to office staff

After becoming familiar with common product features and functions, it will not be difficult to find the EHR features/functions that match to steps in your process flowchart. The "Review of Labs" process appears in Table 16-5 along with EHR functions that support each step.

When gathering requirements it is not necessary to determine exactly how each feature works for any specific EHR product. The goal at this stage is simply to get a complete list of all the features and functions an EHR must have in order to support important practice tasks. If done properly, the total number of key processes listed for an average practice of three to five providers should be in the range of twenty to twenty-five. For most process steps there is usually at least one EHR feature that will support that step. Often two or three features can be identified that support each step. Do not limit requirements to those derived solely from current processes. Review ancillary needs such as interactions with hospitals and practices (data exchange requirements), HIPAA, remote access needs, and regulatory (pay-for-performance) requirements for inclusion in your requirements document (and do not forget your wish list items and other bells and whistles) (Table 16-6).

Often practices move to demos and sites visits too early in the EHR selection process and come away dazed and confused. Site visits should be postponed until you have narrowed the number of products down to maximum of three or four. However, once you have a preliminary set of requirements, demos can be quite useful (Chapter 20). Use demonstrations to see how common features such as prescription writing or documenting a clinical encounter work. Demonstrations should not last longer than one

Table 16-6

ADDITIONAL USEFUL REQUIREMENTS/EHR FEATURES

◆ Use of informatics standards (SNOMED, DICOM, HL-7)
◆ Application service provider model (ASP) availability
◆ Biometric user authentication
◆ Sub-specialty support features:
  1. Documentation templates
  2. Clinical Research support
  3. Video/ picture galleries
  4. Specialized order sets
◆ Interfaces to specific software systems (e.g. practice management)
◆ Hardware interfaces (EKG, PFT, etc.)
◆ Remote access options
◆ Languages other than English
◆ Clinical decision support
  1. Electronic books
  2. Guidelines
  3. Calculators
◆ e-prescribing
◆ Voice recognition support
◆ Data exchange and report generation capability

hour and should cover common functions. Never attend a demonstration without a list of specific questions for the vendor. Otherwise, the demonstrations will become a blur of colors and jargon. Do not allow yourself to be taken in by what you are seeing and prematurely sign a contract: these are window shopping excursions. I suggest each team member attend no more than five demonstrations (not all team members need to see the same demonstrations).

Requirements Document

The final requirements specification document consists of a detailed list of requirements that are cross-referenced to process steps and EHR features. However, a lengthy list is cumbersome for decision-making unless the requirements are organized in some meaningful way. Grouping requirements by function and then prioritizing them according to how important they are to the practice makes the document much more useful as a product evaluation aide. As you move on to product evaluations you will need a way to pare down the number of products to be evaluated to no more than two to three and you will require a much more detailed manner of interacting with potential products. The request for proposal (RFP) and test scenarios respectively fill these roles.

Step 5: Request for Proposal

An RFP (Chapter 19) is a document that lists all of the requirements that you have identified for an EHR that will meet the needs of your practice. The RFP consists of a practice profile (Chapter 14), information taken from the requirements document, and questions that aid in vendor analysis (Chapter 18). The average RFP is a lengthy document that requires a good deal of effort on the part of the vendor to respond. Therefore, send RFPs only to those vendors whose products you are seriously considering (no more than four, ideally two).

Step 6: Product Evaluation

Test scenarios (Table 16-7) are detailed scripts used to test EHR products that are based on specific real-life scenarios. They help to ensure that product evaluations are methodical and focused, permitting "apple-to-apple"

Table 16-7

TEST SCENARIO: NEW PATIENT VISIT

A 63-year-old female patient with a history of osteoarthritis and gastroesophageal reflux disease presents for an initial visit.

Front Desk
1. Enter demographic information
2. Check insurance plan/eligibility
3. Check duplicate name alert
4. Enter Visit type

Nurse
1. Enter vital signs
2. Enter past medical history
3. Enter social history
4. Enter allergies
5. Enter chief complaint

Provider
1. Enter encounter note
2. Create a problem list
3. Create medication list
4. Write prescriptions
   ♦ drug interactions
   ♦ allergies
5. Order test/x-rays
6. Set up preventive medicine profile

Nurse
1. Patient education

Front Desk
1. Schedule next appointment

product comparisons. The complexity of the product being evaluated will help to determine the number scenarios to be used and the level of detail that each will contain. For office-based EHR products, generally three scenarios that cover a majority of common office functions is sufficient. In test situations, scenarios might take anywhere from forty to sixty minutes to complete. When creating your scenario make sure that you account for all important requirements. Create a form based on your requirements specification document that contains your complete list of prioritized requirements and the name of the product being evaluated. As you are moving through a scenario, note on the evaluation form how each feature or function performs. Also note the overall look and feel of the product. Finally, unlike window shopping demonstrations, all team members should test each product.

Final Product Selection

Final product selection will depend on a number of factors: price, comfort with the vendor, and of course, team evaluations. However, if the approach outlined in this chapter is used, you will maximize the likelihood of buying just the right product to meet your needs.

References

1. Workflow Management Coalition Terminology & Glossary. Available at: http://www.wfmc.org/standards/docs/TC-1011_term_glossary_v3.pdf, accessed January 12, 2008.

17

Evaluation of Product Features

Jerome H. Carter, MD

E valuating the various types of electronic health record products and their features is never easy. A major impediment is the sheer number of available products. At last count, more than 250 companies offered products in this category. Therefore, selecting a product to meet your needs requires a careful, well-thought-out strategy. A sound evaluation policy should occur on two levels. The first level involves the analysis of your practice's clinical and business processes. A review of product features and functions constitutes the second level. Once the results of these analyses are available, then and only then, should attention be given to evaluation of specific products. If you have skipped this vital step, save yourself future headaches; go back and complete it.

The Role of Process Analysis

The lack of a standard definition for an EHR and the desire of vendors to differentiate their products has had the practical effect of encouraging significant variation in products' functions, features, interfaces, and technical quality. (CCHIT criteria focus on core requirements, which leaves room for significant product differences). Comparing apples to apples is nearly impossible. What is possible, and very doable, is comparing your process support needs to the features and functions of an EHR product. The previous chapter offered guidance on performing process analyses and using the results to create a "Request for Proposal" (RFP) and test scenarios. The RFP serves two purposes. First it provides a formal means for telling vendors what you need their product to do for you. Second, it may be used as a resource document for conducting formal product evaluations, demonstrations, and site visits. After all, it contains a statement of what you think is important in a product. This is a very key point to remember. Too often, organizations spend months creating an RFP and use it only to solicit a response from vendors. Avoid this common mistake and treat it as an active on-going statement of your needs. Keep a copy handy and refer to it often during the evaluation process.

Getting a Handle on Electronic Medical Record Features

The features and functions incorporated into EHR products are derived from product designers' understanding (or lack thereof) of the features, functions, and potential uses of the medical record. Your ability to effectively select and use an EHR product will also depend upon how well you understand the many ways that medical records are used. For example, there are undoubtedly some current activities that you wish to speed up (determining all current medications a patient is taking) that would be faster using a computer. However, with an EHR, new capabilities not available with paper charts (quickly finding all patients taking a specific drug) are possible and may not be obvious if your list of desired features is formed solely from interactions with paper records.

Uses of the Medical Record

The Institute of Medicine Report on computer-based patient record systems divides medical record usage into two categories: primary and secondary (1). Looking up an old EKG, checking a medication list, reading a progress note, and so on are primary uses. Primary uses are those which involve direct patient care. Clinicians tend focus too narrowly on primary uses when evaluating products. Secondary uses may be thought of as non-clinical analytical uses (outcomes analysis, cost studies, regulatory reporting, etc.). Secondary users tend to be researchers, educators, and regulatory bodies. However, with the increasing emphasis on quality improvement, patient safety, and pay-for-performance, secondary uses have become very important for clinicians as well When using paper records, primary and secondary users have specific forms or processes that they use to maximize the value of the chart to them. Thus, if a doctor wishes to record more preventive health data, a form is added to the chart, and a protocol for using the form is created. Administrators attempting to meet regulatory reporting requirements often take a similar approach.

Obviously, the paper chart with all of its shortcomings is quite flexible and useful. Unfortunately, the ease with which one can expand the uses of the paper chart can make it difficult to appreciate its true complexity. The failure to appreciate the true complexity of the paper chart is one of reasons that EHR selection is so problematic. A good EHR product makes allowances for the needs of both primary and secondary users of the medical

Table 17-1

PRIMARY USER AND REQUIRED EHR FEATURES AND SECONDARY USES

Primary EHR Uses

Progress notes

Problem list

Medication list

Drug information/Rx management

Lab/test reports

Preventive health support

Referral creation

Guidelines and protocols

Patient education

Secondary EHR Uses

Provider profiling

Patient utilization information

Quality report cards

Performance reviews for practice guidelines, protocols, and pathways

Outcomes analyses

record. Because adding new features is not simple, a good deal more fore-thought is necessary to build a good product. Similarly, selecting a product will be difficult unless *all* potential users have a good understanding of their needs and can articulate those needs sufficiently to vendors, consultants, or information systems professionals. Table 17-1 provides a list of primary and secondary uses of the medical record that should help formulate a good conceptualization of the various uses of the EHR.

What Features Should an Electronic Health Record Product Have?

Until the creation of the Certification Commission for Health Information Technology (CCHIT) in 2005, no formal set of criteria for judging EHR functionality existed. The CCHIT set criteria for core EHR features in three categories: functionality, security, and interoperability. The commission instituted a formal process for product review and certification, and a list of certified products and current certification criteria are available at www.cchit.org.

The discussion of features that follows is offered as an educational tool to help readers understand the range of features available in EHR products. (The evaluation criteria and checklist are adapted from *Electronic Patient Records for the Office-Based Practitioner*, copyright 1998-2006 by Jerome H. Carter, all rights reserved.) This listing of features/functions was compiled by the author and is derived from two sources: feature lists of currently available products and a review of common office and clinical processes. They are not based on the CCHIT criteria.

Using the Evaluation Aide

The criteria offered in this chapter are intended to act as a aide to understanding common EHR product features. Core features that are deemed essential are listed in the tables in regular type. Advanced features and "wish-list" items listed in italics.

The proper time to use this set of criteria is after all process analyses have been completed. The criteria may then be used to aid in the development of a formal list of requirements that will be used to create an RFP and test scenarios. Look through the criteria and for each feature area (e.g. medications), determine which are *required* for your needs. It is your personal list of required features that will determine the ideal product for you. It is very important that the needs all potential users be addressed when deciding on required features: be mindful of this during the product evaluation. Whenever possible, make determination of feature requirements a team activity with all parties represented.

Medications

Medication management is an important part of clinical practice. At a minimum, an EHR should provide the ability to maintain a medication list and an allergy list, write prescriptions, and automatically alert the practitioner to any drug allergies (Table 17-2). If a prescription writer is present, then automatic drug interaction checking would be a very desirable additional feature. Note that if this feature is available, one must ensure that the number and types of interactions reported are adjustable. Advanced medication features would be formulary tracking by insurance plan, provider-specific medication lists, the ability to e-mail or fax to pharmacies, and on-line drug information concerning side effects, adverse reactions etc., and the ability of the user to add new drugs/prescriptions to the system. Provider-specific medication lists allow each provider to create a list of drugs and dosages that he/she uses most often. This saves time by removing the need to scroll through long lists of medications each time a prescription needs to be written. Minimal report capability should offer the ability to search by patient, drug, and provider. Finally, a link to an online PDR or other drug databases for reference is a desirable feature.

Laboratory/X-Ray/Pathology

Perhaps the most useful lab-related features in an EHR is automatic downloading of labs and other test reports from outside facilities. Most major independent laboratory companies offer an automatic download feature. The

Table 17-2

MEDICATION FEATURES*

1. Medication list
   - Long-term
   - Per episode
   - Active/inactive
   - *Failed after trial*
2. Allergy list
3. Automatic allergy warning
4. Prescription writer
   - *E-mail or fax to pharmacy*
   - Rx history
5. *Maintains formulary information*
   - *By insurance plan*
6. Drug interactions
   - Drug-drug, drug-food
7. *Practitioner specific medication list*
8. *Drug information*
   - *Side effects*
   - *Adverse reactions*
   - *Overdose*
   - *Dosages*
   - *Forms supplied*
9. Reports by
   - Patient
   - Medication
   - Provider

---

*Core features that are deemed essential and listed in the tables are printed using regular type, and advanced features and "wish-list" items listed in the tables appear in italics.

minimal lab/X-ray/pathology feature set consists of test history by provider and patient, automatic flagging and tracking of abnormal results (panic values and delta checks: warnings for significant changes in parameter), and the ability to create specific test panels (Table 17-3). Advanced features in this setting provide more decision support during the ordering process, bi-directional interfaces that support order uploads, alerts for redundant tests, guidelines-based ordering, and the ability to generate reports by patient, provider, and test.

Telephone Calls

Telephone call management features are geared toward improving documentation (Table 17-4). These features are increasingly found in many EHR products. They can reduce potential liability risks. Call management features can aid in reducing unnecessary office visits by helping to monitor patients via tracking functions.

Table 17-3

LABORATORY/X-RAY/PATHOLOGY FEATURES*

1. Maintains test history
   - Patient
   - Provider
2. *Permits automatic data download from outside facilities*
3. *Permits uploading of orders to other facilities (ex: lab orders)*
4. Maintains profile of available tests/indications
5. Flags abnormal results
   - Permits tracking of abnormal lab follow up
6. *Permits creation of panels*
   - *Disease specific*
   - *Patient specific*
   - *Population specific*
7. Alerts for redundant testing
8. *Guideline-aware order entry*
9. Reports by
   - Patient
   - Medication
   - Provider

*Core features that are deemed essential and listed in the tables are printed using regular type, and advanced features and "wish-list" items listed in the tables appear in italics.

Table 17-4

TELEPHONE CALL FEATURES*

1. Maintains call history
   - Patient
   - *Site*
   - *Provider*
   - *Number called from*
   - *Automatic dialing*
2. *Captures call reason and action taken*
3. *Provides alerts and reminders for required follow up*
4. Report by
   - Patient
   - Provider
   - Call reason
   - Call action

*Core features that are deemed essential and listed in the tables are printed using regular type, and advanced features and "wish-list" items listed in the tables appear in italics.

Table 17-5

DIAGNOSIS FEATURES*

1. Problem list
   - Long-term
   - Per episode
2. *Guideline-based advice*
3. *Access to knowledge resources*
   - *Internet*
   - *Practice guidelines*
4. Report by
   - Patient
   - Provider
   - Diagnosis

*Core features that are deemed essential and listed in the tables are printed using regular type, and advanced features and "wish-list" items listed in the tables appear in italics.

Diagnosis Features

The problem list is the most important feature in this area (Table 17-5). The ability to list and view long-term problems separate from those that are acute and limited is a potential time saver. Guideline-based advice or access to decision support and other forms of clinical knowledge resources (e.g., electronic textbooks) are advanced features.

Referrals

Referral management features (Table 17-6) can greatly increase practice productivity. Aside from providing the ability to monitor patients' adherence to referral advice, features that provide insurance plan-specific referral guidance are particularly helpful in managed care environments. All systems should provide a list of referral sites and providers. Insurance plan features and provider preferences constitute advanced capabilities.

Preventive Medicine

Managed care and pay-for-performance have made preventive medicine features (Table 17-7) a major reason for buying an EHR. Patient intervention histories (list of all interventions done for the patient to date), provider-defined alerts, and the ability to create user-defined protocols by age, sex, and disease state are essential. Similarly, reporting in this area has to be fairly sophisticated and should provide multiple reporting views.

Table 17-6

REFERRAL FEATURES*

1. Maintains list of referral sites/Providers by
   - Specialty
   - Reason for referral
   - Location
2. Maintains referral history
   - Patient
   - *Provider*
   - *Site*
   - *Reason/Diagnosis*
3. *Maintains list of approved providers/sites by*
   - *Insurance plan*
   - *Provider preference*
4. Report by
   - Patient
   - Provider
   - Reason/diagnosis
   - Referral site/provider
   - *Reports by email attachment*

*Core features that are deemed essential and listed in the tables are printed using regular type, and advanced features and "wish-list" items listed in the tables appear in italics.

Table 17-7

PREVENTIVE MEDICINE FEATURES*

1. Maintains patient intervention history
2. *Permits design of intervention protocols by*
   - *Sex*
   - *Age*
   - *Disease state*
   - *Insurance plan*
3. *Permits guideline-based protocols*
4. *Provides user-defined alerts*
5. Report by
   - Patient population
   - Patient
   - Provider
   - *Diagnosis*
   - *Protocol*
6. *Health Status reports*
   - *SF-36*

*Core features that are deemed essential and listed in the tables are printed using regular type, and advanced features and "wish-list" items listed in the tables appear in italics.

Table 17-8

CLINICAL ENCOUNTER FEATURES*

1. Progress note
   - Plain text
   - Encoded and searchable
     - ○ Vital signs
     - ○ *Clinical findings*
2. E&M Templates
   - *Defined by end-user*
     - ○ *Specialty specific*
3. *Disease-based guidelines/protocols*
   - *Defined by end-user*
     - ○ Specialty specific

*Core features that are deemed essential and listed in the tables are printed using regular type, and advanced features and "wish-list" items listed in the tables appear in italics.

Clinical Encounter

Two very important needs collide here: creating an accurate description of the encounter in a readable form (primary use) and creating a searchable description of the encounter that can be easily analyzed (secondary). Most EHR systems handle progress notes as plain text, which is not suitable for analysis. Notes may be typed into the system or imported after transcription. Even systems that permit voice or pen-based input usually capture notes as plain text. Templates provide a boost in productivity for those who are comfortable with their use. Ideally, a number of templates for common problems should be provided with the system. Also, creation of templates by providers should be supported as part of the basic product. Coded, searchable notes are advanced features found in very few products.

Patient Education

Patient education materials, especially drug information, can be very useful in a busy practice (Table 17-9). If patient education materials are provided with a system, make sure that they are derived from an authoritative source

Table 17-9

PATIENT EDUCATION FEATURES

User definable
Preloaded
Updated regularly
Web access to educational materials

and are updated frequently. All materials provided should be modifiable by the user.

Population Health Management

The information needs associated with population-based care spring from the need to aggregate patient data. In order for a system to provide useful data analysis and reporting capabilities, it must be designed with certain features. Foremost among the required features is a database that stores discrete, coded data items. Note that the presence of a relational database alone is not sufficient to guarantee that a system offers useful analysis and reporting capabilities. In addition, the data must be coded using a standard vocabulary or terminology and the database must capture the true relationships that exist between items in the database. For example, if one wishes to analyze the average cost of antibiotics for patients diagnosed with bronchitis, the database must contain links between diagnosis, medication, demographics and billing data. Unfortunately, it is not possible during a demonstration or site visit to determine whether the underlying architecture

Table 17-10

POPULATION HEALTH MANAGEMENT FEATURES*

1. Profiles of provider activity
   - Profiles of provider activity
   - Medications
   - Labs
   - Referrals
   - Preventive health

2. Profiles of practice site activity
   - Medications
   - Labs
   - Referrals
   - Preventive health
   - Patient

3. *Disease Registry*

4. *Reports by*
   - *Guideline/protocol*
   - *Provider*
   - *Disease*
   - *Site*
   - *Pre-defined reports*
     - *HEDIS*
     - *JCAHO*
   - *Data exchange and reporting*
   - *Create P4P data sets*
   - *Quality Improvement Reports*

*Core features that are deemed essential and listed in the tables are printed using regular type, and advanced features and "wish-list" items listed in the tables appear in italics.

of the system is able to support a full range of analyses. In order to determine whether the system that you are considering is capable of performing useful analyses, it is best to request a demonstration using data from your practice site or discuss this issue with other practices already using the system. Another approach is to obtain a working copy of the program and use it for a brief period of time to see if it performs as desired (this is not a canned demo, but an actual working copy of the commercial software product). Advanced features include support for health status measures, disease registry or disease management functionality.

Communications and Infrastructure

The technical issues involved in selecting an EHR can be somewhat intimidating (Table 17-11). However, it is not as difficult as it may seem. There are a relatively limited number of acceptable options, and knowing what they are and why they are important is not difficult to learn.

Communications

Remote access allows one to access a computer without being physically present (e.g., calling into your office computer from a computer in your den). Remote access is a desirable feature and along with e-mail, fax, and Internet capability, greatly increases the utility of an EHR system. For practices hoping to conduct in-depth analyses of data, the ability to export data to statistical analysis programs or other systems is an essential feature.

Data repositories and warehouses are very large database systems that may have links to EHR systems and help to support patient care and data analysis. Both repositories and warehouses are suited for only the most sophisticated information systems environments. The ability to import data is also a very desirable EHR feature. However, import of structured data between EHRs from different vendors is not usually possible.

Operating Systems

For much of the history of the EHR market, Unix and Novell were the dominant operating systems. The Windows operating system now appears to be the platform of choice for ambulatory EHR vendors.

Client/server is a mode of computing in which the database and applications reside on a central computer (server) and other computers (clients) make requests to this server to either save or retrieve information. Client/ Server is the environment most commonly found in ambulatory sites.

Web-based systems are available that use the Application Server Provider (ASP) model. ASP EHRs tend to be less expensive because they do not require practices to own servers and other expensive hardware. ASP-based EHRs store their data remotely and are accessed via a web browser. The

Table 17-11

COMMUNICATIONS AND INFRASTRUCTURE*

1. Remote access
2. FAX support or linkage
3. Word processor support or linkage
4. Provides e-mail support or linkage
5. *Internet*
6. *Decision support*
   - *Statistical analysis*
   - *Knowledge resources*
     - ○ *MEDLINE*
   Permits data export
   - *Support for clinical data repository*
   - *Data warehouse*
   - *Statistical analysis packages*
7. Supports varied data formats
   - *Sound*
   - *Video*
   - Graphics
8. File Format
   - Proprietary
   - Commercial standards (Oracle, SQL Server, etc.)
9. Standards
   - HL-7
   - SNOMED
   - ICD
   - CPT
   - *MEDCIN*
   - *LOINC for lab data*
10. Interface
    - *Pen*
    - *Voice*
    - Keyboard
    - Graphical
      - ○ User modifiable
11. Security
    - Audit trail
      - ○ Permits audit trail analysis
      - ○ Automatic activation
12. Passwords
    - *Biometric*
      - ○ *Fingerprint*
13. Role-based access
14. Data validation
15. Back-up process
    - *Encryption*

Continued on next page

Table 17-11

COMMUNICATIONS AND INFRASTRUCTURE* (CONT'D)

16. Operating systems
    - Unix
    - Macintosh OS X
    - Windows XP/Vista
    - Novell
    - Internet based
      - ASP
17. Technology
    - Database
      - Relational
      - *Object-oriented*

---

*Core features that are deemed essential and listed in the tables are printed using regular type, and advanced features and "wish-list" items listed in the tables appear in italics.

downside to this arrangement is the lack of control that the practice has over its data. If the ASP provider goes out of business it is possible to lose all of your data.

Data Types and Storage Formats

Although not essential to EHR functioning, the ability to store sound, video, and graphics may increase the utility of an EHR product for some practices. If these types of data are accepted by an EHR, be sure that they can be searched and indexed. EHRs store data in databases. Each vendor decides the database "layout" for their product (referred to as a "schema"). There are no rules for what constitutes an acceptable EHR database schema. Therefore, even when vendors use the same database management system to support their EHR product the schema invariably differ. This is one of the factors that makes moving data between EHRs difficult. Keep this fact in mind because practically it means that generally you will not be able to move your data to a new EHR if you change products.

Standards

There have been a number of attempts to make the sharing of medical information easier. Health Level-7 (HL7) is a standard promoted as a means of permitting easier communications between computer systems. Any EHR system under consideration should support this standard. ICD and CPT codes are standards for billing and recording diagnoses and represent the most widely used coding standards. SNOMED Clinical Terms, released in 2003 has become the standard reference terminology for EHR systems.

MEDCIN, a terminology for recording the information that appears in the progress note, is also becoming more widely adapted by EHR vendors.

Data-Entry Interfaces

Pen-based computers and voice recognition systems may prove to be a boon to those who cannot type with sufficient skill to use a computer during patient encounters. Pen-based systems no longer focus mainly on handwriting recognition as their main data input mechanism. Instead, more often they act as pointing devices with the same functionality as a mouse. The most important feature of pen-based systems is their portability. Both Tablet PCs and PDA systems fall into this category.

Voice recognition systems have improved significantly over the last few years, with the appearance of clinical systems that accurately recognize continuous speech. Voice recognition, despite recent advances, is still very sensitive to accents and other individual speaking traits. The best advice is this area is to try the system out under normal work conditions (background noise, different users) before deciding that it will work for you. Voice recognition systems are relatively inexpensive and worth evaluating. Should you decide to try a pen or voice-based system, inquire about the availability of medical dictionary or spell-checker add-ons. They will make the job of correcting mistakes less time-consuming and frustrating.

Security

Access

Putting data into electronic form always raises the possibility of tampering or misuse. In order to ensure proper security for patient information, specific policies and procedures should be implemented to complement intrinsic EHR security features. Passwords are the most common security feature found in EHR systems. They offer an acceptable level of security when properly handled. Recent gains in computer technology have made user-authentication more reliable and may one day make passwords obsolete. Biometrics, the use of biologically unique markers to provide secure access, has made significant gains recently. Fingerprint, face print, and voice pattern recognition systems are available, relatively inexpensive, and make unauthorized access to data files very difficult.

Role-based access offers additional protection by restricting access to data files based upon the "need to know". In such systems, each type of file is coded to permit access only to certain classes of users. The internal code for billing clerks would be different than that for doctors, thus allowing the system's administrator to easily prevent access to lab data by clerks while permitting unencumbered access to physicians.

Audit trails provide an additional security measure. They maintain a record of all file access attempts and authorized usage. Many EHR packages permit the audit trail feature to be disabled; this is a bad idea. Security features are also important to assure that electronic records are deemed acceptable as legal documents. In order to pass legal muster, you must be able to demonstrate that your records cannot be altered, deleted, viewed or otherwise accessed improperly.

Validation and Storage

Security issues are not limited to unauthorized access. Data validation is equally important. For example, does the system check data input for unlikely values (e.g., temperature of 300°F, or a blood pressure of 400/300 mm/hg)? All data stored in an EHR should be validated prior to storage. Because patient information may be shared between sites or with other business entities, some form of encryption should be available either within the EHR package or as an add-on utility. Automatic encryption of files saved to disk is a valuable form of data protection.

A final security matter is that of file preservation. Here again office policies are the most important component. Back-up, file storage, and disaster-recovery procedures must be set by the systems administrator. This is an area where many businesses fall short with painful results. Look for EHR packages that permit on-line back-ups (i.e., copies of all files stored on the computer's disk drives can be copied for storage while the computer is being used). Other measures such as mirroring (using two separate drives or servers to hold identical data) and real-time off-site storage are available. These measures help to keep your practice up and running through many types of computer problems. Give serious consideration to making them a part of your EHR set-up.

References

1. Dick RS, Steen EB, Detmer DE. The Computer-Based Patient Record: An Essential Technology for Health Care: Revised Edition. Washington, DC: Institute of Medicine; 1971.

18

Vendor Evaluation

Sarah T. Corley, MD

This chapter will help you to identify and analyze information about electronic health record (EHR) vendors to narrow the field to a manageable number. It will cover topics such as where to locate information about a vendor, the importance of learning the certification status, the financial health and stability of the company, whether their product is suitable for your specialty and what the customer experience has been.

Vendor Evaluation

Vendors should be evaluated in a systematic fashion using similar criteria for all vendors. A worksheet is included in this chapter that may be used as a template to start your own practice's worksheet (Table 18-1).

The first step in evaluating vendors is to identify those who make products suitable for your specialty and practice situation. Professional meetings are an excellent opportunity to meet established vendors who have products designed for your specialty. Medical journals often review different software packages. Many web sites and search engines provide links to EHR vendors as well. Web sites that have links to or lists of vendors as of publication date include:

♦ www.emrconsultant.com

♦ www.telemedicalrecord.com

♦ www.elmr-electronic-medical-records-emr.com/

A number of magazines provide reviews or lists of software. Healthcare Informatics, www.healthcare-informatics.com, has a resource guide in their December issue. Many specialty societies have resources to assist you with

Table 18-1

VENDOR WORKSHEET

Company
URL
Contact name
Phone number
E-mail
Fax number
CCHIT certified
Years in business
Operating systems supported
SQL, oracle licenses required
Number of installed sites
Number of users
Specialties supported
Medical record software
Appointments
Billing
Decision support
Frequency of updates
Customizable by user
Web browser interface
SNOMED for structured data entry
Drug-interaction checking, frequency of updates
Lab interfaces
Device interfaces
Practice management interface
PACS interface
Cost of interfaces
Hardware required
Local support available
System cost per user and per workstation
Cost of upgrades
Cost of support
Cost of training
Frequency of upgrades
User groups: Frequency, number of attendees
Data entry modes: keyboard, mouse, voice dictation, handwriting recognition
E-mail and messaging

narrowing the scope of your search. The American College of Physicians Practice Management Center has a number of resources for members at http://www.acponline.org/pmc/index.html?hp. The AAFP's Center for Health Information Technology also provides resources for its members at http://www.centerforhit.org/. If you belong to a different specialty society, be sure to check with them early in the process. State quality improvement organizations (QIOs) also can provide a number of free resources to physicians in their state. To locate your state QIO, follow the locator link on the American Health Quality Association web site: http://www.ahqa.org/pub/connections/162_694_2450.cfm.

Length of Time in Business

It is useful to find out how long a company has been in business. Some vendors may have long established businesses selling other products, but are just starting in the EHR business. While a vendor who has been making electronic medical records for many years may not necessarily be more stable than a newly established one, there will be a better opportunity to evaluate how well the company responds to the changing needs of users. Established vendors have long-term users who can objectively provide feedback on their product.

Next determine how long the vendor's EHR product has been on the market. For each EHR product it is important to determine number of actual copies sold and the number of users at each site where the software is installed. These are important distinctions. It is possible for a vendor to have sold only one copy of an EHR package to a very large practice and truthfully state that they have more than 500 users. Which is, of course, quite different from having sold 500 copies of the software. In the former example, local users of a single product copy may be referred to as "seats" or "licensees".

Certification of Electronic Health Records

The Certification Commission for Health Information Technology (CCHIT) was started in 2004 by a consortium of HIT industry leaders who felt that adoption of EHRs would be accelerated if there was a neutral certifying body that identified core functionality, security, reliability, and interoperability and tested for compliance with this set of features. The three organizing groups were the Health Information and Management Systems Society (HIMSS), the National Alliance for Health Information Technology (Alliance), and the American Health Information Management Association (AHIMA). They were joined with financial support by many other organizations including the American College of Physicians and the American

Association of Family Physicians among others. In September 2005, HHS awarded CCHIT a three-year contract to develop and evaluate certification criteria and create an inspection process for HIT in three areas:

- Ambulatory EHRs for the office-based physician or provider
- Inpatient EHRs for hospitals and health systems
- The network components through which they interoperate and share information

Certification criteria add additional requirements each year, so it is important to ascertain in which year the product you are evaluating was certified. Certification testing for a given year begins in May, with results generally announced mid-summer. Specialty certification will begin in 2008 and will certify products that meet additional criteria for a given medical specialty or clinical setting. It is anticipated that many of the proposed pay-for-performance programs and government initiatives will require the use of certified products. A list of certified vendors can be found at their website: www.cchit.org.

Customer Profiles

Request a list of clients with practices of a similar size and composition to yours and request three references. Find out the total number of software licenses *sold* each year over the last three years and the total number of software licenses *installed* each year over the last three years. Some software that is sold is never installed, so these lists may be different. If there is a significant discrepancy between the number of systems sold and the number installed, this can be a red flag that the company has a problem with its support and training divisions. A final question in this area: are annual sales increasing, decreasing, or flat? Mature products may have flat sales, but they should have a large market share. If a product is new on the market, then increasing sales may be the only means available for estimating market share or customer base.

Obtain the name, address, and telephone number of clients representing the ten most recent sales and the ten most recent installations. Often they can provide information about how smoothly the current sales and training force is working. Ask for a complete list of all clients utilizing the product with name, address, telephone number, date purchased, date of first productive use. These users can provide historical information about how the company has met their needs over the years. Many vendors may be unwilling or unable to provide this information because some practices do not wish to be contacted by potential customers, but you should still try to get this information. If you personally know any users of the system, call them as well as the three recent references for similar products already given. Determine whether there is a users group and whether the reference sites attend meetings. If so, ask for an appraisal of their usefulness. Well-developed user group meetings can be an excellent source of helpful advice in making optimal use of the EHR. Medical software is very complex, and software developers write manuals; full-time medical practitioners do not. Experienced physician users can help a new user use the software more efficiently. Beta testers can offer insight into the latest releases. Some physicians may have written programs that are compatible with the product and may offer it as shareware. Find out if there is a regular newsletter published with useful tips, or whether there is there a web site or a Listserve available.

Public or Private Corporation

Request audited financial statements for the last three years as well as a banking reference. If you are making a large monetary investment in a software package, you want to be sure that the company will be in business for years to come and able to provide upgrades and technical support. For publicly owned companies, you should search the records for details on finances, funding, and profit and loss statements. SEC reports are available on line at www.sec.gov. For privately held companies, bank references must be requested and checked.

Upgrades

Compare the major releases planned for each of the software packages and also compare release and implementation time frames. Check with users to confirm that information that the vendors have provided about the frequency of past upgrades is accurate. A major upgrade at least once a year is desirable in an EHR product to keep up with changes in technology and medical practice. References should also be asked about the utility of the upgrades: whether they provide valuable features or just cosmetic changes.

Mergers

Inquire about mergers; inquire in particular about whether the company has purchased or merged with any other companies within the last two years. If so, try to determine if all software products have been supported during this period and whether current users were offered upgraded products. The EHR market is rapidly evolving, and as companies purchase other complementary products to speed the development/product releases process, they have left users of orphaned systems without any support or upgrades. Buyer beware.

Litigation

Ask for details of any current litigation. Is this litigation involving users, corporate partners, or the government? Litigation can take away money and time that would otherwise be spent improving the product. Do not buy products from companies that are having legal difficulties with customers. This is never a good sign. Other types of litigation must be judged on a case-by-case basis.

Corporate Partners

Obtain a listing of all technology and/or distribution partnerships and alliances in which the vendor participates. Obtain the names of all partners along with name, address, telephone number, and a brief description of the nature of the relationship. If partnerships involve software packages that are intended to work together, ascertain the level of integration (users groups and client references are helpful here). These partnerships can be detrimental if the partnerships restrict the types of operating systems or peripherals supported. For example, if you already have a UNIX or LINUX operating system and your vendor institutes a partnership with Microsoft, your operating system may not be supported in future releases. Other examples could be limited interfaces with EKG machines, blood glucose monitors, or electronic claims warehouses. Problems can also arise if the second company becomes financially unstable or starts requiring concessions from the vendor you have selected.

Development and Technical Support

Determine the total number of employees within the organization that are directly and exclusively associated with the EHR product. Break this down by department and quantify the average tenure of employees in marketing and sales, research and development, maintenance, quality control/quality assurance, technical support, client services/installation, field service, and end-user support.

Tenure in the sales and marketing department is much less important than in support and training. Try to ascertain whether the company has adequate resources to train new users. Are there well-written user manuals? Have the trainers had experience with sites similar to yours? A longer tenure will have given them more opportunity to work with disparate practices and improve training material. Computer software support, in general, has a high turnover rate but, again, the longer the average length of employment, the more likely they are to have encountered your particular problem before and have a rapid solution for you.

Product Viability

A product, even a great one, is only as good as the latest version. Research and development (R&D) spending is very important to the continued viability of a product. Look at the budget dollars set aside for R&D, as well as the number of personnel working in that area. Often when companies are strapped for cash, R&D spending is one of the first areas to be cut. Insufficient spending for R&D translates into a product that will not be kept up to date. Avoid products with poor R&D support. You should look for at least as many employees involved in support and R&D as there are in sales. An average tenure of at least one year in support and two years in R&D should ensure that the employees are familiar with the product. The longer the length of employment, the more likely it is that the company can devote energy to improving the product rather than training replacement staff.

Ask about annual research and development plans in the area of EHR systems for the next three years and current and projected (three years) expenditures for R&D activity, in both absolute terms and as a percent of gross revenues. Investment in R&D will ensure that the product will continue to keep pace with changes in the field and with the needs of the users.

Compare various data entry modes and determine whether they are currently functional, in development, or planned for the future. These may include speech (voice) recognition, graphics- or icon-based interfaces, touch screens, handwriting recognition, light pens, or dictation files. If you have a large practice, you may want to have many different options of data entry. If the practitioners have always dictated, the ability to use voice recognition in the program can keep dictation costs down and allow direct data entry without physician revolt. Ask what methods the vendor uses to make sure that clinical decision support and embedded guidelines are kept up to date. Do they have physicians on staff to research this, do they use third-party products, or is the software static once shipped? Practices with residents or medical students may be more interested in the decision-support features and up-to-date guidelines.

Interfaces

Is the company's software HL7 compliant? What data interchange standards does the vendor adhere to? Which lab companies have functional interfaces with the software? In order to save time on data entry, a complete EHR should be able to download lab results directly from the lab into the individual chart in an EHR. If the EHR does not employ a standard such as HL7 it may be impossible or very expensive to download labs or exchange information with others. Which medical management packages have successful interfaces with the software? If a practice plans on keeping its current medical management software, an interface can eliminate the need to enter demographic data twice. You would want to know the cost of the interface with your practice management system because this is usually an additional charge. Find out if this is a total turnkey price or if it is hourly. Expenses can increase rapidly when custom interfaces must be written. Ask about interfaces with hospital systems if a large part of your practice is inpatient. For practices dealing with a lot of images, find out which PACS systems they interface with. If you use a lot of medical devices such as vital signs monitors, EKG machines, spirometry, holter monitors, or ophthalmologic testing devices, you should enquire whether interfaces to these are supported and at what cost.

Cost Comparisons

When analyzing costs, be sure that you are comparing comparable proposals. It is helpful to separate out the costs of hardware, software, installation, training, technical support, and upgrades. That way you can estimate the total costs of each system.

If a vendor requires that you purchase hardware from them, list the exact specifications of what will be provided and the total cost. Compare that to the cost of commercially available hardware. Hardware costs are dropping rapidly and bargains are easily available. If hardware is provided, what is the length of the contract? Is it leased or purchased? Most equipment is adequate for three years, but improvements to both hardware and software can render the hardware obsolete after that time. It is very important to have service costs included. A practice that is "paperless" must have guaranteed immediate service on the server and at least next-day service on the workstations.

When evaluating the costs of the software itself, you should list the total cost per user. That way if the practice grows, you will already have the dollar amount needed to increase the number of licenses. Most vendors will have a lower cost if more licenses are purchased so you may wish to group the prices such as 0-10 licenses $3000 per user, 11-25 licenses, $2500 per user, etc. Compare the costs for regular updates on the drug interaction package and software updates. If this is a flat rate, note whether the rate is guaranteed for any period of time. If you are considering separate components in addition to an EHR such as a billing and scheduling package, those prices should be itemized separately.

Training Services

Training costs can be very expensive. You should itemize training costs by the number of hours and number of users to be trained. You should list the number of hours of training the vendor suggests and whether any training is included in the cost of the software. You should also note if the training is on site or off site. If it is to be off site, you must factor in travel costs for those attending the training, and if it is to be on site, you need to include the costs of the trainers' expenses if they are to be paid by the practice. You should check references on the assigned trainer before confirming the training dates. The quality may vary widely between trainers for the same company. It is extremely important not to try to save money by shortening the amount of training. Because of the richness of features of most certified EHRs, they are not intuitive to use without formal training, and many of the advanced features that make the user more efficient and practice higher quality care need to be taught after the user is comfortable with the system. Optimal training would include initial training followed by additional training in six weeks to three months to learn more advanced techniques once you are comfortable with documenting progress notes, writing prescriptions, ordering medications, and the other, more day-to-day features. Too much information in a short period of time will not be retained. Ask if the company has any web-based or electronic training. This is useful for reinforcing what you have learned and for training new office staff who may join the practice later.

19

Creating a Request for Proposal and Negotiating a Contract

Sarah T. Corley, MD

This chapter will provide information about what a request for proposal (RFP) is and why you might want to create one. It will provide details on the steps you will need to take to do a thorough evaluation of your internal needs so that you can create an effective RFP. The chapter will also discuss contract negotiation, asking for discounts, what to make sure is included in the contract, and ways to protect yourself in the event that problems occur.

What Is a Request for Proposal?

An RFP is a document constructed to allow for side-by-side comparison of different products. It must include detailed information about the needs of the practice so the proposal can be tailored appropriately. The process of designing an RFP will help in assessing and setting priorities for product features. Responding to an RFP requires a significant time investment by the vendor, so the practice should strive to present a concise document to a few select vendors.

Why Do You Need a Request for Proposal?

The intent of the RFP is to specify *exactly* what the practice is looking for in a product, including hardware, software, maintenance, and training. The vendor's response will indicate whether the desired features are available in their current product, and if not, whether the desired features are in development.

The reply should also provide detailed cost information. Because responding to an RFP may be very labor intensive for a vendor, they may be unwilling to complete one if they do not think the buyer is serious. To prevent that appearance, the practice should complete a rigorous self-evaluation before designing the RFP (see Chapters 14, 16, and 17). You also should narrow your search to two to four companies before submitting an RFP to a vendor. A sample RFP is included (Table 19-1) that may be used as a template to design your own.

Table 19-1

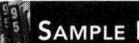 **SAMPLE RFP**

SECTION I: PRACTICE AND COMPANY INFORMATION

Practice Information

1. Main contact at the practice: Name, Title, Address, Telephone, FAX, and Email.
2. Person (if not the main contact) who will negotiate terms of the relationship: Name, Title, Address, Telephone, FAX, and Email.
3. Provide total number of physicians, advanced practice providers, nurses, and administrative staff.
4. Provide total number of exam rooms and workstations.
5. Provide details on software that will need interfaces designed.
6. Provide the name and contact person for outside lab(s) information system.

Company Information

1. Main contact for this proposal: Name, Title, Address, Telephone, FAX, and Email.
2. Person (if not the main contact) who will negotiate terms of the relationship: Name, Title, Address, Telephone, FAX, and Email.
3. Address of company headquarters and main telephone number if different than the contact address and telephone.
4. Provide the name, address and phone number of your parent organization and any specific division or subsidiary company completing this proposal. Provide the name and a current resume for the President/CEO, Development Director, Marketing Director, Maintenance Director, Installation Manager, and Support Manager.
5. Provide the total number of employees within your organization that are directly and exclusively associated with the EMR product. Provide the number and average tenure of the employees in Marketing and Sales, Research and Development, Maintenance, Quality Control/Quality Assurance, Technical Support, Client Services/Installation, Field Service, End-User Support.
6. Provide information concerning your annual research and development plans in the area of EMR systems for the next three years. Indicate current and projected (3 year's) expenditures for research and development activity, in both absolute terms, and as a percent of gross revenues.
7. Describe the major releases planned for the proposed platform we would use, with release and implementation time frames.
8. Describe your progress and plans to incorporate the following into your products: Speech (voice) recognition, graphics- or icon-based interfaces, touch screens, handwriting recognition, decision support, Internet, wireless transmission, CCHIT requirements.

Continued on next page

Table 19-1

SAMPLE RFP (CONT'D)

9. Brief description and history of the company.

10. Please provide copies of audited financial statements for the last three years. Please provide a banking reference.

11. Please provide the number of clients in a practice of a similar size and composition to ours and three references including name, address and telephone number.

12. Please provide the total number of software licenses sold each year over the last three years.

13. Please provide the total number of software licenses installed each year over the last three years.

14. Please provide the name, address, and telephone number of clients representing the ten most recent sales.

15. Please provide the name, address, and telephone number of clients representing the ten most recent installations.

16. Describe your three most successful and three least successful installations for the proposed system within the past two years. Please highlight those that are similar in size and scope to ours. Include the following information:
    * Client name, address, phone, and contact
    * Number of users
    * Date of contract commencement
    * Brief hardware configuration, including the number and type of workstations, scanners, printers, and other system components.

17. Please submit a complete list of all clients utilizing your system: Name, address, telephone number, date purchased, and date of first productive use.

18. Please describe any current litigation the company is involved in.

19. Please list all technology and/or distribution partnerships and alliances including the partner name address, telephone number, and a brief description of the nature of the relationship.

20. Is the company's software HL-7 compliant? What data interchange standards does the vendor adhere to?

21. Have there been any objective studies of your system's benefits reported in journals? If so, please include a copy.

22. Do you have a users group? How often does it meet? Do you have a regular client newsletter? How often is it published? Include all copies for the past year.

SECTION II: FUNCTIONAL REQUIREMENTS

1. For each numbered area below please indicate a current status of the feature as follows:

   C = Current feature supported in a commercially available release.

   P = Planned feature for a future release - include the expected month/year of the commercially available release.

   N = Not planned.

   O = other product: the feature is available in another product either from your company or from another company with which you have a distribution relationship. Please include any cost information or future date information that might be relevant.

2. Also include a narrative description for each numbered area below that describes the capabilities of your product in this feature area. Please keep responses to each question under a page in length. You may include additional information in a separate appendix.

Continued on next page

Table 19-1

SAMPLE RFP (CONT'D)

1. Chart Summary
   Status: _____ Date/Other Info: _____ Narrative Description:
2. Links Among Chart Elements
   Status: _____ Date/Other Info: _____ Narrative Description:
3. Flexible Data Collection
   Status: _____ Date/Other Info: _____ Narrative Description:
4. Results Display
   Status: _____ Date/Other Info: _____ Narrative Description:
5. Health Maintenance
   Status: _____ Date/Other Info: _____ Narrative Description:
6. Intuitive Interaction Model
   Status: _____ Date/Other Info: _____ Narrative Description:
7. Standards-based Encoding
   Status: _____ Date/Other Info: _____ Narrative Description:
8. Scheduling
   Status: _____ Date/Other Info: _____ Narrative Description:
9. Intra-office
   Status: _____ Date/Other Info: _____ Narrative Description:
10. To-do Lists
    Status: _____ Date/Other Info: _____ Narrative Description:
11. Rapid User Interaction Model
    Status: _____ Date/Other Info: _____ Narrative Description:
12. Referral Management
    Status: _____ Date/Other Info: _____ Narrative Description:
13. Order Entry
    Status: _____ Date/Other Info: _____ Narrative Description:
14. Client-Server
    Status: _____ Date/Other Info: _____ Narrative Description:
15. Oracle, Sybase, Informix (For larger practices)
    Status: _____ Date/Other Info: _____ Narrative Description:
16. Communications Manager
    Status: _____ Date/Other Info: _____ Narrative Description:
17. Scalability
    Status: _____ Date/Other Info: _____ Narrative Description:
18. System and Data Security
    Status: _____ Date/Other Info: _____ Narrative Description:

SECTION III: SUPPORT AND SERVICES

1. How are new releases handled? Please be specific about costs and time frames.
2. How is routine technical support handled? Please be specific about costs and time frames.
3. Please provide address and telephone numbers for support locations nationally and the closest support available for our practice.
4. Please attach a standard contract and describe any exclusions.
5. Please list any procedures expected from clients to ensure smooth system operation.

Continued on next page

Table 19-1

SAMPLE RFP (CONT'D)

6. Describe all hardware and software maintenance options.

7. Describe any additional services offered if hardware is purchased as part of the transaction.

8. Describe your approach to providing appropriate clinical content and knowledge bases for the specialties in our practice.

9. List all third party products your system has been interfaced to.

10. Describe your problem escalation policies in general and specifically for: software errors, hardware errors, and disasters.

SECTION IV: COSTS

1. Detail the proposed hardware including manufacturer, model numbers, unit prices, quantities, and total cost.

2. Detail the proposed software including module name, unit prices, quantities, and total cost.

3. Detail the proposed implementation and training services including costs per day, number of FTEs from your organization, number of FTEs recommended from our practice, number of service days, number of calendar days, and total services cost.

4. Detail the proposed hardware maintenance services including costs.

5. Detail the proposed software maintenance services and technical support including costs.

6. Describe the fee structure for: help/questions, trouble shooting: general release enhancements: upgrades, bugs/ fixes technical support, system performance fine tuning, training (at vendor and on-site), custom development/ modifications.

SECTION V: APPENDIX

1. Respondents are encouraged to supply additional material considered relevant to their respective proposal in this section.

Gathering Background Information About Your Practice

Before you select an electronic health record (EHR) system to speed or fix the problems identified in your practice, you must know how the current system is working. Start by collecting information about how well your practice functions. The information gathered needs to be very detailed and should involve several months of self-examination and study (see Chapters 14 and 16). This information, along with desired product features, should be provided to the vendor as part of your RFP.

Number of Users

How many staff will be using the system? Most software packages are sold by the number of licenses. You should know the maximum number of users who will require access to both software and hardware at any given time. Do not make the mistake of underestimating future needs; plan for all potential users and not just those who are present initially.

Number of Workstations

Remember that a paperless office usually needs more than one workstation per user. Physicians will need terminals in the exam rooms as well as in their offices. The staff will need access throughout the office. As with the software, do not underestimate the total number of workstations required. Consider whether wireless tablets are a viable option for your practice. Decisions about this need to include the ability of the physicians to see the smaller screen and document with a touch pen or small keyboard. Barriers to wireless communication such as lead-shielded walls also need to be taken into consideration.

Computer Experience of Users

In order to accurately estimate training costs, the degree of computer literacy of all staff must be taken into account. Training costs are based on an hourly rate, and you do not want to spend expensive training time going over the basics of learning how to log on/off, use a mouse, and other basic computing skills. If few staff have even minimal computer skills, it may be cost-effective to pay for those staff members to attend basic computer classes at a local community college (if the practice is large, on-site training is a reasonable alternative). This approach will ensure that money spent for on-site EHR training will not be wasted.

Degree of Computerization of Tasks

Consideration of how the EHR system will be used should be an early part of the selection process. Will the practice be paperless? If so, then each staff person must have his or her own terminal and user license. It will also require workstations in the exam rooms, labs, and other areas where the staff must have access to the information. A paperless office requires other changes in the office work flow as well. Instead of filing documents from outside sources, they will have to be scanned into the EHR. Labs will require an electronic interface so that results can be downloaded automatically into your EHR system. If computerized EKGs will be used, the computer station in the exam rooms must be close enough that the lead from the EKG machine may be attached to the computer adapter. Will scheduling be included with the EHR? Will phone messages be handled through internal e-mail? Will the nurses be entering their own notes for procedures such as immunizations, allergy shots, and ear washes?

Existing Software

Integrating current software with the newly arrived EHR can be a difficult and time-consuming process. In many offices a practice management system (PMS) will already be in place. You may be able to avoid duplicate entry of demographic data if it is possible to interface your EHR to the PMS. Interfaces exist for many popular PMS systems. Be sure to ask EHR vendors for which PMS they provide interfaces. If there are other programs you wish to keep, you must be sure that the platforms are compatible. Incompatibilities may arise because of operating system (UNIX vs. Windows) or hardware differences. If you plan to change operating systems, you will need to know which current programs will be compatible with the new operating system. Also, be sure there are programs available for the new operating system that are capable of meeting all of your needs. Even when new software is found, problems may occur due to differences in how files are handled. For example, if you are changing your word processing program, you may need to plan for time and money spent reformatting documents.

Existing Hardware

If you plan on keeping existing computers, they will need to be itemized by processor speed, hard drive size, and amount of RAM. All software programs will have minimal hardware requirements and optimal hardware requirements. It will aid in a smooth transition if your new hardware meets the optimal requirements of the EHR systems, as minimal requirements often result in frustratingly slow response times.

What Is the Budget?

EHR software varies widely in cost, and the practice budget should be used to narrow down the choice. Be realistic about budget issues: it is much too easy to take on an unmanageable debt load. Keep in mind that new systems tend to make offices less productive for a period of time following installation, so do not assume that income will increase: it is more likely to decline slightly or stay flat in the short term. Larger practices generally see a bigger return on investment as they can afford to cut more support staff. Try to avoid being seduced by features for which you may have little need. Twenty-five features that you use often are a better buy than one hundred for which you have only an occasional need. The vendor should know your budget range so that realistic proposals can be made.

Who Will Decide on Needed Components and Select the System?

The practice needs to decide who will make the final decision. Will there be one individual or will it be a committee decision? Some techniques for arriving at a consensus in a group are detailed in an article by Chocholik et al (1). Ideally the RFP should reflect what has been learned from the analysis of your practice and the goals that you have set (Chapter 14). The decision-making mechanism should have been created and tested during the problem definition and process analysis. If this is the case, the decision as to which system to buy and what features are essential will be a natural outgrowth of the completed analysis. If you have not created a formal process for analyzing your practice and arriving at product-related decisions, then go back and do so. Otherwise, it is likely that you will pay a stiff price in dollars and disruption of the practice.

Typical Components of a Request for Proposal

An RFP should have four basic sections: practice information, vendor information, product features required, and support and services (Sample). Provide the vendor with detailed information which reflects the size, scope, and future plans for your practice. The vendor will use this information to determine if you are really a potential customer. For example, if your budget is too low or your practice is smaller than what the vendor is accustomed to working with, then earlier in the process the vendor can remove himself from consideration and save everyone time and frustration.

Just as the vendor may use practice information to determine that you are not a good prospect, you will use the information provided by the vendor the make the same determination (see Chapter 5). Length of time in business, financial stability, percentage of dollars spent on R&D, and available support, are very helpful in determining the viability of the vendor as a continuing enterprise.

Assuming that the vendor appears to be profitable and stable, you may turn you attention to reviewing product features. Be detailed and specific when identifying desired product features. Use the feature list provided in Chapter 4 to create a list specific to your practice.

Familiarize yourself with the core features for CCHIT certification. If a vendor is certified you will know that they have demonstrated that their product has that functionality and you may simply focus on any additional requirements that your practice may have. This will save both you and the vendor time.

A smooth installation requires attention to support and services. Use the RFP process to identify vendors who will provide the level of support that you require. Typical issues are training, technical support, provision of interfaces, updates, etc. Ask if the vendor provides physician-to-physician training. Some physicians learn better from peers and if this is the case you should be sure your vendor of choice offers the service. Each of these should be spelled out in detail and, once agreed upon, should be written in the contract (Chapter 8).

Negotiating a Contract

The contract often becomes a source of misery for many practices. Much too often a practice will trustingly sign a standard contract, which is usually written to favor the vendor, without reading the contents. This is a serious mistake. Always read the contract carefully, then have your attorney look at it. Also, do not accept any terms that are not favorable to you. When negotiating a contract consider your areas of strength as well as the vendor's weaknesses. If you have a large, high-profile practice, you should be able to negotiate a discounted rate based upon the visibility and marketing advantages that accrue to the vendor if the implementation is successful. If the company is just starting out and has no existing installations, you should never pay full price (your practice will be a beta test site whether or not it is labeled as such). If the vendor has a product with functional installed sites but is moving into a new geographic market, you may be able to negotiate a discount based on the uncertainties of local support and the benefits to the vendor of your practice being a local reference for other interested buyers. If you are buying a large number of user licenses either for your practice or as part of a local consortium of physician buyers, you should ask for a volume discount because installation and training costs can be shared.

Everything that is being purchased should be listed in detail in the contract. If you are purchasing hardware from the vendor, you must detail, exactly, the manufacturer, the model, year, hard drive size, memory, network card speed, modem type and speed if any, size of monitors, and types of keyboards. Nothing should be assumed. Hardware service contracts should also be spelled out in detail, including the time frame for service on both the server and the workstations, as well as whether this is on or off-site. The contract should specify the costs of the hardware and any service costs and whether this includes installation/setup costs.

The contract for your network should include the type of cable to be laid, the speed of the network cards, the type of hub, any routers to be used, and the type of network software to be used. It should specify the maximum number of network users and the costs of increasing network connections. If network maintenance is to be included, this should detail the costs and time frame of support as well as the contacts for service on weekends and holidays.

The contract should specify any pre-implementation services to be provided along with the time frame for such assistance and any costs for those services. All software should be itemized in the contract by the modules included, number of concurrent users, cost per user, and total system cost. It should identify the maximum number of users and the incremental cost of adding users. If the company makes other modules, which the practice is not currently purchasing, the costs of acquiring them later should be set at the time the contract is signed. The costs and frequency of upgrades should be listed in the contract as well as the length of time that upgrades will be available at that price. Try to negotiate a set price for the next three to five years if possible so that you may budget appropriately.

Training costs should detail the number of trainers to be provided, the number of trainees allowed, and the number of hours of training included at the agreed upon price. The contract should specify the cost of additional training at a daily or hourly rate. Make sure this price is valid for the next one to two years because employees often require additional training. Additional training after three months will often improve their efficiency once they are familiar with the system. If the trainer is traveling from a distant site, the contract should specify the maximum amount that will be paid for living and travel expenses.

If the software requires customization, the fees should be listed along with the services to be provided. A practice should always try to negotiate a flat fee for the customization of office forms, billing, and demographics information. You should also try to negotiate a flat rate for lab interfaces, and the contract should specify that final payment will not be made until the interface is completed and functional. If progress note templates cannot be created or amended by practice staff, have the cost for this service clearly stated in the contract.

Technical support is crucial to successful EHR implementation. The contract must identify who will be providing these services, at what hours (9-5 or 24/7/365), and at what cost. If the vendor provides support outside of regular business hours, determine whether these services are charged at a higher rate than those rendered during business hours. Be sure that you have phone numbers, e-mail addresses, fax numbers, and pager numbers so that you can contact technical support at any time.

Remember, if it is not in the contract, it is not binding. Read all contracts carefully and do not be timid about negotiating the best deal possible.

References

1. Chocholik JK, Bouchard SE, Tan JK, Ostrow DN. The determination of relevant goals and criteria used to select an automated patient care information system: a Delphi approach. JAMA. 1999;6:219-33

20

Gathering Information: Site Visits and Demonstrations

Bruce Slater, MD, MPH

Site visits and product demonstrations are some of the most enjoyable parts of working with a vendor. They are vitally important to the evaluation of a product and offer a welcome change of pace for the team. The excitement of a road trip or welcoming a visitor can liven up the even the dullest vendor/product evaluation selection process.

Site Visits

Why Make a Site Visit?

The purpose of a site visit is to see the vendor's product in use in an environment very similar to yours. The two operative features are making sure that 1) what you are seeing is very similar to what you are buying, and 2) the group you are visiting is very similar to your group.

Who Should Attend the Site Visit

The team leader should be a knowledgeable person who has leadership overall within the vendor selection process at your institution. The team size should be relatively small. Three to five people are reasonable unless your site is very small or very large. If your team size is larger and there are no "non-essential" members, consider making two visits or visit two sites rather than imposing a large group on the host site. It is quite possible to overwhelm the visiting site and create problems for the vendor who has asked the indulgence of the host for this visit.

In choosing your visitors it is important to keep compatible personalities in mind. It might be better to have a knowledgeable yet socially competent person rather than one of your "experts" who doesn't play well with others.

The team should involve a physician leader, administrator or managerial person, or a user of the system. If this is a physician system that nurses also use, then inviting a nurse is wise. If the system involves administrative systems such as scheduling, then having a front-line person who deals with patients and schedules visits is appropriate. Similarly if there is a telephone interface piece, then a receptionist is important to have present. If the product has a patient interface, then you could consider bringing along your favorite patient, although the patient should have some computer experience so he or she can give you the best evaluation. In fact, team members should be very comfortable with computers.

The people who you bring should have a history with your organization so that they know people who will be using the system and can represent their views. In addition, members of the site visit team should be very comfortable working with each other. Each person chosen for the team should bring a level of knowledge or expertise that can be brought to bare when evaluating a product. There may be a time when you can only take one person to represent two different functions. Such can be combined into a single visit, but the representative should have a full set of questions and issues from both of the sectors they are representing. Avoid making your team lopsided. Since team size must be limited, it is rare that you can afford to bring two people representing the same function. Even though physicians have a lot of clout, it would be a bad idea to take two doctors on a site visit. The same thing should apply to administrative personnel.

The team has a specific function and in building it you should be very careful about your choices. Once members are selected, team composition should be reviewed by relevant decision makers. To make sure there are no surprises when the team is announced, you should confirm availability before finalizing membership. Most importantly, team members should be fair and not go into the evaluation with a pre-conceived notion about the outcome. It is possible to have "leanings" without prejudicing the evaluation. Team members should be made to understand that they are not being sent to render opinions but rather to objectively gather information. There should be an opportunity for a global assessment in which any member may voice subjective assessments of all visit-related findings. Be careful that an outspoken member does not insult the host organization by "explaining" the faults of the host's system to the host in the middle of the visit.

None of the team or their family members should have any financial arrangement with the vendor. Likewise, team members should not receive any direct support or gifts from the vendor. The team should be able to leave its current work for a day or two without untoward results. Support from the institution should be given to the team in the form of time for preparing for the site visit and subsequent write up. Be careful to select members whose workload permits adequate preparation for site-visit related duties and activities. Site-visiting expertise is a rare but valuable skill. Potential team members who have conducted site visits in the past may be able to provide useful insights even though their present job functions are not directly applicable to the product investigated. Site visiting is an anthropologic skill. Being a professional stranger is a valuable ability.

People to Interview at the Site

Choosing people to interview at the site is more problematic. Always include line-users to aid in assessing user interface and workflow issues. Managers and administrators may help with understanding the effects of system implementation on job performance, job functions, cost-savings, etc. Request a list of people with whom you will be allowed to visit. This is to ensure that you are not being given personnel who cannot answer your operational questions or those who don't understand the higher administrative aspects of the installation. It is important to get the correct balance between users, managers, and administrative personnel. You want everyone to be comfortable with the kinds of people they will meet and the questions they need to ask.

When to Make a Site Visit

The site visit should not come at the beginning of the selection process or at the very end. The site visit is allows the team to evaluate how a specific product works in a production environment. Therefore, it is essential that the electronic health record (EHR) selection process be far enough along to have resulted in a narrowing of the field to a few very desirable products. Do not wait until after you have settled on a single product. Site visits conducted at this point serve simply as rubber stamps, and it is too easy to gloss over deficiencies because team members would not be inclined to "disagree" with what amounts to a foregone conclusion. Except for the most complicated multi-function systems, a day should be adequate for a site visit. If travel issues are a consideration, arriving mid-day and leaving the following mid-day can accommodate a complete visit.

Where to Go for a Site Visit

Always select sites that will allow you to answer questions pertinent to your evaluation process. If system response time is an issue, try to visit a site that has a high patient volume or a large number of workstations. Vendor-support quality issues are also good site visit topics. However, the best rule to go by is: visit sites that are most like your own in terms of patient volume, revenues, technical expertise, etc. There are several determinants of destination for a site visit. If money is no object, then the sites most like your own with the products most like the one you are considering, regardless of location are the places to go. Usually a compromise will have to be made. By limiting the scope and cost of your visit, you limit the number of potential of host sites. Usually a reasonable compromise can be made in the number of visitors and number of sites so that a good representative visit can be arranged. Vendors often make arrangements with sites to allow site visits. This may include a monetary payment to the site and/or to selected individuals at the site. Always ask those at the site if they have any form of quid pro quo arrangement with the vendor.

Questions to Ask During a Site Visit

Divide the functionality of prospective systems into logical groups. For each group develop questions that address process and ease-of-use for each aspect of the system. What follows is a sample list of functional groups and potential questions. Study and modify them according to your needs. If the questions generate questions about your installation, these must be answered before a site visit. For example, if you have a robust, secure e-mail system at your institution but you have not thought about using e-mail in your clinical system, perhaps this should be addressed in the project design.

1. **Front end.** This includes patient contacts (in person, over the phone, or via a messaging system), check-in processing for visits, financial verification, insurance confirmation, managed care processing (verifying correct network, co-pays, deductibles, referral verification, and other managed care issues), check-out processing, taking payments, and making follow-up appointments or referral appointments (Table 20-1).

2. **Clinical pre-processing.** Clinical staff take over and escort the patient to the examination room, take the initial history, vital signs,

Table 20-1

FRONT END

1. Is patient look-up easy? Are you prompted with a list of pre-scheduled patients to choose from?

2. How are patients identified? Is a soundex feature available?

3. How are potential mis-matches dealt with? How do you resolve incorrect matches?

4. Does the system prompt you with financial details for each patient?

5. Does the system integrate with your phone system to use caller ID to bring up the caller's record?

6. Does the system follow your workflow? Can it be made to?

7. How much managed care information does it supply? Is it accurate? Up to date?

8. Is simple cash collection quick and intuitive?

9. Is the scheduling system easy to use?

Table 20-2

CLINICAL PRE-PROCESSING

1. Is patient look-up easy? Are you prompted with a list of pre-scheduled patients to chose from?
2. Are templates provided to enter data? Are they easy to use?
3. Is the system used in the exam room? Can patients "peek" into their record?
4. How easy is it to enter medications or allergies?
5. What are provisions for security? How long does it take to log in? How often do you have to log in?
6. Are there any features that patients can use? Are they easy to use? Do patients like them?
7. Does the system make it easy to check on immunizations?
8. Can you easily look up lab and imaging results for patients?

check medications and allergies, and prepare for the provider. In some systems clinical personnel assist patients in using data collection and education software in the waiting room or exam room (Table 20-2).

3. **Clinical visit.** During the clinical visit the provider takes a history, reviews past records, examines the patient, plans treatment or further evaluations, documents the visit, creates a super-bill, and plans follow-up (Table 20-3).

Table 20-3

CLINICAL VISIT

1. Is the system used in the exam room? Is the patient pre-selected by the aide before your visit?
2. Is there expert advice built into the system? Is it easy to use?
3. Does the system help with documentation? How much time does it take?
4. Does it fit into your workflow? What changes did you have to make?
5. Does it enable ordering labs or images or referrals?
6. If available, are templates easy to create or change?
7. Can you schedule the patient for a return visit or to see other specialists in your organization?
8. Are clinical guidelines or informal local information available through the system?
9. Does the system enable electronic communication? With patients? With staff? With other providers?
10. What do you like best about the system? What part of the system do you interact with most? Least?
11. Does the system perform as expected? Does it respond fast enough?

Table 20-4

CLINICAL POST-PROCESSING

1. Does the system help with immunizations?
2. How does the system fit into your workflow?
3. Does the system save time?
4. Is the system connected to managed care information to make referrals easier?
5. Is there patient education material available?
6. Does the system make it easier to order labs or images?
7. Does the system offer an appointment option/feature?
8. Does the system provide for electronic communication?

4. **Clinical post-processing.** Clinical staff do procedures, immunizations, treatments, collect specimens, and may help facilitate referrals or lab tests by filling out forms or getting approval from managed care organizations (Table 20-4).

5. **Pre-visit triage.** Clinical personnel, usually nurses, handle messages from patients, most often on the phone, but increasingly via e-mail or web interfaces. They give advice and/or reassurance and pass the message to a physician to approve before or after the fact or for the physician to contact the patient directly (Table 20-5).

6. **Back office.** Billing, collections, finance, accounting, and other administrative and management functions constitute the back-office activities that do not directly deal with the patient (Table 20-6).

Table 20-5

PRE-VISIT TRIAGE

1. Does the system pop up with the patient's clinical information when a call comes in?
2. Can you record telephone consultations directly into the system?
3. What decision-support tools are available while you are on the phone with a patient?
4. Does the system enable you to message to physicians for assistance? During a call?
5. Can you make appointments for the patient while on the phone?
6. Can you order labs or images through the system?
7. Does it help you with prescription refills?
8. Can you make a managed care referral for a patient while on the phone?

Table 20-6

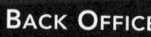

BACK OFFICE

1. Can you view bills easily to answer questions for payers or patients?
2. Does it make it easier to perform the usual functions of your previous accounting system? Harder?
3. Is the accounts receivable module easy to use and intuitive?
4. Does it fit into your workflow? How much do you have to change to fit into the new system?
5. What features exist to edit claims before they are sent to the insurance company?
6. Can you access clinical records to correctly code visits?
7. How are the managed care functions interfaced with the managed care companies?
8. What other administrative features does it have that make it easier to use than the alternative?

7. **General system questions.** There are some questions that either do not apply to a specific sub-system or apply equally to all parts of a system. In Question 6 (of Table 20-7), the functional model refers to how the system represents concepts. That is; do you select the data first then indicate what you want to do with it? OR do you decide first what you are going to do before you select data? In Question 7 (of Table 20-7), the information model refers to

Table 20-7

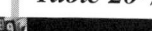

GENERAL SYSTEM QUESTIONS

1. Does the system force the use of redundant data entry procedures (enter the same information twice or in two different places)?
2. Do the users find themselves "going in then backing out" of menu systems to get where they need to go, or is navigation simple and straightforward?
3. Does the system make you write down information on paper and transfer it or use it in another section?
4. Does the system offer a consistent look and feel? Do all dialog boxes operate the same way? Is printing similar in all places that printing can be done?
5. Do the keys do the same thing in all places in the program? Are they standard for the platform or idiosyncratic? Does the system require a template for the keyboard?
6. Does the system operate with the same functional model in all places?
7. Does the system operate with the same information model in all places?
8. Is the vendor responsive to problems and inquiries?
9. Are you generally pleased with the functionality and value from the system? What do you not like about the contract with the vendor?
10. Would you go with the same system and installation consultant next time?

Table 20-8

TRAINING AND INSTALLATION ISSUES

1. Did you receive adequate training? Was it from the company or a train a trainer model?
2. Was the training logical and did it fit into your workflow model?
3. In situations in which the system didn't fit your current workflow model, did you get adequate explanation of the model it uses and why?
4. Were people present to help you when you went live? How is phone support?
5. How long was productivity decreased after installation before back to normal?
6. What is your local support model? Do you have/need a help desk?
7. Is there on-line training and help functionality?
8. Are there wizards to help with complex functions?
9. What was/were the worse mistake(s) you made during installation?

how the system represents data or information. For example, is the name represented the same way in all places? ((FirstName Last-Name or LastName, FirstName) (Table 20-7)

8. **Training and installation issues.** Some issues can be brought up in all interviews regarding training. The "train-a-trainer" model is a good idea ((a company trains a cadre of trainers who then train end-users to be peer trainers). It can be a cost-effective training method (Table 20-8).

9. **Technical issues.** Technical issues may not be addressed sufficiently if all members of the team are users and administrators. If the team leader has access to technical personnel on-site, then the leader should ask these questions. If the answers are not understood by the team arrange for a follow-up contact from a more knowledgeable person at your home site. (Table 20-9)

Logistics of the Site Visit

The site visit team should review the list of potential questions for completeness. Ideally, each team member should talk to several people at the site. The team may have to divide and conquer so that physicians interview MDs, nurses, and other direct users, while an administrative person talks to managerial and other administrative front-line users. The visit matrix should be worked out well before the visit. Confirm in advance which personnel you will be given access to and that they will have time set aside to answer your questions. Keep in mind that quiet observation of site personnel going about their usual activities can be quite helpful. If possible try to

Table 20-9

TECHNICAL ISSUES

1. Were the hardware and utility functions adequate for your purposes?
2. Were the sizing calculations by the vendor realistic?
3. How often does the system go down? What is up-time percentage?
4. Is the vendor responsive to problem inquiries?
5. Did the vendor stay on schedule for installation and training?
6. How hard is it to interface to new systems?
7. Has the vendor ever deceived you?
8. Were there hidden or unexpected costs?

arrange for actual use of the system by team members (register a patient, log and make a phone call, make a referral, etc.).

The objectivity of host personnel is very important. It is okay to ask what, if anything, was given as a quid pro quo (by the vendor to the visit site) for granting the visit. While it is not ethical to specifically snoop around and ask questions of people to whom you have not been given access, there are ways to get confirmation of your host's opinion. While in your host's presence, it is considered fair game to strike up a conversation with a hosting coworker by asking the coworker to confirm your host's recently voiced opinions of the system. You may not get a full answer, but if there are hidden issues that your host has overlooked, a few passing comments may suggest further direct questions to your host about aspects he/she is less pleased with.

Parting Advice

Extensive planning before the visit is required in order to ensure a fruitful visit. Try to anticipate activities that might make team members unavailable (vacations, project deadlines, etc.) and plan accordingly. Keeping everyone on schedule, while being able to change the schedule to accommodate unanticipated opportunities, is a balancing act that only experience can finely tune.

Project Demonstrations

Why Have a Product Demonstration?

Product demonstrations usually occur at either of two stages of the evaluation/ selection process. During the earliest stages you may want to show your constituents a few of the leading products in the field so the project becomes more real. Later, the definitive product demonstration occurs as a part of a systematic evaluation of several products (finalists) and should be scripted.

The initial free-form demonstration may be open-ended and run completely by the vendor sales team. It may include information about the company, how the product fits into the "bigger picture", and why it is better than the competition. It should take an hour or more and end with a session which permits hands-on access to the product.

The scripted demo may be a multi-day affair. There may be several scripts, lengthy interactions, multiple users and de-briefing sessions at the end. The scripts (these are scenarios created by the practice—see Chapter 16) must be carefully chosen before considering which vendors to invite to participate. The scripts must entail tasks that are commonly done and those that are critical. Physician data entry is the heart of an EHR system and must be addressed during any demonstration.

Participants in the Product Demonstration

Vendor Personnel

The vendor usually determines the make-up of the initial free-form demonstration. Typically a number of sales staff are included in the initial group. Generally, the more senior the company personnel who attend, the more you as a customer will get out of the demo. Sales people can only offer so much insight into the past and future development of the product. The vendor should bring a substantial team for the short-list scripted demonstration. You should meet with senior-level personnel who have the authority to negotiate. Insist on having a physician from their staff, usually VP level, attend the demonstration. If there is no such person available, an early physician-user can suffice if accompanied by a vendor VP level representative. The other vendor personnel should be experienced users for each module featured in the product.

Personnel from Your Institution

On the customer side, who attends will depend upon on the purpose of the demonstration. In the early stages of EHR promotion, a series of sales presentations can be opened to the general audience of all potential users. Open presentations of this type can help in generating enthusiasm and momentum for the project. The clinical and administrative opinion leaders should be invited, as well as the decision-makers. For a scripted short-list demo, a much smaller team should be involved. The lead physician and key administrative personnel should be present, and one of them should sponsor the demonstration. A few persons on the project steering committee should be invited so that three to five might attend the demonstration of each module.

In addition, there should be a team of required attendees who would use the module in your institution. You should aim for at least three users in order to have enough for a balanced opinion (but not so many as to bog down the proceedings). The criteria for selecting persons to participate in a demonstration are similar to the site visit criteria. Level-headed individuals who have a history with your institution are better than very computer savvy but socially dissonant individuals.

When to Have a Product Demonstration

The pep-rally type of demonstration should take place early in the process. As soon administrative approval is given and a team is assembled, demonstrations may be used to perform a limited survey of products and vendors providing a stimulating beginning to your selection process. The scripted demo should occur after the field is limited to about three finalists. The sequence of demo and site visit is not critical and may depend on local factors such as availability of the vendors and the site visit team. If you have a formal set of questions and tasks for the site visit and a script and variations for the short list demonstration, you could intersperse these as schedules permit.

Where to Host a Product Demonstration

The early sales demo is best done in an auditorium or small conference room depending on the size of the audience. You will want to consider power, video monitor projection, and network or phone connections, as well as the typical audio projection depending on the needs of your presenter. For political reasons you should consider the impact of a sparsely attended demo in a large auditorium versus the standing-room-only effect of a medium-sized room. The setting of a scripted demonstration would ideally be a clinical area. However, you will not usually be able to secure a real clinical or patient area unless you do it during non-patient hours. Since workflow can be critical to success or failure of a system, it is definitely worth the trouble of creating a mock-up that represents the physical realities of your clinical area. For example the mock-up reception area, waiting area, clinical area, and checkout areas should represent the physical realities of your situation. You should supply mock patients to move through the system and interact with vendor personnel using the product.

What to Do During a Product Demonstration

The sales-type demonstration requires only a brief introduction of the vendor personnel conducting the show. The audience will usually not be interested in the history of the company, although the company will frequently want to tell you how many years they have been selling this product and why their company is better than the competition. While there may be some merit to a limited review of company make-up, philosophy and history, this should not be more than a few minutes. An overview of how the product fits into the overall information and patient care system is appropriate at the beginning. What the audience really wants to see is how the product works, what the screens look like, how data entry is accomplished, how easy it is to navigate through the screens and how it is going to improve their daily lives or increase the quality of the care that they give to patients.

The success of the scripted demo depends heavily on the script. The script should take at least one patient from initial problem discovery through contacting the provider, receiving care, and the follow-up. Other patients can focus on smaller areas of the spectrum of care. Separate patient scripts could involve extensive telephone dialog, changing insurance or demographic information, a nurse protocol, a single-problem primary care visit, single-problem specialty visit, a multi-problem primary care visit, a surgical procedure, and various administrative tasks and reports. The vendor should bring a system mocked up with adequate clinical data to make these realistic. Be wary of data that has already been entered to "speed-up" the demo.

Addressing Important Issues During Demonstrations

The vendor primarily drives the sales demo. Sales demonstrations are usually in response to a request for information or request for proposal. Therefore, the client should provide specific guidance on what is desired during the demonstration. Failure to properly target a sales demo should reflect poorly on the company or at least the sales force. Scripted demonstrations are much more formal and more is at stake. Preparation of a scripted demo involves several steps: (Table 20-10)

Evaluating Site Visits and Demonstrations

For each site visit and each scripted demo of a system, it is important to objectively quantify your appraisal of the system's performance and how well it meets your needs. This information combined with the cost of the system will significantly enhance one's ability to calculate the value that the system could bring to your enterprise. To organize the evaluation, a formal evaluation document should be developed with questions grouped into categories based upon the results of a needs assessments and wish list.

Where possible, study documents used by other organizations making similar decisions. When perusing other organization's list of survey documents, consider how closely the other organization's situation resembles your own. As much as is practical avoid open-ended questions. That is, create yes/no or multiple-choices questions. It is important that a means of

Table 20-10

ADDRESSING IMPORTANT ISSUES DURING DEMONSTRATIONS

1. Determine what problems the system is to address/solve.
2. Talk to your users to get the details of their needs and workflow issues surrounding these problems.
3. Get a specific list of steps a system must do to in order to provide the functionality that you require.
4. Get users to suggest scenarios that address the full range of functionality issues.
5. Write up detailed scripts of what the patient says for each scenario.
6. Make this list available to the companies that you invite to conduct scripted demonstrations.
7. Discuss misunderstandings ahead of time to make sure the products address the areas correctly.
8. Modify, if necessary, the scripts and deliver the final version to each company.
9. Schedule demos.
10. During the demo have your people play the part of the patient or other outside person.
11. Be prepared to change details slightly to be sure the demo hasn't been "hard-wired" into the program beforehand to make data entry appear easier than it really is
12. Create and use a weighted grading tool for the demo.

scoring responses be created. Scoring may be on a 0-1 scale or a more conceptual essential/non-essential feature format. For example if you are a predominately but not exclusively Unix network environment, you might make a question concerning network platforms have a value of .8 for a Unix friendly system and .2 for a system that will run, but is not designed specifically to take advantage of Unix's features. Alternatively, you may choose to make Unix compatibility a requirement, in which case you would arrive at a score by determining the total essential-features for all products considered.

Systems with equivalent essential-feature scores would then be compared using non-essential (wish-list) items. To record this quantification, a spreadsheet is a good idea. The spreadsheet follows the outline of the survey. On the spreadsheet record the importance of each question in a category to the overall category assessment. For each category, in a similar way, assign an importance factor for the category to the overall decision. When you fill in answers for each question you can transfer a numeric value to the spreadsheet and a score will emerge representing an objective measure of the value of a particular system. To facilitate multiple users contributing input to these decisions, you should develop a survey guidebook explaining the importance of each question and the significance of each answer choice.

Summary

"To do" checklist for site visits and demonstrations:

- Do your political homework first to be sure you have support from practice leadership
- Make sure the system fits in the practice/enterprise strategic plan
- Make sure you get a feeling for start-to-finish functionality
- Be prepared with a questionnaire for each area
- Look for common real-life uses
- Search for time savers and time wasters
- Think about installation, training and back-office issues
- Keep tone even handed
- Make sure you evaluate all important features quantitatively
- Do ask about a work-around plan if a feature is not present
- What "*not* to do" during site visits and demonstrations:
    1. Don't get caught up in unimportant details
    2. Don't get drawn in by hard sell tactics
    3. Don't let logistic mistakes detract from the evaluation
    4. Don't keep your script exactly as advertised; change details
    5. Don't invite problem personalities
    6. Don't pass judgment during the evaluation
    7. Don't let overly solicitous salespeople sway you
    8. Don't accept vendors advice on the relative merits of features
    9. Don't accept unproved bromides like "Everyone Loves It"
    10. Don't allow the flash of the presentation to obscure critical dysfunctions

21

Planning Your Implementation

Jerome H. Carter, MD

The decision to implement an electronic health record (EHR) is a decision to change every major aspect of your practice. EHRs are change agents because every product is designed to work in a specific manner and the practice has to adapt to the EHR's notion of how a practice should function. If you thought that you were simply replacing the paper chart with an electronic version, then you are in for a very rude awakening. Failure to appreciate the abruptness and extent to which an EHR will alter your current practice environment can be very jarring, and in extreme cases may lead the practice to abandon the implementation. An article from the December 11th, 2006 issue of *American Medical News* chronicles two such cases (1). It details the removal of an EHR system from a physician's office after only two weeks' use. The article went on to state that industry estimates are that between 20% and 33% of EHR systems installed in physician practices are removed within the first year.

While no formal studies exist that detail the exact failure rate for EHR systems, stories of failed systems are not uncommon. De-installation represents a **total failure** and is easily recognized. However, failures can take other forms as outlined by Heeks, Mundy, and Salazar in their paper "Why Healthcare Information Systems Succeed or Fail" (2). In addition to total failures, they cite partial failures, sustainability failures, and replication failures.

Partial failures are more common than most would like to admit. A good example is the practice in which an EHR is installed but not all providers use the system, resulting in a mixture of paper and electronic charts. Another good example of a partial failure is an implementation in which one or more key features are never used by anyone (e.g., preventive medicine or lab download never worked). In either case the benefits of using an EHR are never fully realized. **Sustainability failures** occur when an EHR is implemented but is never really embraced by the users and after a while is replaced. As the name implies, **replication failures** are those in which an implementation worked well in one practice but failed to work at all in an ostensibly similar practice. All types of failures result in wasted time, effort and money.

A very insightful study, concerning "runaway" computer projects was published in 1995 (3). Conducted by KPMG, the study defined a **runaway project** as one that "has failed significantly to achieve its objectives and/or has exceeded its original budget by at least 30%". It was based on a survey of information systems managers conducted by KPMG in which respondents were asked to list the most important reasons that computer implementation projects become "runaways". The survey was conducted across major industries and included in-house developed as well as commercially purchased software. The results of the survey listed the top six reasons as:

- Project objectives not fully specified
- Bad planning and estimation
- Technology new to the organization
- Inadequate/no project management methodology
- Insufficient senior staff on team
- Poor performance by suppliers of hardware/software

Interestingly, there were no differences in problem implementations noted between commercial systems and in-house built systems. After having spent more than 12 years reviewing the troubles encountered in implementing healthcare information systems, I find these reasons to be right on target. In fact, it has been my experience that if one of these issues is present during an implementation, it is in serious danger of failure. If two or more are present, the project is usually doomed.

Ensuring a Successful Implementation

As the KPMG study clearly demonstrates, successful implementation of any complex computer system requires clear objectives, planning, leadership, and adequate resources. Successful organizations rely on the team approach. The number of teams required, along with their size and composition, depends on the type of practice. In a practice of three to five providers, a single team with representatives from each job position is usually adequate. However in a hospital or an IPA, four or more teams are frequently used. (Table 21-1).

Horizontal and Vertical Teams

Teams come in two basic flavors: policy-focused (horizontal) and workgroups (vertical). Horizontal teams are composed of personnel from differ-

Table 21-1

TEAM TYPES

Teams (horizontal)	Function	Practice Team Members (3-5 providers)	Hospital/IPA Team Members
Executive	Oversees change management, budgeting and resource allocation, policy changes, and conflict resolution.	MD, nurse, office manager, front desk, project manager	CEO/Executive VP, chief information officer (CIO), chief financial officer (CFO), chief medical officer (CMO), nursing director, director of health information management, and project manager
Clinical	Oversees workflow changes and standardization of clinical practice and policies	Same	CMO, chief medical information officer (CMIO), nursing director, and additional clinical personnel, and project manager
Administrative	Oversees administrative workflow, administrative policy and procedures, and billing issues	Same	CFO, COO, human resources director, project manager and other administrative personnel
Technology	Oversees technology infrastructure (networking, servers, security, etc.) policies and procedures	Same	CIO, project manager, and additional technical personnel

ent organizational units and are designed to permit input from all affected areas of the organization when policy decisions are being made. Vertical groups, on the other hand, are used to get work done. Vertical groups are composed of personnel with similar job roles and have as their main task the design, analysis, and testing of new processes/workflows. Generally speaking, vertical groups propose and test new workflows while horizontal groups set policy and review the work completed by vertical groups. Vertical groups may be created based on a patient care service (ICU nursing), medical specialty (cardiology), workflow (medication order entry), or staff group (respiratory therapy). The key fact to remember is that vertical groups address issues at the level of the end-user.

Four upper-level teams (horizontal: executive, clinical, administrative, and technology) are typically formed to preside over major EHR implementations (Figure 21-1).

Executive Team

The role of the executive team is to guide the organization through the significant changes that the EHR implementation will trigger. This team consists of key members of upper-level management and to be effective it must be involved with the project on a daily basis. It is not a committee that meets once per month to hear about the progress of the implementation: that approach is too "hands-off" and does not provide the steady executive leadership required for a complex software implementation. All other teams report either directly or indirectly to the executive team. Here is where issues related to budgeting, new positions, conflict resolution, new policies/procedures, and organizational restructuring are discussed and decided.

Clinical Team

The clinical team has the job of overseeing standardization of care processes and clinical workflow redesign. This is the lead clinical team

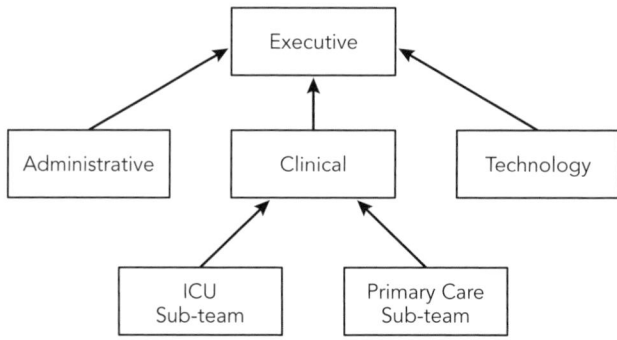

Figure 21-1 Team relationships.

where polices/issues are debated and finalized before presentation to the executive team. Sub-teams that tackle special problems of clinical domains are often formed and report to the lead clinical team. Standardization issues are the main source of friction and resistance from providers. Amiable resolution of care process matters is more likely when everyone feels that they have a voice in shaping the outcome. Therefore, promote open membership in order to ensure that as many members of the medical/nursing staff participate as is practical.

Administrative Team

An EHR affects all aspects of an organization. Administrative policies and procedures must be changed to adapt to the new way of doing things. This may mean changes in charge capture, billing, job descriptions, adding new staff positions, and other administrative adjustments.

Technology Team

Depending on the size of the organization, administrative and technology teams may be combined. In any case, the role of the technology team is to ensure that the technical infrastructure of the organization is sound. The focus here it is on "wires" and "boxes" (e.g., network throughput, server capability, security).

Teams in Small Practices

Even though by comparison, the complexity of small practices is considerably less than that of hospitals, the decision-making requirements for a successful implementation are not proportionally diminished. Therefore, in small practices the work required of EHR team members to achieve a successful implementation is greater. The imposition of implementation tasks along with the lack of expertise are major barriers to EHR adoption in small practices. One way to address these issues is through the selection of a vendor that targets small practices. Generally they provide more in the way of services such as project management and workflow redesign to clients than do vendors who target larger practices (larger practices hire consultants). The Doctor's Office Quality–Information Technology Project (DOQ-IT), provides free consulting services to practices that want to implement EHRs. The project is sponsored by the Centers for Medicare & Medicaid Services (CMS) and is available through state-level quality improvement organizations (QIO) (4). Keep in mind that even with a helpful vendor, consulting expertise, and/or what you learn from this book, there remains a lot of work for the practice's EHR team. For an in-depth look at how various organizations use teams to manage EHR projects try reviewing a few of the case study from Davies Awards winners (the award is given for excellence in EHR implementation) (see Appendix B).

Avoiding Common Mistakes

The factors cited in the KMPG study provide an excellent starting point for self-review and goal setting when you start your implementation.

Project Management

An EHR implementation consists of a number of interdependent activities (workflow redesign, staff training, chart migration, hardware installation, interface testing) that require painstaking attention to detail and constant monitoring to make sure that everything is on schedule and on budget. This is what project managers do. Project management is a professional skill but one that can be developed by a highly motivated staff member. Vendors often provide some project management support; however, the bulk of daily project management tasks usually falls to a member of the practice staff. Even in a small practice, project manager responsibilities can require up to 0.5 FTE over the course of an implementation (four to six months); in large practices it is a full-time job.

Project management (Chapter 22) should be approached in a formal manner. Software such as Microsoft Project, Excel, or other spreadsheet is required to keep track of the many tasks, dependencies, and deadlines associated with an implementation.

Planning and Estimation

The biggest planning task for a small practice is workflow redesign. If the EHR selection process outlined in this book is followed, then the workflow redesign simply picks up where process analysis left off. If no process analysis was done, then it is best to go back to the beginning (Chapter 16) and start from there. Workflow redesign is absolutely crucial because the software system and the practice'smanual way of doing things have to be seamlessly integrated. This requires intimate knowledge of the software as well as intimate knowledge of the practice, neither of which can be obtained without study. Failure to pay attention to workflow redesign will almost guarantee a failed implementation.

Budgeting is another problematic issue for many practices. There are many costs associated with EHR implementations that do not necessarily show up in the contract. Keep in mind that a successful implementation never ends (5). Therefore, some costs will recur. For example, updates, monthly maintenance, equipment upgrades, new employee training, interface updates, new staff (e.g., the information technology staff), disaster recovery/backup solutions, and security protection are ongoing. In fact, some vendors charge as much as 20% of the cost of the original purchase price yearly for maintenance and support. Obviously some of this will be offset by the savings from being paperless (or nearly paperless), but be aware that there will be ongoing costs and budget accordingly.

Technology New to the Organization

Be very careful not to get carried away by gadgets. Tablet PCs are great but they are expensive and can be easily damaged by dropping them. Also, they are easy to steal. Wireless networks are very convenient, but the security for them can be difficult to set up properly. Cutting-edge technology may seem like a good idea until it breaks and there is difficulty finding someone knowledgeable to repair it. Use technology (and this applies to software as well) that has been battle tested, is widely available, and that does not require expertise that is not readily available from your local information technology vendor. Buy EHR products from CCHIT-certified vendors that have been properly qualified (Chapter 17). Verify that they are financially sound and are known for good customer service.

Insufficient Senior Staff on Team

Effective implementation teams have the authority to act. Whether this means spending money, hiring new staff, changing policy, or redesigning workflows, these teams have the authority to get things done. This requires that senior clinical and administrative leaders participate actively in the implementation. In a small practice this means getting as many people involved as possible, especially the key decision makers.

Poor Performance by Suppliers of Hardware/Software

Be wary of offers to beta-test a product in return for free or reduced-price licenses. Beta-testing is an agreement to allow the vendor to experiment with their product using your practice. If things do not work out well, the vendor simply removes the software and leaves. Meanwhile you are stuck with cleaning up the aftermath. Always keep in mind that a failed implementation can leave you worse off than when you started. Leave beta-testing to hospitals and large groups who may have "test sites" that can afford to endure a beta-test.

Be sure that the product you purchase is actually shipping. This is not a problem with CCHIT certified systems. When evaluating vendors determine whether they have the expertise required to support your practice. This means asking about project management capability, programming expertise, technical skills and R&D activities, etc.

Finally, buy workstations and servers from either major national vendors or stable, local vendors with whom you have a long-term relationship.

Implementation Start-Up

Implementations are complex endeavors that require careful planning and thoughtful execution. Often, knowing just where to begin can be a challenge, so the following pointers are offered to help you manage your implementation.

Assemble Your Team

Team Composition

If your practice has five or fewer providers, then you need only one team. The members of the team should be all the providers, a medical records representative, the office manager, a nursing representative, a front office representative, and the project manager. This usually results in a team that consists of four to nine members. Once teams get to be larger than nine to ten members they become unwieldy. At that point is best to have a representative group of providers as team members rather than all providers. If there are more than five providers consider creating a separate clinical team to mange workflow redesign. This will allow all providers to be involved in implementation planning.

Appoint the Project Manager

The project manager may be any of the members of the team. However, because at least 0.5 FTE will be devoted to project management for at least a few months, this job will likely fall to one of the non-clinical staff. Make sure that the project manager has time dedicated daily to work on implementation. The vendor will also provide a project manager who will work with the practice on major aspects of implementation. However, be clear that the major burden for the implementation will fall to the practice

Attempting to manage an implementation without using the proper tools is a common mistake. Excel or another spreadsheet program will work for a practice with one or two providers. However, Microsoft Project is the better way to go for larger groups. There are at least five parallel paths that occur during implementation: workflow redesign, budget management, training, chart migration, and security. The activities along each of these tracks are interdependent, and it is the project manager's job to make sure that everything happens on schedule and on budget. That is why a good tool is so important. Choose your project manager as early as possible so they have time to master the tools and techniques for project management.

Schedule Regular Meetings

There is a lot of work to be done. Set aside at least two hours per week for meetings and strive for 100% attendance. These are not meant to be "committee" meetings; rather, the focus is on getting work done. Create and post the meeting agenda at least two days in advance and assign tasks to team members. Set a meeting format and stick to it. Use the pathways listed previously as the basis for deciding the tasks to be completed as well as a basis for agenda items.

Review Your Budget

In smaller practices the budget is fairly straightforward and can generally be finalized at the time that the contract is signed. In larger practices additional hands are often required to help get work done (e.g., data entry, document scanning, etc.). Also, consultants are frequently hired to help with implementation details such as workflow redesign and other common tasks. Of course these extra items are not included in the contract signed for software and hardware. Therefore, it is wise to set aside an additional sum, usually no more than 20% to 30% of the overall project budget, to help with items that appear along the way.

Review Staffing Needs

An EHR represents a significant change in the way practice functions. There is a much greater dependence on information technology, and new concerns arise that were not previously present. The reliance on new personnel such as systems administrators for the network, computer support personnel, and security staff will be much greater. These job functions can be obtained through new employees or by contracting for these services through a third-party. Either way, be sure that you have access to these skills when you need them.

Set the Project Timeline

Work with your vendor to set a project timeline. Implementations can be emotionally draining and seemingly never-ending; therefore, setting a timeline helps to focus everyone's attention on the ultimate goal while providing a way of measuring progress. This can be very helpful when things seem to be completely out of hand and the work seems to be endless. A timeline also helps the team maintain focus because it provides a list of milestones that can be used by everyone to see the overall progress of the project. It is easier to keep going when you can see the light at the end of the tunnel.

Select a Chart Migration Plan

Chart migration is a difficult topic for many practices because they do not settle on a formal way of accomplishing this task. The most important decision is what will be taken from paper charts to the electronic system. Typically practices either create an abstract of the old chart, decide on specific documents to be moved, or scan the entire chart.

Abstraction of the old chart is probably the best way to go. Here specific data (e.g., problem list, medications, preventive health) are selected for migration to the EHR. These data are then entered into the system prior to the patient's next appointment. Key reports (labs, radiology, and EKGs) are scanned. Often a final summary note is created for inclusion in the EHR. Scanning the entire old chart is rarely worth the effort.

There are two approaches to moving the entire patient population to the EHR. The first is the "big bang" in which all patients are moved to the EHR in a very short period of time: days to weeks. The most common incremental approach is to add patients to the EHR within a week or so of their next appointment. The usual deciding factor is cost. Doing a big bang migration requires extra hands. Whatever the approach taken, always ensure that is easy for staff members to predict whether a patient's chart is on paper or has been moved to the EHR

Set Up a Test/Training Lab

Once the EHR is in place training will be a recurring need. All new employees will require a period of training of a week or so prior to being able to do their jobs. This means that you will have to develop some type of training capability for the practice. A good way to do this is to set up a small network of one to two computers as a "training lab". This does not have to be an elaborate setup; a corner in a back room will work fine. This is also a good way to test upgrades before bringing them up on the live system. Workflow redesign has to be done with the EHR's features and functions in mind. Having a test/training lab provides staff members with the ability to test out workflow redesign ideas on actual software prior to the go-live date. This helps to take the guesswork out of what will work best and also provides a way for everyone to become familiar with the software prior to beginning formal training. It is also helpful to have one or two staff members receive training very early on in the implementation so that they can become expert users by the time of the go-live date.

Initiate Workflow Redesign

Workflow design will be the biggest challenge of implementation. Every process that is supported by the EHR will have to be redesigned with the EHR in mind. This can be very tedious work, but it is very necessary. EHRs have a significant impact on provider work habits and workflow, so every provider should be involved in workflow design at some point in implementation planning. One of the outcomes of workflow redesign will be standardization of care processes across all providers. This can be very jarring and the earlier in the implementation that this discussion begins, the more likely it is to be resolved with as little acrimony as possible.

One of the most important issues is provider data entry. Hopefully, you have chosen an EHR that allows for a variety of data entry mechanisms: pen, voice recognition, transcription download, and typing. This points to another use for the training lab, allowing providers to practice data entry in advance of going live.

Review Security Policies and Procedures

Data security is often overlooked during implementation planning. Keep in mind that data security encompasses more than simply preventing unauthorized access. It also covers disaster recovery, backups, and business continuity planning. Data security planning is usually limited to passwords for authorized users and daily backups of the EHR system. This is really no security at all. Create a formal set of security policies and procedures and stick to them.

Conclusion

The final four chapters of this book will help you understand each of the above points in greater depth. Read them, discuss them with members of your team, resolve to succeed in your implementation, and then go for it.

References

1. Chin T. Avoiding EMR meltdown: how to get your money's worth. AMNews. 2006;49.
2. Heeks R, Mundy D, Salazar A. Why healthcare information systems succeed or fail. Institute for Development Policy and Management; 1999.
   http://www.man.ac.uk/idpm/idpm_dp.htm#isps_wp, Accessed June 25, 2007.
3. Glass R. Software runaways: some surprising findings. ACM SIGMIS Database 1997;28:16-19.
4. http://www.joindoqit.com.
5. Chin HL. The reality of EMR implementation: lessons from the field. The Permanente Journal. 2004;8:4. http://xnet.kp.org/permanentejournal/fall04/reality.pdf . Accessed June 25, 2007.

22

Project Management: Concepts and Methods

Thomas C. Tinstman, MD

<p>A project is an ambitious plan to change. The magnitude of change as an organization moves information from "atoms to bits" (1) is transformational. In health care organizations, a patient's medical history is used as the starting point for each encounter, to study populations, and to support the payment process. The electronic health record (EHR) transformation will involve changing culture, process, knowledge, skill, tools, and even the facility in every corner of the organization. In this chapter we will provide an overview of an approach to managing clinical information system projects based on change management principles, project management methods, and the author's own twenty-three years of personal experiences.</p>

Defining the Project

The first step is to define a project. Projects come in all sizes, but projects large and small share the same defining characteristics. These characteristics describe what will change, who is responsible for the change, and when the change will occur. More important than what, who, and when is why. When you are in the middle of the project and there is a long list of issues, the budget is tight and dates are in question, everyone involved needs to believe in the *why* and use the *why* as a rallying cry to move the project forward. In the language of professional project people, the *why* is the goal or objectives, *what* is the scope, *who* is the resources, and *when* is the date.

A clear and concise statement of the project objectives in order of priority will be one of the most important and long-lasting decisions that will be made. If this statement of the objectives is well formulated and communicated, it will be used hundreds to thousands of times to guide the thousands of small decisions and hundreds of large decisions that are made during a project. The first major decision the objectives should guide is the selection of the EHR supplier. If all those involved in the project, including the software supplier and any consultants, do not have the objectives at the top of their minds and use them to guide their actions, it is unlikely that the objectives will be achieved.

With EHR projects, the objectives typically fall into three major categories: quality of care, service levels, and financial. The executive sponsors of the project should prioritize these three categories as the first step in creating the objectives. Next, the leadership must decide if there will be an objective(s) representing each category. Some organizations choose to keep the objectives very simple and high-level. Others choose to have more specific objectives. As an example, the objective could simply be "Improve the quality of care" or it could be as detailed as "Reduce the preventable adverse drug events that, as a result of appropriate laboratory test use, are predicted or identified early". In between these degrees of specificity would be "Improve the quality of care" with a short list of bullets, one of which would be "Reduce adverse drug events". Another alternative is to set the high-level prioritized objectives and add specificity at certain places within the project. For example, for the high-level objective of "Improve the quality of care" more specificity could be associated with important steps in the workflow of a clinic visit. For rooming the patient it could be accurate recording of weights and calling attention to an increased BMI. For ordering it could be preventing adverse drug events with sensitive and specific alerting for possible drug-allergy and drug-drug events. Remember, if the project team does not use the objectives to guide their actions, it is unlikely that the objectives will be achieved.

A project has three variables to be managed on the road to achieving the objectives. The variables are scope, resources, and dates. If during the project one variable is changed, then the other two must be reexamined and appropriately adjusted. Failure to do this evaluation and adjustment adds a new risk to the project that will most likely result in last minute changes or collapse of the project.

Scope defines what will be changed by the project. When the change is being led with an implementation of software such as an EHR, scope is commonly described by software module, i.e., orders, documentation. The definition of scope may begin with the process or workflow that will be automated followed by the listing of the applicable software module(s) and external sources of data. External data can be added to the EHR with an interface, by file transfers, or integrating another system. Scope will be used to set the users and define expectations. Scope is so important that project charters frequently have an "out of scope" section that calls out the things that users might assume to be included, but are not. Failure to be clear and consistent in defining and communicating scope will result in increased resource consumption (direct cost) or delays in deployment (indirect cost).

Resource is the term used to represent what will be consumed to complete the change identified in the scope. It includes the organization's staff time, purchased services, tools, software, hardware, and facility changes. Determining the resource requirements of a project accurately requires knowledge and experience with the software selected and implementations in organizations with similar processes, infrastructure, and legacy systems. To get the experience, one must rely on the software supplier, purchase consulting services, or hire an experienced project manager. By using this knowledge and experience, a plan of work is created. This plan estimates the number of hours of work required from the organization's staff, supplier's staff, and consultants.

Dates are determined by selecting a date that work will start, sequencing the work plan, and deciding how many people with appropriate knowledge and skill will be working at each step of the project. Using the estimated hours from the work plan and the estimated number of people, the duration of each step is calculated. Summing the duration of each step and correcting for any overlap in the timing of the steps gives you the date the project will be complete.

It should be clear that if the scope of a project is increased and resources are not increased, it will take longer to complete the project. If the resources are not available on a timely basis, completion will be delayed or scope must be reduced to keep the completion date. If someone wants to finish the project sooner, resources would need to be increased or the scope of the change reduced.

Managing the Project

The sponsor and project executives (management) must have a process for overseeing the project to ensure its success. Management is responsible for the cost of the project. Typically total project cost is three to five times the cost of licensing the software and buying the hardware. Thus, most of the cost is people's time (project team, supplier's services and the organization's staff). Variable costs are well-managed if time is managed. Time management requires a sound process for making decisions, identifying risks and mitigating the risks so they do not become issues that delay the project.

The project team will want all decisions to be perfect. In pursuing this goal they may invest too much time in analysis to develop options or hesitate in making decisions. It is management's job to be certain that *perfect* does not become the enemy of *good enough*. On the other hand, the project team may be concerned that frequent user participation will slow the project process. It is management's responsibility to be certain there is adequate user participation. Management review of all the important Design Decision Documents is the best way to ensure good, timely decisions.

The quality of decisions will be improved if management, the project team and the user community all agree on principles and objectives for the project. The principles and objectives for the project should be reviewed in the context of each major decision. Examples of guiding principles for an EHR project are:

- Encourage participation
- Challenge the current ways
- Design for best practice
- Bend workflow to meet the application
- Clinician's time is highly valued
- Typing is a required skill
- If you oppose, you must propose
- Perfect is the enemy of good enough

The possible objectives might be:

- Improve the quality of care
  1. Improve access to the medical history
  2. Reduce medication errors
- Reduce cost of care
  1. Decrease repeat visits
  2. Complete all preventive care at each visit
- Best service
  1. Increase the rate of first phone call fulfillment

For example, if the question was whether workstations should be at the point of care and one were to read through the above, it should be obvious that the point of care location aligns with valuing the clinician's time, improved access to the history, and completing preventive care at each visit.

In the ideal project all issues will have been anticipated and mitigated, thus there would be no issues that delay the project. Unfortunately, this is not possible so when an issue arises it must be called out immediately, faced squarely, options for resolution developed, and a decision made. All issues should be brought to management's attention when they are identified so management is prepared to act if required to make an important decision.

During the planning process management should work with the project manager to establish milestones throughout the project plan. On a weekly basis the project manager should report in writing the status of the work to reach the next milestone, expressed as per cent of completion. If the work is falling behind the schedule, the project manager should explain in an exception statement what is being done to return to the schedule. Reporting the work to be done for the next reporting interval creates time-based objectives for the team that will be used in the next per cent completion report. In Figure 22-1, the top quadrants and the left lower quadrant are used to summarize the above. That is how decisions are managed. The lower

Weekly Status report

TEAM: *Team Name*   Date: *Date*

Overall Project Status Ⓖ

Accomplishments & Key Findings

- TBD

Activity/Deliverable	% Finished	Due Date	Status
• TBD			Ⓖ Ⓨ Ⓡ

Upcoming Work

- TBD

Risks, Issues, Points of Discussion

Risk/Issue/Discussion	Proposed Solution/ Decision Needed	Status
• TBD	• TBD	

Status: O - Open   C -Closed   P-Pending

© Thomas C Tinstman, MD

Figure 22-1 Status Report.

right quadrant is used to manage the risks through risk mitigation plans and actions.

The most common causes of project delay and increased cost are increases in scope, delayed decisions, and loss of the time and attention of key project staff. Increases in scope are referred to as "scope creep". As the term implies the project gets bigger and/or more complicated in a series of small steps. No one "calls the ball" on a per step basis and suddenly all discover the work has increased beyond the capacity of the project resources and the dates are unachievable. The best defense against scope creep is everyone asking with each decision, "does this increase work and/or delay the dates". When there is no easy answer or a subject is politically sensitive there is a natural tendency to put off having the challenging discussion that gets to a solution. We all intellectually know that the most difficult issue should get first attention. Management needs to remind and support the project staff to push forward. A project counts on the knowledge and expertise of a small group. Typically these people are valued by others too. Allowing key project personnel to be "loaned out" to other projects usually causes delays. Avoid this temptation.

Project Charter

Once you have determined the objective, defined the scope, aligned the resources and set the dates for the project, it is time to combine this information in a single document called a Project Charter. The level of detail can vary. Use the Project Charter Summary (as shown in Figure 22-2), as an outline for the document. The Charter Summary is used to deliver the message and obtain commitment. The Charter Summary describes the project concisely and asks the involved parties to sign indicating that they understand and agree with their role in the project.

Budget

The budget is next. The process of creating the Charter document and the signing of the Charter Summary gives a clear view of the resource requirements for the project and focuses all the participants on the known risks. These risks can become issues that increase the resources required for the project. With the signing of the Charter Summary, the participants are agreeing to work to mitigate the known risks and thus complete the project with the resources identified in the Charter. The resource requirements are monetized and added to the cost of hardware, software, facilities, external professional services, and training for your project staff and the users, thus completing the budget (Figure 22-3).

Project Charter Summary:
<Enter Project Name>

Start Date: <enter date>
Est. End Date: <enter date>

Project Executive Leadership

Member	Role	Telephone

<Project Team Name> Members

Member	Role	Telephone

<Project Team Name> Responsibilty
<enter responsibility statement>

Project Objective Statement
<enter project objective statement>

In Scope
1.
2.
3.

Out of Scope
1.
2.
3.

Assumptions
1.
2.
3.

Customer Benefits
1.
2.
3.

Dependencies/Constraints
1.
2.
3.

Risks
1.
2.
3.

Critical Success Factors
1.
2.
3.

Major Milestones

Milestone	Planned	Actual

Charter Review and Approval

Member	Signature	Date
<enter name>		

Figure 22-2   Project Charter Summary.

Discoveries during the project frequently increase the work required beyond the initial estimate. The number and size of the discoveries vary greatly with the type of project and from one organization to another. The best way to estimate what might be discovered with your project is by talking with similar organizations about their discoveries and how the

Resource Planning Template

Project Staffing[1]	Salary (Annual FTE Salary)	Benefits (Salary* .22)	Total Costs (Salary+ Benefits)	Year 1 FTE	Year 1 Cost[5]	Year 2 FTE	Year 2 Cost	Year 3 FTE	Year 3 Cost	Year 4 FTE	Year 4 Cost	Year 5 FTE	Year 5 Cost
Management					$0		$0		$0		$0		$0
Clinical Staff[2]					$0		$0		$0		$0		$0
Technology Staff[3]					$0		$0		$0		$0		$0
Support Staff[4]					$0		$0		$0		$0		$0
TOTAL	$0	$0	$0	2.75	$0	1.35	$0	1.35	$0	0.00	$0	0.00	$0

Input Cells — Numbers are required in these cells
Calculated Cells — These cells contain formulas and will update automatically based on inputs

Notes:
1. This spreadsheet supports the resource planning template referred to in the CIS Lifecycle documentation
2. Clinical staff may include: physicians, clinical nurse managers, clinical staff RN, practice managers, clinical managers, radiology and medical records
3. Technology staff may include: application managers, analysts, architects and network support
4. Support Staff may include: facilities/engineering and other non-clinical positions
5. Annual costs equals salary and benefits for each group multiplied by the estimated number of FTEs per year

Figure 22-3   Resource Planning Template.

discoveries affected resources. Sometimes the software supplier can also offer good insight. Based on this input it is advisable to add a contingency to the budget. The alternative to a contingency is to revise the budget when the cost of each discovery can be calculated.

One of the most common causes of increased project cost is delay in making decisions. If decision delays result in the loss of one day of productive work a week, the project will be two and one-half months behind at the end of a year. For most projects that would increase the total project cost 10% to 15%.

Typically the budget will go to the funding authority. After approval the budget should be presented to the signatories of the Project Charter Summary along with a final warning about the cost of failing to mitigate risks and delay of decisions.

Managing Change

Managing a large change that is being led with the introduction of technology to replace a paper system is similar to managing the care of a very complex case in an ICU. Many things have to be planned, coordinated and monitored. The stakes are high. There is a foundation of science and a great deal of art required to get a good outcome.

Moving from the current state to the future state requires planning, analysis and a design that coordinates changes in people, process, knowledge, skill, tools, and sometimes even the facility. The management of an EHR project begins with a focus on the tool, in this case the medical history. The project will move the patient history from "atoms to electrons". Most information systems build the record by automating the processes of registration, ordering, scheduling, and documentation. These processes produce the results, reports, clinical notes and messages that become the medical history of a patient. With the information in an electronic format it is possible to integrate knowledge into the context of the process. Obviously, new skills will be required to use the EHR. Last, facility changes will be required to support the network, workstations, and printers.

Managing this requires a "change architecture". In Figure 22-4A the elements of this change architecture are listed on the vertical axis. Projects seldom leap from a current state to a future state so the horizontal axis allows the organization to designate steps or a series of transitional states of change for each of the elements to achieve the future state over time. Since health care is an applied-knowledge service business, most processes to be automated involve multiple roles, so the change architecture is role based. The content that describes the change in an element in each step is role specific. Figure 22-4B proposes the current state to future state changes for each element of the architecture for physicians.

Change Architecture-Physicians
Transition

	Current State	Step 1	Steps...	Future State
People Leadership Language Communication Measurement Recognition Learning	"I can order anything I want. I can document any way I want."			"I want the most appropriate order. I will document for measurable quality and to optimize the financial health of the organization
Process Next Collect Decision Actions	Complex, multiple handoffs, errors, rework, miscommunication			Simple, coordinated handoffs, measurable without chart abstraction
Knowledge Viewable Actionable Executable	• Experience • Articles • Books • Best guess			• Policy and procedure • Protocols • Order sets • Reminders • Alerts • Medline • Patient Education
Skills Training	• Write • Dictate • Forms			• Windows • Browser • Mouse • Keyboard • Applications
Tools	• Pen • Prescription pad • Order sheet • Progress note			• EMR • Computer • Cell phone/ PDA • Printer • Scanner
Facilities	• Writing counters • Form holders • File cabinets • Medical record files			• Computer and paper • Printers • Paper storage

Elements

© Thomas C Tinstman, MD

A

Figure 22-4A   Change Architecture-Physicians.

EMR Program Roles

- **Sponsors** — Responsible for resolving escalated issues that involve the clinics and/or across the enterprise.
- **Project Executive** — Accountable for operating results during and following the project.
- **Project Manager** — Leads project planning, workflow analysis, and application configuration; works with the Project Executive to develop training and the implementation.
- **Business/Clinical Analysts** — Responsible for analysis of current workflow and work activity; lead development of future process.
- **Content Analyst** — Responsible for systems integrated knowledge.
- **Systems Analysts** — Responsible for knowledge of data model and definitions; understands how configuration interacts with the data; leads test planning and testing.
- **Domain Expert(s)** — Works in role being automated and acts as consultant for workflow analysis, design, validation configuration, testing, communication, and training.
- **Domain Advisor(s)** — Works in role being automated and participates in validation, content development, acceptance testing, communication, and deployment support.

B

Figure 22-4B   EMR Program Roles.

Organizational Culture

The element People is a code word for behavior. The official boundary on acceptable behavior should be detailed in organizational policies. Policy is the tool that the leadership uses to codify and communicate the organizations expectations for roles and employees. The informal boundary of acceptable behavior is culture.

All organizations have a gap between expectations set in policy and the behavior that the culture will tolerate. It should be obvious that the project must be completed within the boundary of policy or the policy should be changed in advance to align it with the future state. An example would be the delivery of care by e-mail. Policy may be silent on this subject or there may be a policy that allows care to be provided by e-mail. If the EHR will provide a secure web messaging service which provides improved security and privacy, then a new policy should be created that says when the EHR and web messaging is available, physicians must move their patients from e-mail to the secure web messaging service.

Culture is the unofficial boundary of acceptable behavior in an organization. We have all seen a someone where they did not. First they are isolated by their colleagues and then subtle pressure is applied. Eventually the person transfers or leaves. Look to the history of your organization. Have there been changes proposed that succeeded and more importantly changes that eventually failed? Examine the failures carefully. Learn from them. Apply these lessons to the project. For additional study I would suggest Daryl R. Conner's book, *Managing at the Speed of Change* (2).

Process and Workflows

My preferred definition of process is the one proposed by Michael Hammer in his book Reengineering the Corporation (3): "A business process is a collection of activities that takes one or more kinds of input and creates an output that is of value to the customer". Applying this to an EHR project, one could define the visit care process as beginning with registration and scheduling and ending with collection of the fees. Within this process there are workflows for registration, scheduling, visit, and patient accounting. The visit workflow would typically involve check-in, rooming, clinician visit, and check-out. A variable would be how follow-up with the patient about test results should be represented. Should it be shown in the visit workflow or a separate follow-up/messaging workflow?

Software is designed to follow an idealized workflow. Most of the project work will be focused on the analysis, design, and configuration of the software to automate a workflow. The project team and, to a lesser degree, the sponsors assisted by the supplier must develop a good understanding of the workflow for which the software was designed. There are some software changes that the supplier creates to allow the team to adapt the software to workflow variations. These are called configuration changes. The project team's job is easiest if the organization changes its workflow to fit the workflow for which the software and its configurable variations were designed.

The organization's ability to align workflow with the software is where culture can collide with process redesign and determine project success and cost. The more the organization insists on adapting the software to the organization's current workflow, the longer the project will take. If there is a shallow agreement to change the workflow to meet the project, culture may cause a delayed rejection of the new workflow and the associated EHR. This, in my experience, is the major cause of high project costs and project failure.

Health care is a service that applies knowledge to answer a health question. The great hope for EHRs is that they will improve the quality of care by integrating the best knowledge at the point of care (POC) and at the time of decisions. Just making the complete medical history available at all POCs is the first step of integrating knowledge into the care process. Other less apparent forms of integrated knowledge are terminologies such as ICD-9 and CPT. Pharmaceutical safety has received a lot of attention. Using the EHR to alert the provider to possible drug-allergy, drug-drug, and drug-lab situations to reduce preventable adverse drug events is a quality improvement objective of many EHR projects (Chapter 9).

The changes in skill by role will always include basic computer use, typing, and the ability to use the applicable modules of the EHR and associated new workflow and work activities. Do not overestimate the staff's ability to use a computer and type. Test the staff, including all physicians, and provide either individual or classroom training with assessments and remedial training if indicated. A simple way to improve typing is by use of e-mail to automate administrative process and encouraging the staff to adopt e-mail at home for personal correspondence with family and friends.

The major tool change will be the EHR replacing the paper medical history and most or all of the forms used for orders, documentation, and charging. To use the EHR, most clinicians agree that a computer at the POC is essential. This means one in each exam room and maybe at other places such as vital signs stations. Printers will be necessary at points where your electronic process will need to transition information back to atoms. This might include patient education, instructions and charge information. If the physicians will continue to dictate, a new device interfaced to the EHR may be indicated. Frequently this is a PDA or a cell phone/PDA that manages the patient identification using a copy of the office schedule and sends the voice file wirelessly or when docked to transcription.

Changes in the facility need to be planned in conjunction with the design of the future state workflows. Pay particular attention to the best location for the workstations that will be used at the POC and printers which will be required to convert EHR information to paper to give to the patient. Unfortunately, there is an extended need to work with both paper and the EHR so be certain there is enough space for the computer, printer, and necessary paper. It is best to walk-through the new workflow with staff acting as patients and family. Do not forget the patients with walkers and wheel chairs. Each device will require an electrical outlet and data port. Many times the electrical outlets are the most problematic. One key decision will be whether printing should be done at all POCs or at central locations. There are role, workflow, and cost factors in this decision that each project needs to consider carefully. Remember to have paper storage and secure disposal conveniently located relative to the printers.

Project Roles

Successful projects are sponsored at the executive level of an organization and involve a dedicated team focused on managing the change by working with those who will use the future state to care for patients and operate the business. The roles that will be discussed are sponsor, project executive, project manager, business (process) analyst, content (clinical) analyst, system (technical) analyst, domain experts, representatives, super-users, and users.

Sponsor

Project sponsorship is critical. Generally the sponsor has the political position and organizational authority to initiate the project and sustain it to completion. This means selling the EHR to the organization, approving or assuring funding, dealing with competing priorities, and leading the decision process for EHR issues that are escalated because there is the perception of a win-lose result. Using their political skill and authority, the sponsor must lead the management of the behavioral changes required for project success.

Executive

The project executive(s) are the managers who are responsible for the operating results for the areas the project will affect. In an organization with multiple clinics this would be the clinic managers, support service leaders, and patient accounting. You need the managers of everyone whose staff's work will be changed by the EHR as project executives. At a high-level, the project executives must understand and commit to the changes that their part of the organization must make in each of the change architecture elements throughout the transition to the future state. Most of the decisions elevated from the project team to the project executives will require that the project executive understand current state process and workflow and how it must transition to the future state with the EHR. The decisions will be presented to this group by the project team as a design decision in a format shown in Figures 22-5A through I.

Domain Experts

Domain experts work in a role where the process is being automated by the EHR. They serve as a "Let's be real" connection for the project team to their units' operations. In this role they may participate in, and should review, all workflow analysis, design, validation, testing, training, and deploy-

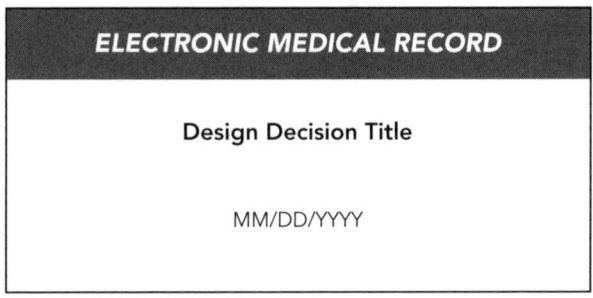

A

Figure 22-5A   Design Decision.

Design Decision: Name of Issue

Table of Contents
- Issue Summary
- Issue Description
- Options and Considerations
  - Option A: Description of Option
  - Option B: Description of Option
  - Option C: Description of Option
  - Option D: Maintain Status Quo
- Recommendation Design Implications
- Participants

B

© Thomas C Tinstman, MD

Figure 22-5B   Design Decision: Name of Issue.

Issue Summary

Summary of Issue	Research and Analysis
This is an executive summary of the issue	This section outlines the high level approach for researching the issue

Summary of Options	Recommendation/ Decision	Summary of Design Implications for Recommendation
Listing of options	Recommended Option	Impact on other design/ .build activities and/or operations/workflow

C

© Thomas C Tinstman, MD

Figure 22-5C   Issue Summary.

Issue Description

Issue Description

• Provide a detailed description of the design issue under consideration

Background Information

• Provide a list of detailed bullet points that provide context for the decision to be made; include system requirements or limitations, workflow implications, etc.

The following slides outline the options for resolving this issue and include a one-page comparison of the options and a recommended solution

D

© Thomas C Tinstman, MD

Figure 22-5D Issue Description.

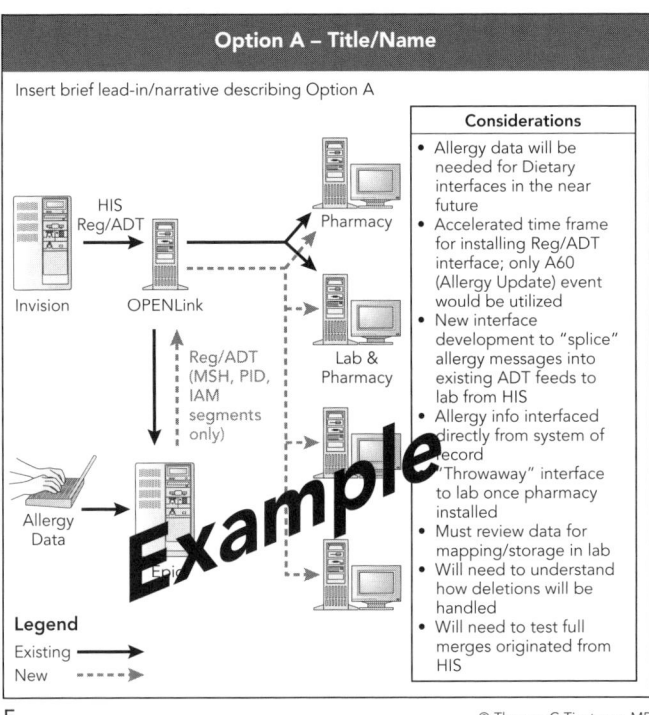

E

© Thomas C Tinstman, MD

Figure 22-5E Option A: Title/Name.

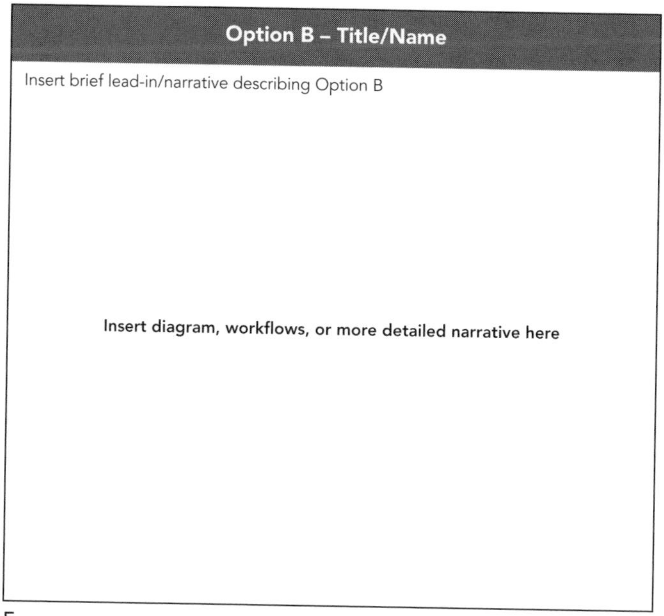

Option B – Title/Name

Insert brief lead-in/narrative describing Option B

Insert diagram, workflows, or more detailed narrative here

F

© Thomas C Tinstman, MD

Figure 22-5F   Option B: Title/Name.

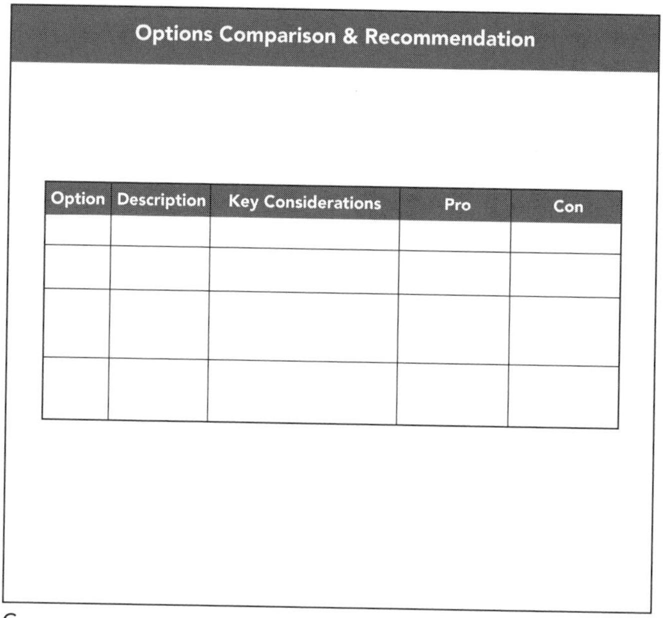

Options Comparison & Recommendation

Option	Description	Key Considerations	Pro	Con

G

© Thomas C Tinstman, MD

Figure 22-5G   Options Comparison and Recommendation.

Recommendation Design Implications

	Best Case Scenario	Worst Case Scenario
Workflow Implication		
System or Interface Build		
Vendor Involvement		
Timeframe (Some Tasks Can be Done Concurrently)		
Estimated Cost		

H

© Thomas C Tinstman, MD

Figure 22-5H   Recommendation Design Implications.

Participants

Area	Participants
CIS Tecnical Team	
EMR Team	
Training	
SMEs	

i

© Thomas C Tinstman, MD

Figure 22-5I   Participants.

ment support. It is best if the domain experts are jointly selected by the project executive and the project manager with their project-related performance reviewed jointly at frequent intervals. Domain experts should be dedicated to the project, usually at least 25% of their time, but not full-time. If they don't work at least 40% of the time in their own role, they have become a project analyst. To be a domain expert the person must be a fact-based decision maker who is capable of representing their peers effectively in the design decision and deployment processes.

To ensure good design and successful deployment, additional users need to be involved early in the project. These are domain advisors. The advisors are recruited from interested users. The advisors participate intermittently at key points in the project. They will review design decisions before and after the application has been configured to be certain they are realistic. Before configuration, this is design validation. After configuration this is called user acceptance testing. The advisors will become the nucleus of the superusers for training and deployment.

Representatives

Representatives meeting as a group may be important in larger projects. There should be a person representing each department or unit. These persons are selected by the operating manager. They should meet for a specified time on a regular basis, weekly, biweekly, or monthly. During the design steps, they review current state policies and procedures and determine what might need to be changed to align with future state. The group's involvement increases with user acceptance testing. The representatives may be the testers or they may recruit other staff from their unit to participate in testing. Most importantly, this group is responsible for communicating with their manager about how the unit/department will be affected and actions to be taken as the work progresses.

Project Manager

The project manager leads the project planning, workflow analysis, application configuration and successful deployment of the EHR. The project manager is responsible for convening the project executives and appropriately involving them in the project process. This includes the identification, recruitment and management of the domain experts and advisors. The sponsor is kept informed and engaged by working with the project executives to identify and mitigate the project risks.

Project Team

The project team is responsible for implementing the EHR successfully. The team is led by a project manager who should always be full-time to ensure success. Other members of the team are project analysts. One analyst should have special expertise in workflow analysis and workflow automation, referred to as the business analyst. One analyst needs to understand the data model, data definitions, and how the configurations interact with the data in the EHR. This person is referred to as the systems analyst. For large projects there may be a separate content analyst who is focused on the terminologies integrated into the application, order catalogs, protocols, orders sets, and documentation tools. In smaller projects this work will be divided between the systems analyst and business analyst. In the project methodology all the analysts come together with the domain experts for the design and configuration of the application with its future state workflow. After this, the principle focus of the systems analyst is application testing, and workstation and printer configuration. The business analyst is focused on training and deployment support.

If staff are not available to fill a specific project role discuss this with the software supplier. Compare what the supplier can offer with staff from an organization that schedules individual independent contractors. With extra effort you can find contractors with more experience and less supplier bias to fill the knowledge and skill gaps on the team.

End-users

The users are the project's customers and will need to become the future owners of this electronic patient history and its associated workflow automation. To support this objective, a subset of users is identified who will work in an over-staffed model during the deployment to support and assist the users as they learn the future state. This role is the superuser. It is best if superusers are recruited from the user community, but it is possible to use people from other roles, the supplier, or consulting companies. The superusers receive standard training and then additional training and time to practice so they can answer most user questions or know who to contact to get the answer. The superuser role may continue after the initial deployment to support standardization and optimization.

Project Methods

Project management is a profession with a number of widely recommended methodologies. All software suppliers should have a project methodology that they recommend for implementing their EHR. If the project manager is a supplier employee, then it is best to use the supplier's methodology. Similarly, if you will have a third party consulting firm or a contracted project manager, you may want to use their preferred methodology. If your organization has been or will be doing projects on an ongoing basis, then the organization should adopt a project methodology with standardized tools for managing the project and documenting the work.

What follows is an adaptation of a supplier's methods and generally recognized information system project methods. Many of the adaptations are based on the need to incorporate change management and a content management method since health care is an applied knowledge service.

The first step is to develop a model for project participation. Management, the user community, and the project team need to agree on how the user will participate in the project and take ownership after the deployment of the EHR. Additionally, management must agree with a process for project oversight. Oversight usually includes reviews of key design decisions, schedule status, budget review and risks/issues updates.

For modeling participation it is useful to separate the work required to configure the application, workflow redesign and the content development at each step into three flows while remembering that all three must function as one for testing, training and deployment. The sequential steps of work for each flow are shown in Figures 22-6 A, B, and C. The project manager is responsible for assigning the project analysts the duties for the steps in each flow. The analysts are responsible for appropriately engaging the experts, advisors, and representatives individually or in workgroups to provide advice and make decisions. How each role aligns with the flows and steps is shown with the circles overlapping the steps in Figure 22-6.

Design decisions that are sound produce successful implementations. A project consists of hundreds of decisions that must be made on a timely basis. Good decisions result from good analysis, the development of viable design options, followed by timely design decisions that do not have to be revisited. This may be an iterative process (Figure 22-7). It is essential to have appropriate user participation. This participation is best done using workgroups. A workgroup should be three to seven users referred to as domain advisors. The workgroup should be led by a domain expert and supported by a project analyst. The workgroup should review the analysis and proposed design options in the first meeting. In the second meeting an

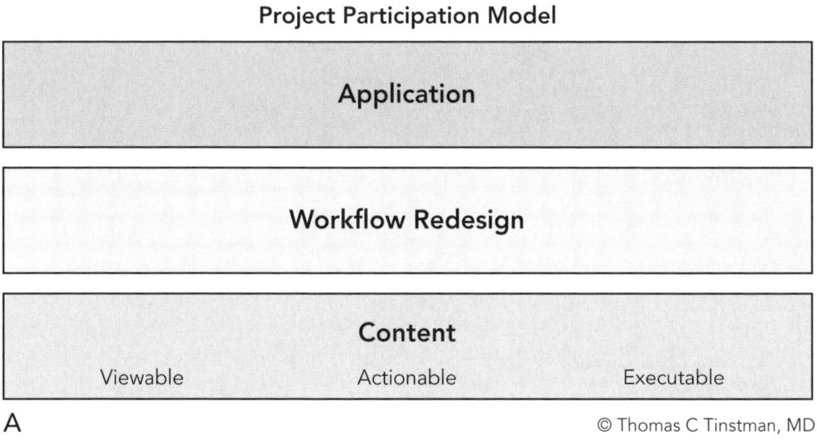

Project Participation Model

A   © Thomas C Tinstman, MD

Figure 22-6A   Project Participation Model.

Project Participation Model

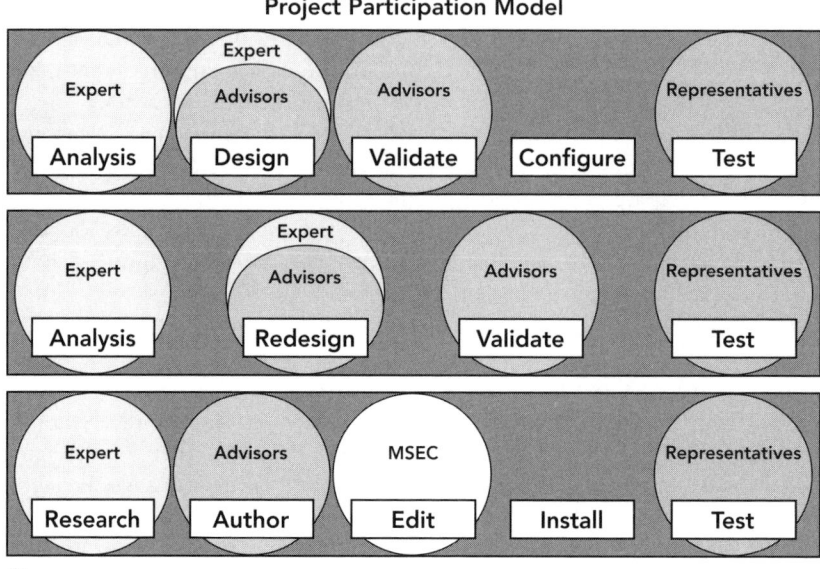

B

© Thomas C Tinstman, MD

Figure 22-6B Project Participation Model.

Project Participation Model

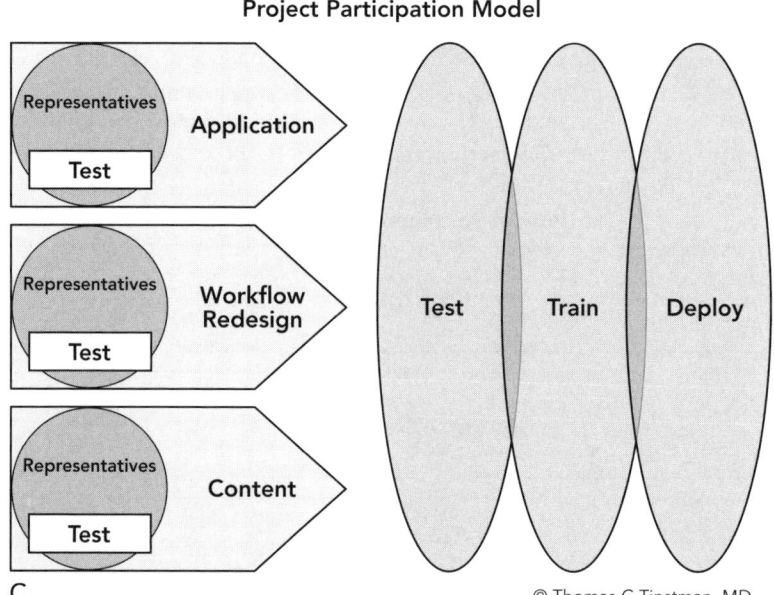

C

© Thomas C Tinstman, MD

Figure 22-6C Project Participation Model.

Decision Process Model

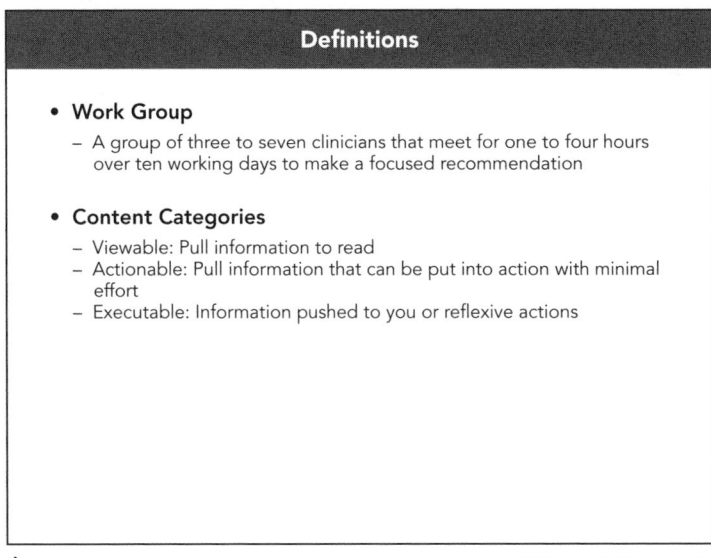

© Thomas C Tinstman, MD

Figure 22-7   Decision Model.

option should be selected. In the third meeting the same group or another group of advisors should validate the decision. The workgroup's task is complete. The group is disbanded and new groups are created for future decisions (Figures 22-8 A, B, C, and D).

Definitions
• **Work Group**
– A group of three to seven clinicians that meet for one to four hours over ten working days to make a focused recommendation
• **Content Categories**
– Viewable: Pull information to read
– Actionable: Pull information that can be put into action with minimal effort
– Executable: Information pushed to you or reflexive actions

A   © Thomas C Tinstman, MD

Figure 22-8A   Workgroup Model Definitions.

Project Participation — Roles

- **Representatives of Unit, Clinic or Department**
  - Zero to two hours per week
  - Test configurations and integrated solutions
  - Communicates with clinic/department and recruits advisors
  - Supports training & deployment

- **Domain Experts — Analysis and Design**
  - Ten hours per week plus
  - Reviews analysis, guides design of application and redesign of clinician workflow
  - Leads or facilitates workgroups
  - Demonstrates and trains

- **Domain Advisors — Work Group**
  - Two to three hours per workgroup
  - Workgroup participant for design options & writing content
  - Validates designs and clinician workflow
  - Supports training & deployment

B

© Thomas C Tinstman, MD

Figure 22-8B   Project Participation: Roles.

Work Group — Types & Work

- **Process**
  - Application Design Options
  - Design Validation
  - Best Workflow for application Design

- **Content**
  - Research
  - Author
  - Edit

C

© Thomas C Tinstman, MD

Figure 22-8C   Work Group: Types and Work.

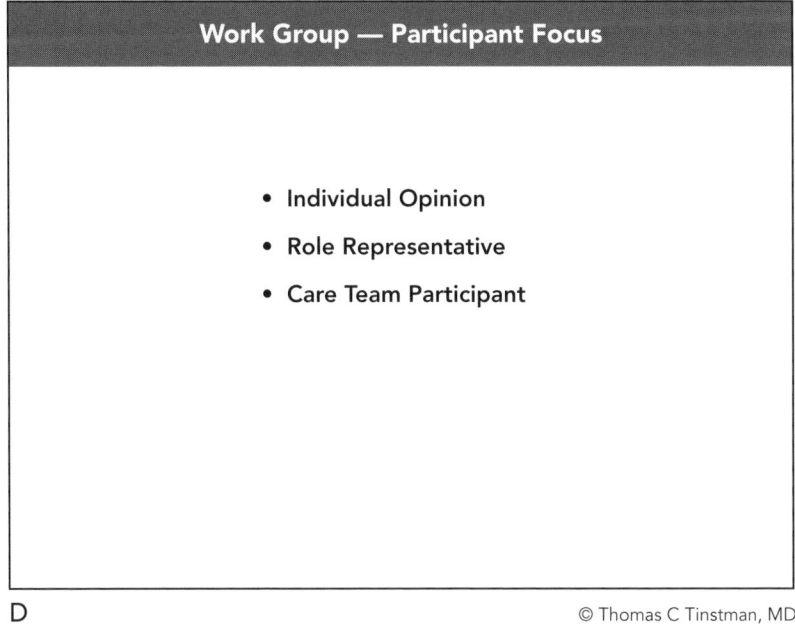

D   © Thomas C Tinstman, MD

Figure 22-8D   Work Group: Participant Focus.

The Project Manager must ensure adequate user participation so that good decisions are made by the correct people while keeping management informed throughout the project process. The challenge is staying on schedule and within the budget when you are dependent on domain experts, domain advisors and representatives who have other full-time roles in the organization. This requires advanced planning and flexible scheduling. The workgroups must end with the participants recognizing the value of their contribution.

Project steps are usually sequential. A version of these steps is:

1. Planning

2. Analysis/Research

3. Design decisions/Author

4. Validate/Edit

5. Configure & Develop

6. Testing

7. Train

8. Deploy/Publish

9. Structured review

10. Operate

Creating content or managing purchased content in an EHR is analogous to the steps for publication. The term following the slash (/) is the word more commonly used to describe that step for the process of creating content.

Many people say the two hardest parts of a project are "getting started and finishing". Getting started requires the completion of a good plan. Creating a good plan before in-depth analysis requires knowledge and wisdom gained from experience. The steps that follow are challenging, but once underway a momentum develops that makes the next step feel natural. Finishing is the completion of deployment and the hand-off to operations. During the project the team develops a desire to produce a perfect result and develops a sense of ownership. Finishing requires the discipline to know when the result is good enough since perfect will never be achieved, or stated another way "perfect is the enemy of good enough". When good enough is reached, the team has to "cut the cord" and hand the EHR off to an operating group.

Planning

Planning the project is sometimes referred to as the start-up or initiation phase. The activities that must be completed were outlined in the first part of this chapter. First the sponsor must define the project by codifying the scope. With that definition, a project manager can outline the required work in an initial project plan. This work plan is used to create the budget. If measured benefits are part of the Charter then an estimate is required during the planning. Figure 22-9 gives an outline of how the benefits could be defined, estimated, and tracked. The Project Charter, Figure 22-2, is a summary of the plan and should be finalized and signed to mark the completion of planning and the beginning of the iterative process of analysis, design, and validation that will produce the EHR.

Analysis, Design, and Validation

The analysis, design, and validation (ADV) process has two major variations. If data is coming from another system such as a lab system or transcription system, an interface is required. For data that will be viewed and entered by the staff, the process must include an intense focus on workflow and content.

ADV for interfaces is best led by a systems analyst with interface design experience. This project analyst will work closely with systems analysts

EMR Methodology
Benefits Realization
Financial Impact Tool

Benefit Name:
Benefit type:
Change source:
Description:
Rationale:

Key Metric	Description	Baseline	Projected	Change (should not = 0)

Fixed Variables	Description	Baseline	Projected (=Baseline)	Change (should = 0)
				0
			0	0
			0	0
		$		0
			0	0
			0	0
			0	0
			0	0

Misc Calculations (if req'd)	Description	Baseline	Projected	Change
				–
				0

Benefit Calculation	Description

Timing and Sensitivity Analysis	0 months (go-live)	3 months	6 months	12 months	24 months	36 months
Conservative	–	$	$	$		$
Medium	–	$	$	$		$
Aggressive	–	$	$	$		$

Annualized Benefit		
Conservative	$	–
Medium	$	–
Aggressive	$	–

Notes - Do not write in shaded areas

© Thomas C Tinstman, MD

Figure 22-9   Benefits.

from the EHR supplier, the sending systems supplier, and interface programmers. The basic steps are the documentation of the business requirements, functional requirements, and a technical specification. All parties will use the technical specification to create the necessary configuration and programming for the data to move from the sending system to the EHR accurately while satisfying the business and functional requirements. Failure to do accurate and complete business or functional specification is a frequent cause of project delay to rework the interface configuration and programming as a result of issues uncovered at user acceptance testing.

ADV to create the views of the medical history and support actions (documentation, orders, and charges) by the staff is workflow automation. To automate workflow, the first step is the documentation of the current workflow. This is best done with interviews and observations. All the paper results/reports should be collected and annotated to the steps in the workflow where the clinician is collecting information from the medical history for the next decision. All forms for documentation should be collected and annotated to their associated workflow step. Take note of the points where forms are given to the patient or sent to third parties. Discuss with all parties where retrospective reports are created. The resulting ADV documentation should describe this current state.

Any changes that the organization knows it needs to make should be added as the first version of the future state. Next, the configuration options of the EHR application are considered along with their associated workflow changes. Where the configuration and/or workflow choices are not obvious or there is disagreement, a Design Decision Document (DDD) (see Figure 22-5B), should be prepared. In the process of preparing the DDD for presentation to the advisors, representatives and/or sponsor, the correct choice frequently becomes obvious to all.

With the final DDDs, the future state ADV documentation should be completed. It should include:

- Business requirements
- Functional objectives
- Application design
- New workflow
- Supporting content
- Paper printouts for the patient and third parties
- Retrospective reports to assist in managing the business and care quality, i.e. HEDIS measures

This future state documentation is used for the advisors to validate the complete future state. At this point ADV should be started and completed for the business continuity plan. The business continuity plan describes how the organization will function when the system is unavailable. This completes the ADV steps.

Configuration

Configuration of the EHR application and development/programming of the interfaces is work done out of sight of all but the project team. Occasionally in this step, previously unforeseen issues will be encountered and an analyst may need to loop back briefly to ADV documentation.

Testing

User acceptance testing should be done with a group of naïve users, if possible. Naïve users are those users who are not domain experts and have only occasionally participated in work groups. The representatives, supplemented with other users covering all roles, are an ideal group. During the ADV the project team should have started creating realistic work scenarios. These scenarios are used to create the user acceptance test scripts. With the most realism possible, the testers go through the scripts stopping periodically to complete evaluation forms and/or participate in a focus group discussion of the strengths and weaknesses of the future state. It is useful to have the trainers observe this testing and review all evaluations to assist the trainers in building excellent training.

A good testing program will improve the deployment and the on-going operation of the EHR. Testing consists of at least four steps: user acceptance testing (discussed above), unit testing, integrated testing, and regression testing. Effective testing finds problems before deployment if realistic, workflow-focused scenarios are used to develop good test scripts. The other secret is accurate tracking of the issues found in testing. The issues must be analyzed, corrected and retested in a tight time frame.

Unit testing is usually conducted as a part of the application configuration and interface development. A unit test shows whether parts of modules operate correctly as they are configured or that data moves correctly from one system to another through the interface.

Integrated testing and regression testing are looking at how the entire application operates after the interfaces are operating and the entire deployable application is configured. This requires workflow-focused scenarios that describe how the application will be used in the future state. It is best if these scenarios are created during or before validation (they are the same ones used for acceptance testing). From the scenarios, test scripts are created. The scripts must test the application as it was used in user acceptance testing, but in addition should test any additional unanticipated actions that could be done by a naïve user on every screen variation. These scripts will be used repetitively for integrated and regression testing.

Things that fail to work properly in the integrated test are referred to as test issues. With a test issue, the first question to answer is whether the application is working as designed by the supplier or the team. If it is not working as designed, the issue must be codified and tracked as it is ana-lyzed, and the system changed. The "fix" is tested with the script that found the issue. If the issue is resolved, then regression testing must be done to check all the associated parts of the application. Regression testing or a complete repeat of the integrated test is required because fixing one soft-ware problem will frequently create new problems.

Before the training and deployment begin, the Business Continuity Plan should be in place. Training must include a section on what the users should do if the system is unusable or unavailable. The plan should spell out how EHR operations communicates system status to the users, and how the users communicate issues to EHR operations. When the system is un-usable there must be prepared forms to support care operations and a process for moving back to the EHR from the paper forms. In general, care providers wait too long to go to paper so it is best to predetermine a max-imum time they can work without the system before going to paper. Twenty minutes works well. Moving back to the EHR is an even larger chal-lenge. Enough of the information on paper must be added to the system so that errors are avoided when the medical history is used to support future decisions. This usually means keying information in from the paper. Most organizations plan for thirty minutes of overtime for every hour the system is down to move the information on paper into the system when the EHR becomes available.

Training

Training is the last step before the users take-over. Unfortunately since it is the last step, it frequently gets too little focus. To be certain training gets the appropriate focus, the process of creating the training should begin when the future state is designed. The gap between the current state and the future state is what must be taught. This includes basic computer skills, new workflow and work activity, possibly new knowledge if a role changes, and how the application will be used in the context of work ac-tivity. Too frequently training consists only of application use by function without work activity context. This increases user anxiety and will make the deployment more problematic.

The software supplier should have excellent training services and mate-rials. If the software supplier does not provide these, you should consider getting assistance from an expert in adult learning.

The best approach to good training is to begin by creating the training as soon as the current to future state gap is defined. The same scenarios that were developed for workflow-based testing should be adapted to form the training curriculum and foundation for the materials and exercises. The key alteration is to add a work activity context to the workflow context. In a clinic, EHR workflow would be the patient flowing through the clinic. For example, check-in, rooming & vitals, physician visit, etc. Work activity would be the flow of the staff person from task to task. For the nurse this could mean rooming a patient, taking a phone message, giving an immunization, rooming another patient, etc. Training with a workflow context teaches process awareness across roles which is very important. Work activity context provides a realistic experience of the "day in the life" for a role. Training by software function usually overwhelms and disorients the users who are struggling to decide how to do their work with the function shown. Avoid this by training with workflow and work activity context.

Deploying the future state in a patient care environment is the "day of reckoning" for an EHR project team. The objectives for deployment are to:

♦ Stabilize

♦ Standardize

♦ Optimize

♦ Operate

The future state workflow and work activity with the EHR. The two critical success factors are scripted answers for frequently asked questions that were identified during training and having trained, confident superusers in adequate numbers so the user is not held idle when they have a question or can not proceed with their work. Busy adults need immediate help and answers when the context of the question is still fresh in mind.

Superusers should be recruited from the domain advisors and representatives. If that does not produce the numbers needed, superusers can be pulled from other areas of the organization, from the supplier, or possibly from the employees of other customers of the supplier. One way to train superusers is to give them a role in the training or create special training with ample scheduled time to practice.

In the first few days of the deployment, the superusers' and the project team's objective is survival and the ability to get the staff home tired, but with the days work completed with limited overtime. Publicly this is called stabilization. During stabilization the users will do anything they can to get their work done. In this rush the user may cut corners, change the workflow, or find another way to use the application. If these are improvements, they should be captured and used during optimization. Usually these survival adaptations are not improvements. Standardization is bringing all users back to the future state design instead of their individualization of the future state. Typically stabilization takes several weeks. Standardization can begin as soon as the superusers have time to observe and coach the users as they are working and will take one to four weeks.

Optimization is the focus after standardization and usually takes about sixty days. During stabilization and standardization the project team learns from the users and the superusers. These lessons are converted into tips and tricks that can be distributed in written format with screen shots and short training scenarios. The training scenarios and scripts can be presented by the team or the superusers at brown bag lunches or distributed as electronic training. These activities should be supported by superusers coaching the new way in the work environment.

There should be no end to optimization; it simply slows down. At the point where optimization slows, usually ninety days post deployment, the project team should hand the EHR over to an operations group. Some members of the project team may move with the application in the future state to operations and others will go on to another project or return to their previous roles. It is best if the hand-off from project to operations is formalized with a Service Level Agreement (SLA). The SLA is an internal contract between the project executives and the EHR operations group. The contract should spell out what the care operations managers should expect from the operations group and what the EHR operations group must have from the care operation.

One of the most important sections of the SLA is the shared Business Continuity Plan. There will be scheduled downtime for system maintenance; hopefully this can be done without disrupting clinical operations. It is an unfortunate reality that there will be unscheduled downtime. There must be a plan. The plan should be in the SLA. The plan should be tested. The plan must be kept up to date as the EHR changes over time.

The technical infrastructure required for the EHR is a requirement. For small projects, the project team may be responsible for planning and installing the technical infrastructure. It is best if the technical infrastructure is planned and implemented by a group familiar with the technology to be used and who will have future operating responsibility for the infrastructure. If it is a separate group, they must integrate their planning with the project team's future state plan.

The technical infrastructure can be divided into three sections:

◆ First 100 Feet

◆ Network

◆ Last 100 Feet

The first 100 feet is the data storage, data base servers, and any middleware. The network connects the first 100 feet to the last 100 feet. The network will be TCP/IP based, operating over wire or fiber to distribution points near the users. From the last router (distributor) to the eyes and finger tips of the users is the last 100 feet. This is, at the least, workstations and printers. It may also include document scanners, bar code readers, and interface medical devices like sphygmomanometers.

The supplier is an essential resource for the design of the first 100 feet and could, in your contract, be held responsible for sizing of this part of

Table 22-1

ADJUSTING FOR PROJECT SIZE

- Large projects are accommodated by creating multiple teams or by adding multiple people in each role. Once the total number of people exceeds five to seven, assigning the work and coordinating within and across roles becomes a larger challenge. It becomes easy for one group to fall behind or for something to "fall through the cracks".

- Small EHR projects are easier to manage, but more stressful for small organizations. The major challenge becomes how to compensate for the added project activities on top of existing work. For a small project it is essential to have knowledge and experienced project staffs who have implemented the specific software in an identical or very similar environment.

- The project manager must have managed projects and should come from the supplier or be a contractor recommended by the supplier. At least one of the project team members should come from the organization. This person should be the organization's best non-physician clinician. In addition, they should be self-starters and comfortable with technology. This person can fill the roles of the business analyst (with the assistance of the project manager), content analyst and domain expert.

- The systems analyst should come from the supplier and might be shadowed by the organizations technical resources if there are any available. In small organizations this team of (along with three the intermittent involvement of other staff) can implement an EHR in an ambulatory practice. The key to success with a small project is for everyone to be willing to learn anything and do anything to achieve the objective (see Chapters 21 and 23).

the system. In some cases it may be best to outsource the first 100 feet design and operations with an application service provider (ASP). An ASP agreement usually works best if the organization retains responsibility for the network and the last 100 feet.

The integration of the design of the last 100 feet with the future state design is essential. Having the best device in the best location will help insure a successful deployment and improve the efficiency of the staff. For workstations there are many device choices and multiple ways to place/mount the chosen device. Having users use samples of the selected devices for things like e-mail is a good test of the device. To test location it is best to put some sample devices in a work area and use the workflow scenarios to walk through the location options to make the final selection (Table 22-1).

Conclusion

With management, a project team, and the organization's staff sharing a common vision and aligned objectives using the methods and processes outlined above, an organization can use an EHR to design and implement a future state that everyone will be proud of.

References

1. Nicholas P. Negroponte, Being Digital, Vintage Books, New York, 1996.
2. Daryl R. Conner, Managing at the Speed of Change: How Resilient Managers Succeed and Prosper Where Others Fail, Villard Books, 1992.
3. Hammer M, Champy J. Reengineering the Corporation: A Manifesto for Business Revolution, Harper Business, 1993.

23

Workflow

Caroline Samuels, MD

ow we do what we do, with what resources, when, where, and under what conditions are all part of workflow. This chapter begins with the generic definition of workflow and covers the workflow support available in electronic health record (EHR) systems. The following sections address information flow, its relation to workflow, and some of the factors to consider before automating workflow in the practice of medicine. The final sections cover workflow constructs and examples that can be helpful in planning for EHR implementation.

For the purposes of the discussion in this chapter the term "EHR" is intended to mean a fully integrated system with practice management (PM) and clinical documentation capabilities.

Additionally, "workflow management system" is a system that defines, creates, and manages the execution of workflows through the use of software, running on one or more workflow engines, which is able to interpret the process definition, interact with workflow participants, and, where required, invoke the use of IT tools and applications. Such systems also typically provide administrative and supervisory functions, for example, to allow work reassignment or escalation, plus audit and management information on the system overall or relating to individual process instances.

Generic Definition of Workflow (Industry-Neutral)

Workflow Definition

The study of workflow is a discipline in the realm of business management. The Workflow Management Coalition defines workflow as "the automation of a business process, in whole or in part, during which documents, information or tasks are passed from one participant to another for action according to a set of procedural rules" (1).

Workflow and Medical Informatics

The study of workflow and development of tools and standards for the management of workflow have largely been the in the business domain. The work in this area is relatively mature, and there are accepted standards for the terms and modeling tools used to represent workflow. There are software applications that explicitly support workflow and are sometimes referred to as workflow engines. Some EHR products are built on workflow engine applications.

Workflow has not been a prominent area of study in medical informatics. Indeed, there are those in informatics who feel that the practice of medicine is too complex to be modeled correctly using workflow constructs. This would probably be true if the object were to model every process in a complex organization like a hospital. However, considering workflow and using simple workflow tools to model well-selected situations can be helpful in the transition to the use of an EHR.

Workflow Support in Ambulatory Electronic Health Records

Typical Workflow Support available in Electronic Health Records with Full Practice Management Capabilities

The workflow support that is often to be found in an EHR includes functionality in four general areas, namely, messaging and information sharing, task completion, resource management, and documentation support.

Messaging and Information Sharing

There are three types of functionality in this category that are included in many EHR systems; simple messaging, document imaging (and routing), and whiteboard functionality. The simple messaging capabilities usually function like e-mail but are integrated with the EHR and are thereby safe (from a privacy protection aspect) to use for clinical information. Document imaging and routing capabilities typically support intake of paper documents (as images) and attachment of these to the appropriate file in the EHR, usually with flagging and messaging to the next reviewer. Whiteboard functionality may be present, displaying (for example) which patients are waiting in what room for what service.

Task Completion

At the most rudimentary level, the workflow support available in ambulatory EHR systems is the presentation of the next logical screens on completion of the steps in the usual progression of care (patient checks in; services are delivered; patient checks out). Shared task list functionality (e.g., post-ing of all patients needing to be checked out, listing of no-show patients to be called, etc.) is another common type of workflow support in this cate-gory. Opportunities to do tasks in parallel (rather than sequentially) can be supported by shared task lists (and/or messaging), and can enable signifi-cant operational improvements. Some EHRs also support task escalation if a task is not completed in a prescribed timeframe, but this function is usually limited to those EHRs with workflow management capabilities (see below).

Scheduling and Resource Management

Appointment scheduling applications are a form of resource management system. The more advanced appointment scheduling applications in inte-grated EHRs have capabilities to manage multiple resources simultaneously. These systems can schedule not only the provider and patient, but ancillary staff, equipment, and rooms, all simultaneously.

Documentation Support

The documentation support available in EHRs evolves as fast as technology can take it. Since capturing correct and complete documentation is such a challenge, there are always new strategies to make this happen intuitively and quickly. Almost all EHRs have templates for capturing information with point and click. Most, if not all, support integration of voice recognition, typing, dictation, and even handwriting recognition. Most allow input from ancillary staff (usually vital signs and chief complaint) to pull forward to the physician note. Some support pulling forward of a previous encounter note, or a note entered by a nurse or resident for editing. Some support pulling forward of patient-entered information to the physician note. A few EHRs explicitly avoid using templates and store the physician's previously entered notes on similar cases, presenting that to the MD for re-use. Some EHRs will populate orders for medications or complete order sets based on previous cases with the same medication used or the same diagnosis.

EHRs with Workflow Management Capabilities

Although all EHR systems support workflow (to a greater or lesser degree), few have workflow management capabilities accessible to the user (2). When using a workflow management system, task sequencing, process constraints, and resource qualifications are all explicitly outlined as business processes and defined. Workflow management capabilities then allow the user to rede-fine tasks, add tasks, rearrange task sequence, and reassign tasks. So, if the practice manager or lead physician identifies a bottleneck in operations, he or she can go into the system and reassign staff resources to eliminate the problem. As noted above, workflow management capabilities typically in-clude task escalation functionality. Workflow management functionality also usually includes auditing capabilities, providing information to guide changes in workflow. Workflow management capabilities provide flexibility for ongoing adaptation of the EHR system to practice operations.

Workflow in the Practice of Medicine and the Transition to using Electronic Health Records

Work Process and Products in the Practice and Business of Medicine

In the United States the practice of medicine operates under a business model. Private institutions, including medical practices, are money-making operations, selling services to customers (patients). To bill and collect, providers have to divide the processes involved in the rendering of care into episodes of care and, within that, billable services. As those who pay for care get more and more particular about exactly what they are willing to pay for, documentation requirements have escalated, and billable services change. To avoid claim rejection, providers have to be able to quickly adapt to these requirements. Increasingly the clinical information is required to render a bill that will get paid, so the systems that support practices can no longer be neatly separated into "business" and "clinical" categories. The clinical information is the billing information; in fact, if these are not the same it can be considered healthcare fraud. Also, payers generally won't pay separately for any of the documentation and coordination tasks involved in patient care. If the physician orders a medication that is not on the patient's insurance formulary, the payer does not pay for the twenty to forty minutes of staff and physician time it may take to get preauthorization for the medication or prescribe an alternative. They won't pay for chart review or physician call to get supporting documentation for authorization of a referral or hospital admission. With stable or falling reimbursements, adding more staff to take care of documentation and care coordination tasks is not an option. Moving to electronic records has the potential to increase the efficiency of these processes. However, there must be some understanding of both the current and desired workflow if essential value is to be preserved and benefits realized. An EHR cannot simply be added on to current operations.

Workflow vs. Information Flow

In developing an understanding of the workflow processes in medicine, it is important to distinguish between workflow and information flow. Often the most significant process improvements that can be made as a result of implementing EHRs are the result of improved information flow. For example, if all ancillary staff are simultaneously notified (by virtue of electronic orders) that the patient needs an injection, a referral, a future appointment, a sample medication, etc., each responsible staff person can begin on his or her assignment simultaneously rather than having to wait for chart and patient to present to each one. The information flow is in the EHR application, but the workflow changes that actually leverage the availability of the information have to be planned and implemented.

In planning for information flow improvements with EHR implementation, it can be helpful to identify what information is needed for each process and when is the earliest point that the information can be captured. Much of the information needed in the outpatient setting comes from the patient. Pushing back the capture of that information to the earliest possible point can mean having the patient enter demographic, insurance, and even clinical information prior to the visit. In-office processes can then be expedited. Some EHRs have patient portal functionality that can support lab test reporting, medication renewal requests, appointment requests, etc. Some payers will even reimburse for electronic visits.

In thinking about the potential advantages of freeing the information from the paper record (such as pre-visit capture of needed information), it is important to also consider potential risks. The paper chart, or parts thereof, are often the visible cue we rely on to see what work is outstanding. A chart on an exam door signals that a patient is ready to be seen. A stack of incoming lab reports are ready to be reviewed, etc. Tasks and review of clinical issues have to be more carefully planned, and cross-coverage more carefully worked out when the stacks are gone, and there is just a list on a screen. Although it can be frustrating to search for a paper chart to enter an order on a patient, there is little danger of putting that order in the wrong chart. In the electronic world, it is easier to make that type of mistake. Information flow changes need to be carefully planned with retention of all the needed review and audit steps so that efficiency is increased, and risk is not.

It is also important to realize that if a physician visit or order documentation in the EHR is required to activate decision support, that documentation can't be delayed. (If the physician can't easily and efficiently do the documentation required, he or she will have to do "work-arounds", double documentation, or be supported to do partial documentation during the visit and completion later.) It may be worth slowing the workflow of patients through the office to get better information in terms of orders and plans; it may not.

Understanding the Value-Adding Processes in Medical Practice and Implications for Electronic Health Record Use

Part of the evaluation of current processes (prior to EHR use) is to identify those processes that add value and to make sure that essential processes are retained as workflow and information flow change. The value-added processes usually fall into roughly three areas: administrative, clinical, and personal.

Administrative Triage

Administrative processing in the usual medical practice includes insurance eligibility verification, referral management, billing and coding support, record management, call processing, and support for messaging. Administrative triage includes verifying that the services sought by a new potential patient are actually offered by the practice, or verifying that the right provider is available, etc. Front office staff usually do a common-sense level clinical triage for patients who obviously need emergency services. For some of the steps in usual office practice, the value added for the administrative staff is to ensure completeness of data in paper forms, and to generally manage the paper records and appointments. Electronic records can substitute for or eliminate the need for some of these clerical functions, but not the administrative triage or messaging support, both of which require some judgment. Although a computer application can constrain the user to complete a given text field before moving to the next screen, it will take supervision of the staff to make sure you are not trying to send the bill to the North Pole.

Clinical Triage and Provider Encounter

The clinical encounter in the usual office visit starts with a nurse intake and vital signs and is followed by the physician visit. Often patients voice issues to the ancillary staff that are not repeated to the physician. It is important to provide for the free-text capture of these items, both in terms of the software and logistically. Escalation based on clinical criteria (rather than time delay or other criteria) often occurs at this point in the visit. Patients may need immediate treatment, testing, or referrals, and the system will need to support these contingencies. The value-added for the physician encounter must be fully represented in the clinical documentation, this function being fundamental to any EHR system. (The workflow challenge for this portion of the visit is outlined above under Information Flow.)

Personal Contacts

In the medical care process, there some types of value-adding processes that are unique. The "customers" we serve are often frightened, worried, in pain, and/or confused. Sometimes the personal comfort, caring attitude, reassurance, or even simple recognition is the most important service we provide at a given point in time. It is important not to lose these unique value-adding processes as we plan future workflow. Although it may appear to be more efficient to have any available staff do patient exit, having the same staff person sign in and exit a patient can not only add to the comfort of the patient, it can help ensure follow-up on all the patient's issues that day.

Recognizing Essential Review, Control, and Auditing Present in Paper and Manual Processes

As we plan for using an EHR, we need to build replacements for the safeguards inherent in our current processes. In most inpatient units, orders written by physicians are taken off and entered into the computer by clerical staff that work under the supervision of nursing. If clerks find unusual or inconsistent orders, they consult with the supervising staff nurse. This can act as a safeguard against making medical errors. Shift sign-outs, both in nursing and for covering residents tend to be done as a group. Presenting to a group, even a small gathering of peers, will give a fundamentally different product than entering text into a computer all alone. Members of the group that are responsible to pick up care are sure to pose questions or think of contingencies that need to be discussed before departure of the outgoing practitioner. Software probably can't completely substitute for doing these transfers in person no matter how good it may be.

Using electronic clinical messaging rather than placing a phone call is easier in some ways for both sender and recipient. The sender can send the message at any time, and the recipient is not interrupted; he or she can do the follow-up as time allows. However, the sender may have no way of knowing that anyone got the electronic message or acted on the message. If a phone call does not get through, the caller knows to try again and keeps the responsibility for that issue until he or she passes it to someone. An electronic message may go to the wrong destination. If the intended recipient is not there, is there back-up? In electronic messaging sometimes messages are sent to a group. Such messages will often arrive as individual messages to each member of the group. Who is responsible? How does person 2 in the group know that person 3 has already responded to the message? How do the messages get deleted from each recipient's list after completion of the requested action? Would it be better to use a shared task list rather than the message function? These questions all have to be addressed, and policies and procedures worked out in advance of implementation. We will need to plan for the time that nobody will see that pink slip of paper stuck to the door or clipped to the chart.

Using Workflow Constructs to Aid in Process Re-design

When to do Workflow Analysis

The usual motivation for workflow analysis in a business process is to optimize production of whatever the business produces. The goal is to produce the most with the least consumption of resources, i.e., money. In an office that anticipates the addition of an EHR, the costs have to be offset, at least in part, by reducing expenses and improving revenues. For the usual practice, an eventual reduction in staff is anticipated to partially offset costs of the system.

The staff who primarily handle paper charts are most likely to be eliminated. In addition, cost savings come from reduction in transcription costs as well as reduced cost for storage of paper records. This being said, the transcription cost reduction will depend on practitioners using the EHR to document. The storage and handling cost reduction may only occur months after starting to use an EHR if old charts continue to be pulled for some time after starting EHR use. Revenue enhancements based on improved coding will only occur if the EHR supports them, and if the practice has not already maximized coding. So, for the usual practice, the financial benefits to be gained by using an EHR are dependent on making fundamental changes in how business gets done. The changes have to be planned, and carefully planned. Analysis of the current workflow is the first step.

Workflow assessment before EHR implementation is also important to improve the over-all process. Many Informaticists would agree with Dr Richard Schreiber when he says "Clinicians (physicians, nurses, respiratory therapists, etc.) must be involved in the process of workflow assessment". "Automating a broken process will make it more broken (put another way, if a process puts patients at risk, an automated process puts them at greater risk). The process must be fixed before it can be automated" (Personal Communication). And before it can be fixed, it needs to be described and that description verified.

Verification of Workflow

The usual way that current workflow is verified is by direct observation, sometimes to include time and motion study. This process can be very enlightening but may take many hours to do well. The level of effort and the amount of detail collected should be driven by the goal. Direct observation for thirty-four hours was needed to develop data for each ancillary staff job at one busy clinic (Table 23-1) (3). The authors estimated that an additional forty-five hours of observation would be needed to obtain sufficient data for computer analysis and simulations of workflow changes. Another similar effort in the recent literature sites fifty-eight hours of direct observation for a specialty clinic (4) to obtain sufficient data. In planning for workflow analysis it is important to decide if you need hard data on actual time spent doing tasks. If so, direct observation for extended periods has to be planned, both to develop the model and to test it. If time-motion study is not needed, a mix of structured interview and observation can provide the basis for a reasonable representation of workflow. Whatever the model or representation developed, it should be re-verified by direct observation.

Finding the Right Level of Detail to be Useful and Feasible

For all of the planning activities, including the workflow redesign, the amount of detail that can be included is nearly infinite. The complexities and possible scenarios can be overwhelming. It is important to find the level of detail appropriate for each planning activity, and be content with documentation that is uneven in its depth of detail. One important factor in deciding the level of detail required is to consider the decision-making capabilities of the actors in a process. For trained professionals doing their usual jobs, it may be adequate to describe functions at a high level, leaving the details to them. For actions being done by those with limited training and discretion, details, especially clinical conditions to be met for diagnostic or therapeutic actions, may have to be explicit.

Given that coordination across groups is always needed, it is important to decide on and construct a summary version of the workflow for each phase of the EHR implementation project (starting at current operations)

Table 23-1

TASK TAXONOMY FOR CHECK-IN CLERK*

Task Code	Task Description	% Time Spent
APT	Clerk makes appointments for consults or tests	0.08%
CHP	Clerk gives the patient their prescriptions	1.10%
CLP	Clerk calls the patient to the check-in window for nurse triage	6.73%
ENT	Clerk confirms address/phone # and other demographics and enters the data into the computer, including any changes to existing data	12.67%
FIL	Clerk fills out specific portions of the encounter form	10.49%
FRT	Free time, because of inter-related workflows, nothing to do	20.85%
IDX	Clerk accesses the IDX registration system, enters username/password	1.70%
INS	Clerk has the patient fill out new insurance information	5.72%
NPT	Non-patient time (photocopying forms, phone calls etc.)	12.47%
PAY	Handling patient co-pays	4.42%
PFC	Clerk takes the filled-in encounter form and places in chart	2.79%
QST	Answer a patient's questions	2.33%
SFC	Clerk makes copies of blank forms and stuffs charts for the next day	6.50%
SIN	Patient sign-ins, helps patients sign-in	5.50%
STK	Places charts on the nurse triage pile for nurses aides to pick-up and triage	2.07%
TYP	Asks patients about visit types (urgent, follow-up, nurse visit, lab draw, med refill, etc.)	0.83%
WLK	Walk-ins, clerk helps the patient fill-out appropriate information	3.75%

*Direct observation of check-in clerks in an urban primary care clinic. (Supplied by Atif Zafar, MD, and used with permission of A. Zataf, MD, M. Lehto, PhD, M. Louthan, BS, S. Carrington, BS, N. Bahamon, BS, and J. Bauer, BS.)

that includes all roles and systems. This forms the basis or infrastructure for the workflow, and each group can create detail around the same framework. (For an example of clinic workflow, see Table 23-2). For each phase it is also useful to make an explicit list of where is the Truth about a patient, i.e., where is the official, recognized version of a given part of the patient record. When we are part on paper and part in an electronic system, this is important. A lawyer's advice may also be needed for help with determination of exactly what is the legal record.

The level of detail needed for workflow analysis and re-design for EHR implementation will also depend to some extent on a few of the fundamental choices made early in the planning process. If the practice is going to make a quick switch over to the EHR (the Big Bang approach) or is going to phase in the EHR over a longer time is one such determining choice. If the practice plans to use a great deal of hired help (from software vendor, or from consultants) to do implementation, the shorter time frame (Big Bang) is usually chosen. If the practice plans to do most of the implementation internally, usually a phased approach is chosen. Neither approach is wrong, neither is painless. From a workflow redesign point of view, the big bang usually requires more in the way of written plans and formal job description construction, whereas the phasing in of the functionality allows the practice to "feel its way" forward, making incremental changes. Less is needed in depth of detail for the phased in approach, but more phases need to be described.

Planning for Future States of Workflow and Information Flow

Most vendors of EHR systems will have no difficulty helping prospective clients to envision the best workflow and information flow that their system can support. Available systems are not equivalent, however, in workflow management capabilities (noted above), nor do they all have equivalent documentation or clinical decision-support features. Both system capabilities and site-specific factors will influence exactly what the ultimate outcome will be. In thinking about the needed changes, it is useful to remember that meeting documentation requirements and improving quality of care are often used as justifications for moving forward with an EHR. System and implementation requirements that support these initiatives have to be factored into the ultimate vision of workflow and information flow.

In general, it is improved information availability and improved information flow capabilities that enable improved workflow when EHRs are implemented. To envision the goal for information flow it is helpful to identify the earliest possible point at which any piece of information can feasibly be captured. The workflow can then be designed around the improved information flow. This type of consideration can be helpful in establishing who captures what data at what point in the workflow. For example, most hospitals collect "quality" data retrospectively, and there is no support for

Table 23-2

OVERVIEW OF CLINIC WORKFLOW*

Event Flow	Admin Staff	Clin Staff	Med Stud	Resident	Amb Resident	Attending, Med Director	Documentation and Tools
Patient Check-in & Pre-visit processing Eligibility checking	First	Back-up Refer				Refer	Sign-in - paper Registration - AcSel Fee collection - paper Demographics - chart Med History - chart
Nursing Check-in Phlebotomy med hx review Triage		First		Back-up	Back-up	Refer	Chief Complaint, wt, vital signs - chart CPT - superbill
Patient Assignment		First				Back-up Refer	Daily roster - paper [chart on MD door]
MD Encounter			First	Report and/or First	Report and/or First	Report	Clinical Notes - chart Rx - Rcopia ICD/CPT coding - E-MDs, superbill Signature - superbill
Clinical Procedures		First		Report	Report	Report	Clinical Notes - paper EKG - file in chart [coding as above]
Referrals	First						Referral form - paper
Exit interview	Report	First					Appointment - AcSel Receipt - superbill
Calls from Patients	First	First			Refer		Clinical Notes - chart Rx - Rcopia

* Workflow at the Glenridge Internal Medicine Practice, June 2005. This overview of the author's clinic operations is used during orientations of new staff, consultants and/or visitors who may need to understand clinic operations

physician data entry aside from a piece of paper. The quality data, however, is the clinical data, and is first known during the care process. It may make sense to re-deploy a portion of the quality nursing staff to act as collaborators, reviewers, and scribes for the physicians. Early entry of the data can enable real-time clinical decision support with quality data derived from the clinical process, also in real time. This model would also reintroduce some nurse review of orders that may be needed in computerized provider order entry (CPOE) information flows.

In thinking about changing information flow, workflow, and people's jobs, it is also helpful to remember that people usually act in their own self-interest. Information quality can be improved if the consequences of making errors fall directly on the person responsible for entering the data into the system. For example, if the person who verifies and enters the patient phone number is the same person who has to contact that patient for follow-up, he or she will take care to get it right.

Using Workflow Diagrams

Accurately depicting workflow is a challenge. As noted previously, the complexity and depth of detail that can be elucidated for medical care processes is vast. It therefore makes sense to focus on one process or one topic at a time. Figure 23-1 and Table 23-3 together depict the diabetes care in-office workflow in a clinic. Table 23-3 is a cross-functional (or "swim lane") depiction showing who does what through all phases of the clinic visit. Cross-functional workflow diagrams can be expanded to include a great deal of detail and can show interaction points between workers (5). This type of workflow diagram is very useful for medical care processes, which usually involve collaboration between numerous parties. Figure 23-1 diagrams the specifics as to how the clinic staff is to handle finger stick glucose results through the full range of values, including escalation and treatments for glucose results that are very high or very low. Note that the staff are constrained by very specific instructions and are enabled to take prescribed actions independently, sharing the clinical workload appropriately. Note also that specifics about the instruments used, the methods, location and all other details are not included in these depictions. That level of detail was not needed and was left out.

Workflow Analysis and Redesign for EHR Implementation: Tools and Example

The example chosen to illustrate these steps is the preparation for a returning medical patient in the setting of a new EHR and is represented in Tables 23-4 through 23-7.

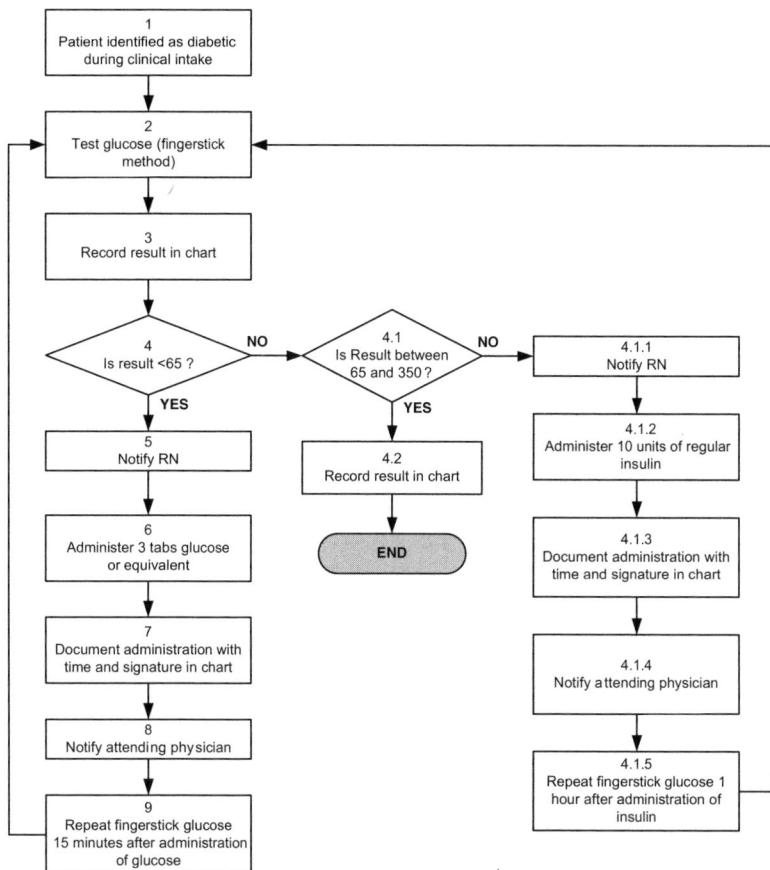

Figure 23-1 Actions needed based on results of fingerstick glucose readings in author's clinic. (Fig. created by Health Care Information Consultants, LLC.)

Table 23-3

DIABETES GLYCEMIC CONTROL CROSS-FUNCTIONAL WORKFLOW (PROCESS OVERVIEW)*

Person/Role	Intake	MD Encounter	Check out	Follow-Up	Comments
Patient	—	—	—	K, T, Rx, D	—
LPN/Tech	K, I, T†, Ed, Rx, D, (Rv)	—	T, Ed	—	Escalate as indicated (see Fig. 23-1)
RN	—	—	—	K, Rv, Ed, D, A, U	—
Physicians	—	K, I, M, D, Ed, Rv	—	—	—
Manager	K, A, U	—	—	—	—

Key:
♦ K; Know standard, understand goals ♦ I; Interview patient ♦ Ed; Educate patient ♦ Rv; Review patient data and compare to standard, review chart for completeness of documentation ♦ T; Do testing (fingerstick, Hgb A1C) (If fingerstick glucose level is low [<65]: 1) Give 3 tabs glucose, notify Attending Physician; 2) repeat fingerstick in 15 minutes and inform Attending Physician. ♦ Rx; Give immediate treatment as indicated or ordered ♦ D; Document ♦ M; Medical Management ♦ A; Audit adherence across patients ♦ U; Update standard as needed ♦ ( ); indicates pending practice

Step One: Context Review

Workflow re-design often requires changing people's jobs and is notoriously difficult to accomplish. Just because a change is sensible, advantageous, and feasible does not mean it will be acceptable and/or doable. Review of the context should be done before even choosing those processes for re-design (see Table 23-4). Context review helps to determine who needs to be included in planning for any changes. It also helps with framing communications about changes to all involved.

Table 23-4

WORKFLOW TUTORIAL: CONTEXT REVIEW

Area	Questions	Comments
Job description and change authority	Who has the authority to set and/or change job descriptions? Are staff members of unions? What are the chains of command and/or supervisory structures?	Needed changes in policies/ procedures and job descriptions take a great deal of advance planning. Those empowered to make such changes have to be included in the planning process.
Regulatory environment	Does the practice fall under regulations governing hospitals, post-graduate training programs or other similar entities?	Changes to practice patterns may be constrained by such regulations. Proposed changes need to be articulated and reviewed by those responsible for regulatory compliance during the planning process.
Care management/ quality reporting	What are the reporting requirements?	There should be opportunities for improved reporting with the addition of information technology.
Resource allocation and budgeting	Who ownes the budget for the area? What is the budget cycle? Will resource requirements change? Will the change be revenue-neutral? If there is financial gain anticipated, will it accrue to those doing the work?	Those who control the budget need to be included in the planning processes.

Step Two: Identifying Specific Processes That Will Be Redesigned

Identification of the clinical processes to be redesigned usually comes from a need to improve an inefficient process and/or an opportunity for improvement that is newly available (as in a new EHR) (see Table 23-5, which includes a list of considerations).

Table 23-5

IDENTIFICATION OF CANDIDATE PROCESS FOR WORKFLOW ANALYSIS AND REDESIGN

Characteristics to Identify Challenges/Opportunities	Possible Instances [Comments]
Process creates a bottleneck in patient flow	Patient Intake processing may create a bottleneck. (Patient self-check-in at a kiosk and vital signs done in the patient room may be allowable for return patients without a history of hypertension).
Process creates a significant delay in patient care	Delays created because patient MD encounter is interrupted to collect data generated subsequent to previous encounter. (Chosen for example). Delays created to do procedures (elective procedures such as EKGs may be better scheduled separately from the MD encounter).
Staff are under-utilized	Staff waiting to do exit processing may be under-utilized (with an EHR staff can open cases being seen and prepare for health-maintenance activities, patient education, disease management, and quality data collection before the MD encounter is completed).
New capability available	Insurance eligibility checking for all patients after arrival (EHRs with practice management capabilities can do automatic elegibility checking for scheduled patients prior to the visit).
Opportunity to increase revenue	Visit evaluation and management coding for higher payments if more patient data is documented (collection of complete review of systems through patient/staff or MD data entry into the EHR can support higher coding, and therefore higher payments).
Process seems to add little value	All patients are called 1-3 days before their scheduled appointment, but no-show rate is still high. (Staff calling have only a list with names and phone numbers. With an EHR available, staff can identify at least one patient-specific clinical need for that patient, thereby demonstrating some commitment to that person's health care).

Step Three: Consideration of Information Flow, Process Controls, and Assessments

As noted previously in this chapter, identification of the best possible information flow informs the plans for the optimized workflow. Process controls are often logistical considerations having to do with capacity, but also include clinical triage, preferences based on administrative considerations, patient preferences, patient disabilities, provider preferences, etc. Any steps in the workflow that require judgment need to be addressed in the workflow analysis. Sometimes a simple and invariable rule can be substituted for an assessment and can improve workflow by allowing participation of support staff (as in Figure 23-1 Table 23-6). For most processes,

Table 23-6

INFORMATION FLOW, PROCESS CONTROL, AND ASSESSMENTS

Area	Factor	Example: Pre-Visit Data Gathering
Information flow	When was the information first known?	Data for review at the visit includes results of any and all orders (mostly diagnostic tests and consultation results). These should be planned based on the orders written at the last visit, but may not have been done. Also, there may be unplanned visits to other doctors or hospitals.
	Who knows of the data, that it exists and where?	The patient knows that tests were done and visits made, hospital admissions, etc.
	What is the earliest feasible point for entering the data into the patient's record at the practice site?	Pre-visit processing and data gathering can be done during the week prior to the scheduled visit. However, unless the patient is contacted, exactly what data exists and where will not be known for certain. Pre-visit calling to patients to confirm appointments should be combined with order follow-up for best efficiency.
	What are the pertinent formats, vocabularies, standards, codings, etc., for this data?	To be able to utilize this data for ongoing patient care and quality reporting, disease management, preventive care, billing, etc., it will need to be collected in, or converted to, the relevant HL7 CDA, ASTM CCR, LOINC, ICD-9, SNOMED-CT or other coding.

continued on next page

Table 23-6

INFORMATION FLOW, PROCESS CONTROL, AND ASSESSMENTS (CONT'D)

Area	Factor	Example: Pre-Visit Data Gathering
Process controls	Clinical triage	Patients known to be sicker, have an unexplained problem that may indicate serious illness, or otherwise have become known to the nursing staff should have priority for nurse pre-visit contacts. All staff and MDs authorized to flag orders for Clinical Priority Follow-up.
	Are there any capacity or regulatory constraints on the process?	Nurse time is at a premium. Patients not identified as having clinical priority for nurse pre-visit contact may have routine appointment reminder calls from any available staff.
	Are there any administrative or regulatory constraints on the process?	None for this example.
Assessments	What administrative and/or clinical judgement is exercised in this process, and is supervision and escalation provided for?	Nursing staff to do follow-up on the priority cases. Nurses already exercise judgement and escalate to MD as needed.
Reporting	Are there any quality, disease management, administrative or financial reporting from this process or the data gathered?	Lab data, referral occurrence, etc., is required for several reports and is dependent on entry into the EHR. For those items without automatic data entry, the first staff to gather the data is required to do the data entry.

the clinical and administrative assessments needed are accommodated by virtue of task assignment. For the current example, review of the clinical results, interim care, and referral notes is done by the nurses, with escalation to the physicians on an as-needed basis. See Table 23-6, which includes a list of factors to consider and the pertinent points relevant to the example process.

Step Four: Outlining the New Process and Changes Needed

The newly redesigned process as well as the anticipated changes can be simply represented as in Table 23-7 for the current example. (A cross-functional depiction as used in Table 23-3 is an alternative format.)

Table 23-7

TASK AND CHANGE DETAIL FOR PRE-VISIT PROCESSING EXAMPLE

Person	Action(s)	Documentation	Change
MD or other provider	Flag patient/orders for Clinical Priority Follow-up	In EHR	New task: flag orders and patients as Clinical Priority
Nurse	Call returning patients before the visit. Obtain and enter data. Review and evaluate with escalation as needed. Complete pre-visit notification and remove from task list.	Shared task list for pre-visit appointment confirmation calls in EHR	New tasks: call returning patients before the visit; obtain and enter data; review and evaluate with escalation as needed; complete pre-visit notification and remove from task list. (Note: nurse usually asked to obtain and enter data DURING visit under previous routine; change does not add greatly to total work done).
Non-Clinical Staff	Make pre-visit appointment confirmation calls for only routine complete pre-visit notification and remove from task list.return patients	Shared task list for pre-visit appointment confirmation calls in EHR	Use shared task list for pre-visit calls, (not appointment schedule as before).

After the process of interest is laid out in detail, it is recommended that all the factors in Tables 23-4, 23-5, and 23-6 be reviewed a final time. A common error in the planning process is to leave out of the final product an element considered early on.

Conclusion

EHRs can enable improvements in operations and documentation. As EHRs are implemented, changes to workflow and information flow have to be carefully planned to maintain and/or improve value and minimize risk.

References

1. Workflow Management Coalition (www.wfmc.org)
2. Andrew W, Bruegel R. Workflow management and the CPR. Advance for Health Information Executives. 2003;7:2:49-53

3. Zafar A, Lehto, M. Workflow Characterization in a Busy Urban Primary Care Clinic. Proceedings, Symposium of the American Medical Informatics Association. 2006:1015

4. Unertl KM, Weinger MB, Johnson KB. Applying Direct Observation to Model Workflow and Assess Adoption. Proceedings, Symposium of the American Medical Informatics Association. 2006:794

5. Poon EG, Blumenfeld B, Hamann C, et al. Design and implementation of an application and associated services to support interdisciplinary medication reconciliation efforts in an integrated healthcare delivery network. J Am Med Informatics Assoc. 2006:13:6:581-600

24

Going Live: Training, Data Migration, and Interfaces

Sarah T. Corley, MD

Once you have selected your system, you should have a written plan for implementation. This should include a time line (Table 24-1) and a list of responsibilities for what will be done by the practice and what the vendor will do. A written plan will ensure that everyone will know what his or her responsibilities are. All services that are to be provided by the vendor should be identified in the contract as to what will be done and in what time frame. This chapter touches on common concerns in this phase of the process and estimated times. As much as possible this should be stated in the contract along with all of the costs. One of the most common causes of poor or failed implementations is a lack of dedicated resources on the practice side. Do not underestimate how much work is involved in the transformation of your practice from paper to electronic. The staff person serving as the internal project manager should expect to spend half of their time on the project in the early phases. The vendor cannot know your favorite diagnoses, what procedures you commonly do, who you refer to, and what pharmacies you transmit to. Plan on physician time to help gather this essential information early in the process.

Pre-Implementation Planning

Physicians should plan on reviewing their paper charts several months in advance of the go-live date. Up-to-date chart summaries should be created if this is not already being done. Data that is important to include on these would at a minimum be problem lists/diagnoses, medications, allergies, preventive health care dates, tobacco, and alcohol use. Once the system is in place an experienced medical assistant or a nurse may abstract this data into the electronic health record so that core data is present when the

Table 24-1

IMPLEMENTATION TIMELINE

Time to Implementation	Suggested Actions
6 months	Start keeping an up to date chart summary and identifying information that must be scanned into the EMR
3-6 months	Finalize EMR contract, work out details of implementation plan. Begin lab interface process
3 months	Order computers, servers. Decide on workstation and server configuration, and non-EMR software Order cabling and set installation date Decide on communications options (Cable, T1, DSL) Request other interfaces required (hospital, practice management system, PACS system) Begin chart abstraction as soon as software is installed
2 months	Set policy for assignment of passwords and other security issues Install software and test system Begin training non-computer literate staff Determine coding systems to be used Review Vendor templates and begin customization Review common office forms to determine which may be computerized
4 weeks	Finalize implementation plans with vendors, consultants, outside facilities Adjust patient/procedure schedules for implementation Set up printers and test Test interfaces
2 weeks	Begin Application specific training Check final systems configurations and specifications In large practices, create an "implementation problem" team to report and review problems which occur after the "go live" date. Review last minute details with staff.

physician first sees the patient using the electronic health record (EHR). Generally one person for every five physicians starting three months prior to physician go-live will be adequate to abstract all active charts. Physicians should also identify any data in the paper record that they absolutely must have in the EHR. Those pages can be flagged with sticky arrows to be scanned in. It is an unnecessary waste of time and effort to scan in the entire paper record.

Physical Plant

If you are adding computers to a space that has already been built out, you will need to consider the wiring layout for your network. Be sure that you are using a reputable, experienced vendor for network installation. Cables can be damaged during installation, and this will slow the network down or cause difficult-to-locate problems. If it is a standard cable-based network, then cable (Cat 6 is minimum; Cat 7 may be needed for certain applications such as teleradiology) will have to be run through the walls into the offices and exam rooms and into a central room where the server will reside. If you are using a radio transmitter network, the transmitters will have to be installed and tested. This may take as little as a day if you have a small space and pop up ceiling tiles to a much longer period of time if you are in an older plaster walled building.

Generally wiring should be completed in two days for a small office and in less than a week for a larger office. (All cables should be tested, found to be functional, and warranted in writing before final payment is made). It will, of course, take time for this to be scheduled so allow for four weeks from when you contact the cabling vendor to completion of the job. During this time of disruption, you should also consider whether the exam rooms will be conducive to the use of a computer and, if not, these should be reconfigured as well. This may involve building small computer stands with pull out keyboards or the purchase of portable computer carts and will very likely increase the time required for design and installation. Proper ergonomics need to be considered. Do not expect users to actually rest their tablet or laptop in their lap. If cable must be run through the walls, you should consider running telephone wires at the same time if you will be using modems. A high-capacity cable internet, T-1, or DSL line will provide connectivity via the server and does not require additional phone lines other than the one to the server.

Computers

In most offices servers and workstations are best custom ordered. This allows selection of server features tailored to your specific needs. If you are leasing your equipment, you should allow at least a month for completion of the lease paperwork, credit approval, and shipping of the computers. If you have an existing lease agreement already, this time period will usually require no more than two weeks between order and receipt. Once the computers have been received from the hardware vendor, they will have to be configured.

Many software vendors will have the server shipped to an installation specialist to configure it before sending it to the office. This can cut down on office disruption. The server will need to be configured for the network first and then for your specific application software. This process will usually take two or three days if all goes smoothly. If there are incompatibilities between the software, network operating system, or server, this can take longer. Each workstation will also need to be configured for the network, and printers will have to be added and configured for users. This

Table 24-2

SOFTWARE INSTALLATION: SUGGESTIONS

Create a policy for assignment of passwords and other security issues
List interface required (lab, hospital, practice management system)
Install required coding systems (CPT, ICD, SNOMED, etc.)
Detailed list of remote access requirements
List common problems for which templates are desired
Review common office forms to determine which may be computerized or eliminated

usually takes about thirty to forty-five minutes per machine. If in addition to an EHR system you are also adding other software applications (e-mail, faxing capabilities, coding software, etc.), installation, and configuration will require a bit more time (Table 24-2). Some specific "helpful hints" and suggestions are listed in Table 24-3.

Software Installation/Customization

It will usually take at least one day to install the various software programs, add users, configure printers, configure scanners, and set up computer shares. The practice should request that data back-up tasks and related utilities be configured to run automatically as a night-time batch file. Remote access will need to be set up in the office and at home sites if physicians will be accessing the system outside of business hours.

Many vendors will supply diagnosis and procedure codes with the software, but there is still a lot of customization that must be done. Lab normal values may have to be added; user names, security levels, and passwords must be created. If prescriptions will be printed, the template and fonts and language of the prescription will need to be configured to fit on the appro-

Table 24-3

HELPFUL HINTS

Negotiate a flat-fee for all training
Have vendor responsibilities clearly stated in the contract
Off-site training may be less distracting and more effective
Begin training of computer illiterate staff well in advance of implementation
Set aside time for additional training a few months after installation

priate size piece of paper and to meet state Board of Pharmacy requirements. Customization will realistically take about two days if worked on
without interruption. For larger practices, this will take longer.

If lab interfaces are to be used you should plan on **at least** three months
and often more than six months from purchase of the interface to the first
test download. This is because a functioning interface depends upon cooperation and coordination with the software vendor, the lab, and the practice. The lab must have the capacity to download labs, design a program
to capture their data and send it to the office, and provide data dictionaries so that the data will end up in the appropriate section of the chart. New
lab requisitions may need to be designed and printed so that the patient's
medical record number and provider ID number are captured by the lab
and reported with the results. If you are purchasing an EHR with a bi-
directional lab interface for both ordering labs and receiving results, the
process becomes more complex (Table 24-4). Your vendor will need to
write or modify an interface to allow the downloaded lab files to be uploaded into the patients' records. There is usually a flat fee for this. The vendor will usually serve as the liaison with the lab and arrange all the
preliminary testing. The practice may be responsible for creating a bridging
data dictionary so that the lab names used in the practice's records can be
matched to the test code numbers used by the laboratory. The matching of
practice test names with formal lab test codes is a task best done by someone with extensive experience (in most instances this will be a physician),
with the lab names used by the practice. Daunting as this may seem, it will
only take about four hours if done by a computer-savvy physician or nurse.

Templates, which can greatly speed entry of progress notes and other
clinical data, may need to be customized for the site. Templates may also
help with quality assurance activities by providing for capture of standard
data sets for certain diagnoses. Templates for common problems such as
"New Diabetic", "New Hypertensive", may speed data entry while ensuring

Table 24-4

ORDERING COMPUTERS: SUGGESTIONS

Written implementation plan

Wiring diagram with proposed server and workstation location

Server specifications for memory, disk drives, communications lines, etc.

List workstations and proposed configuration of each

List software applications and intended users

Contract with detailed listing of specific vendor responsibilities for setup, testing,
    training, etc.

Communications plan (internet connection, FAX, e-mail)

that the same information is gathered on all patients with that diagnosis, making outcomes analysis much easier. Stock templates, provided by the vendor, should be reviewed and changes made to reflect the practice style of each physician who will use them. If the user can customize the templates (a very useful feature), then the templates can be further refined as the need arises. Some specific "helpful hints" and suggestions are listed in Table 24-3.

Training

Training is the most important aspect of implementation. If the users are not well trained, the system is doomed to fail. If at all possible negotiate a flat rate for the training package and be sure that expectations and commitments are clearly stated in your contract. The trainer should be an expert in all of the features of the program as well as a good teacher. The staff needs to have basic computer skills and needs to focus on the training. All hardware should be tested and known to be functional prior to the training session.

Preliminary training for staff members who are not computer literate should be done in advance of the actual implementation phase. It will be difficult for them to focus on software-specific training when they have not mastered the basics of using a computer. Depending upon the size of the practice, training may be done at a local adult education center or on-site (off-site may offer a more distraction-free learning environment). If at all possible employees who have similar work roles should be trained together. This allows the training to be focused on the way that group will be interacting with the software. Receptionists/appointment schedulers will use a system differently from the nursing staff and the physicians.

Allow adequate time for breaks so that the staff can have enough time to absorb what is being taught. One full day of training with each group would be the minimum and preferably a second day could be spent with the trainer to help as the staff becomes acquainted with the system. I recommend setting up another day of training after the system has been in place for three months so that staff members can optimize the way they use the system and also learn more obscure or undocumented features that improve the day-to-day use of the software. Some specific "helpful hints" and suggestions are listed in Table 24-3.

Staff Expectations

Staff should be involved from the beginning of the process and kept informed of what changes will occur that can affect their jobs. People in general are very resistant to change, and it is very important that you consider the needs of the staff and also be aware of their fears. Take time to sit down with each member of the staff and discuss your plans for changes in job duties and employment levels. If you anticipate that fewer staff will be required, make the decisions as early as possible. Staff who will be let go should be given appropriate notice and aid in finding new positions or at least letters of reference (if appropriate). Above all, do not let fear for jobs plague your staff for long periods of time. It may result in unexpected resignations or even malicious acts. If paper records will no longer be kept, the medical records staff may need to be retrained for other functions. While charts will no longer have to be pulled and filed, there will be new tasks. In particular, data entry will become an issue. Outside reports will need to be entered into the new EHR either through file downloads, scanning, or manual addition. Lab results will need to be entered manually until the lab interface has been successfully implemented. If optimal use is made of the new data, there will be work involved in running reports and contacting patients who may be overdue for health maintenance procedures.

The nursing staff will still have the same duties as before but will need to enter and retrieve data from the computer rather than a paper chart. You must be vigilant early on to be sure that **ALL** data are entered in the computer rather than scribbled as notes on the bottom of a consultant's report or a lab sheet. To improve staff buy-in, there should be regular training sessions in the office by "super users" to show other staff members ways to save time and effort using the newly available resources. Physicians should be aware that initially more effort will be required to accomplish the same tasks. However, as familiarity with the new system improves, productivity will increase and patient care quality will be enhanced.

Caveats and Pearls

Try to negotiate a flat fee with your vendor for items that have the potential to be very time consuming. This would include all types of interfaces, billing, scheduling, and lab. All interfaces, even if designed for the exact same versions of the exact same programs, will still require individual changes and unexpected things will always come up. Lab interfaces will always take much longer than you think. Plan for how the data will be entered meanwhile. Do not try to use already busy staff to do this in their free time! It is often most economical to hire a data entry contractor to come in for a few hours on the weekend to enter the labs. If you are not able to change templates or chart format or other items without programming assistance from the vendor, you should try to negotiate a flat fee for a certain number of templates.

Cable wires frequently have flaws, so buy top-quality cable, have it installed professionally, and have it tested and warranted. Get same-day four-hour service for your server. Get next-day office service for your workstations. The peace of mind is well worth the cost.

Try to get your clinical consultants to send you reports on a CD or through encrypted email as an ASCII file to reduce the need for scanning. If this is not possible, try to have them send reports with a large clear font on plain paper, not letterhead. Plain paper will improve the quality of scanned documents using an Optical Character Recognition system. If documents are handwritten, they can be scanned as an image but will take up more disk space and will prevent the text from being searched in a query.

Take the time to plan the exam room layouts so that you can maintain eye contact with patients while using the computer. Ask your vendor for suggestions or, better yet, photos of different practice designs. Plan for the layout of your desk. A traditional desk makes an uncomfortable workstation and often the best solution is all new desks and chairs. Pay attention to the ergonomics of everyone's workstation to avoid lost time.

Spend the money for the fastest, biggest processors and computers available. Once you have a computer in place, you will want to add other software: textbooks, the Gail model breast cancer tool, atlases, patient education material, electronic codebooks, electronic address books, online access, and others. Get an uninterrupted power supply for the server and as many of the workstations as you can afford. There is nothing worse than losing a note or an appointment due to a sudden interruption of power in a thunderstorm. It also prevents the data corruption that can occur with a disorderly shut down. Consider remote monitoring of your server: many vendors offer this service, and they can detect problems before you have a fatal crash.

If high-speed internet access is available to your office, get it. You can save a lot of money in phone calls by emailing lab results and having patients email prescription, appointment, and referral requests to the office and receiving electronic replies. It also makes the office a more peaceful work place with fewer ringing phones. If you have constant access to the Internet, insurance company sites can be visited and claim status checked. Many HMOs allow you to complete referral requests on line.

Consider having a professional design a web page for you. This can include all the material in your practice brochure and serves as a marketing tool. You can include all of your registration materials so they can be completed ahead of time and either printed or electronically sent to the office. This saves a great deal of time for new appointments without the postage and paper costs of mailing forms out ahead of time. You can include links for emailing the appointment, prescription, and referral requests as well.

Do not print out a copy of your notes. This will double costs as you have the computer expense plus chart expenses. Staff will always be tempted to pull charts and put handwritten notes in them if they are available, leaving the electronic record incomplete.

25

EHR, HIPAA, and Security: Practical Implications

Suchit Mishra, MSEE

"**W**riting code is like writing poetry: every word, each placement counts. Except that software is harder, because digital poems can have millions of lines that are somehow interconnected. Try fixing programming errors, also known as bugs, and you can often introduce new ones. So far, nobody has found a silver bullet to kill the beast of complexity." This is a famous quote made by Stuart Feldman in 2001, who was then the Director of IBM's Institute for Advanced Commerce. Looking back, things have not changed much. Information systems security is a very complex area and it requires a collective organizational effort to make it a reality. This chapter will attempt to provide a few pointers and offer general advice on protecting your EHR installation. A key point to remember is that security covers more than preventing unauthorized access; it also encompasses data integrity and prevention of loss.

Vendor Responsibilities

When you sign the contract for your EHR, it should clearly define where the responsibility rests for important security areas such as HIPAA compliance. EHR software should have basic security features built in. Of course it is up to the practice to make sure that they are used properly. There are four major areas to consider: access controls, data validation, audit trails, and data protection during transmission.

Access Controls

Passwords are the most common form of access control. Some vendors offer biometric log-ins (e.g., fingerprint) as well. Passwords are only as secure as people permit them to be. They work well when used properly and are not abused. Systems should support strong passwords (passwords that mix numbers, letters and other characters) and provide hints to users when they are creating passwords. Also, systems should offer the ability to sunset (force expiration) passwords on a scheduled basis.

Role-based access to EHR functions is another common access control measure in which users are given access based on their job functions. When roles are used, nurses, front desk staff, doctors, and others have limits placed on what they are allowed to do and see in the EHR. This is great for restricting access to sensitive information. It may also cause problems. Staff cannot easily fill in for one another as is possible with paper records.

Automatic timeouts for log-ins provide a measure of security when someone forgets to log-out or has to move away from the workstation for an extended period of time. Each of these features should be standard in any EHR system.

Audit Trails

Audit trails provide a mechanism for determining who has accessed data within the EHR. Audit trails are an essential feature for any EHR to be HIPAA compliant. Check to make sure that your EHR system does not permit the disabling of audit trails: this makes them essentially ineffective. Audit trails should not only apply to individual users, but also to all reports and other information that leaves the EHR.

Data Protection

Information stored in EHRs is usually contained within a database. Database management systems provide data access and reporting tools. These tools may be used in certain circumstances to circumvent the EHR user interface and get directly at EHR data. This presents a vulnerability that must be addressed for any EHR installation. One way of getting around this problem is to have all data encrypted while stored or during transmission. Additional measures include password protecting the database and restricting access to no more than two top-level members of the practice. Anyone who gains access to the database management system has access to everything. Vendors should take extra measures to assure that access to the EHR data through the database management system is appropriately restricted.

Vendors should also be asked to execute a business associate agreement to assure that technical personnel and others who have access to the database management system will behave responsibly.

Client Responsibilities

Good security starts with good planning. Understanding how your data may be threatened and current system vulnerabilities is essential to practical security planning.

Threats

Threats come in many forms and may be divided into three groups: intentional, unintentional, and environmental. Environmental threats are possibly the most overlooked. The area in which servers, routers, and other networking equipment are stored must be protected from harm. Typical losses associated with problems such as flooding, overheating, power surges, and fire are preventable with appropriate planning. Rooms that house computing equipment should be properly cooled and constantly monitored for temperature changes. As far as possible they should be interior, windowless rooms away from large plumbing fixtures and pipes.

Unintentional threats are more difficult to address because they often are due to human error and a lack of proper policies and procedures. Data integrity is a key part of data security. The information in patient charts should be accurate and complete. Errors (e.g., incorrect information, information placed in the wrong chart) and omissions (e.g., missing data) compromise data integrity and are difficult to address without proper training and appropriate policies for data collection. Errors and omissions issues can be addressed through data validation features of the EHR as well as through policies and procedures aimed at standardization of data collection and regular audits. Some unintentional threats, such as equipment malfunctions or accidental erasure of a file, are difficult to predict but are ameliorated by a comprehensive security policy.

Intentional threats receive the most attention and are the type of threat to which most security measures are directed. A key point to remember is that most intentional threats arise from inside the organization. Often they are the work of disgruntled employees. Typical examples are vandalism, data theft, extortion, and misuse of access privileges. Access controls do not work unless they are properly enforced. Proper enforcement begins with policies and procedures that clearly outline appropriate conduct by expressly forbidding practices such as sharing passwords. Role-based access to data provides another level of protection. This is true not only for employees who must use the EHR but also for information technology employees. For example, separating systems administration, database administration, and security roles provides an extra level of separation and prevents any one employee for having too much control over EHR data.

Vulnerabilities

Vulnerabilities may be thought of as problems waiting to happen. As with threats, vulnerabilities require a combination of policies, system architecture, training, and actions to address them properly. Many physical vulnerabilities can be removed simply and inexpensively. For example, locks on doors to data centers, secure storage for backup media, restricted access to areas where servers are housed, and a formal process for removing computers from service (e.g., disk scrubbing).

Technical vulnerabilities are often due to security lapses in applications and network configuration issues. A very common technical vulnerability is the failure to change the administrator password on new database deployments. The degree to which technical vulnerabilities are addressed is very dependent on the skills, knowledge, and professionalism of the technical staff in charge of the system.

Security Polices and Training

Security planning has to be a major part of any EHR implementation. Formal policies and procedures should be in place to handle common security issues. Start by addressing common environmental threats and physical vulnerabilities, many of which can be addressed directly in the layout of the data center physical plant. Next, develop strict guidelines for employee behavior regarding data access and use. Make it very clear that unauthorized access and any use of clinical data for other than approved purposes will be swiftly and firmly addressed. Many security issues arise from social engineering (fooling someone into divulging confidential information). Employees should also receive training in ways to recognize social engineering practices. This is actually the way that much confidential information is lost: conversations over lunch, in elevators, and with the friendly stranger dressed as a physician who just has one question about Mrs. Smith (Table 25-1).

Table 25-1

SECURITY BEST PRACTICES (SMALLER PRACTICES)

- Create a policy and procedure manual that outlines clearly all security related issues
- Make security policy and procedures a key part of employee orientation
- All security training provided should be recorded (especially for HIPAA)
- Provide proper training and security related issues to all employees
- Enact disciplinary measures for employee security violations such as password sharing, improper data access and unauthorized disclosures.
- Make security issues a priority for the practice.
- Always use EHR security features such as audit trails, strong passwords, data encryption, and roles-based access.
- Ensure that terminated employees are immediately removed from the list of authorized users

Information Technology Issues

Malware

A major security problem for many small practices is the lack of adequate technical measures for dealing with technical vulnerabilities. Viruses, worms, trojan horses, spyware and other malicious software are a threat to every computer on the Internet. Virus protection, anti-spyware and firewalls for all systems linked to the Internet are a must. These software packages are inexpensive and are very effective in protecting your computers and network (Table 25-2). Antivirus and other protective software should be updated regularly and systems should be scanned on a regular basis. Computers on the network should be configured so that antivirus and other software may not be disabled by the user. Workstations should be secured from snooping by placing them away from well-traveled areas. Screens should timeout within 30-60 seconds when not being actively used.

Computers Off-site: Remote access, Laptops, Repair, Disposal

Remote access is a common reason many practices implemented electronic health record systems. Of course, the convenience of remote access carries with it the threat of security breaches. Remote access to your EHR should be set up only by a professional who is knowledgeable in security measures. The most secure way to provide remote access to your EHR installation is through the use of a virtual private network (VPN). Once in place all access attempts should be monitored closely and there should be a detailed audit trail of all remote use attempts. When setting up remote access keep in mind that you want your solution to be HIPAA compliant.

News stories of lost or stolen laptops containing sensitive patient data are common. Laptops used to house patient data should have at a minimum the following security measures: professional level operating system

Table 25-2

MALWARE	
Virus	A computer program that infects a computer and spreads to other computers via a host (e.g. floppy disk, e-mail)
Worm	Self-replicating programs that spreads itself over computer networks. Can damage files or cripple a network by creating copies of itself
Trojan Horse	File that masquerades as a safe program but once activated is dangerous. Trojans must be activated by user action before they become effective.
SpyWare	Computer software that resides on a computer and collects information about the user.

(e.g. windows XP professional), strong password or biometric access control (e.g. fingerprint) and encryption of all stored data. These measures will go a long way to protecting data if the system is stolen although they are not foolproof. The best idea is not to store sensitive data on mobile devices—it is just a bad idea.

When computers that are removed from the practice for repair or to be discarded, they should be checked to make sure that they house no sensitive data. This is an important policy matter and should be addressed by requiring a formal process to release computers for repair or disposal. Disk drives can either be destroyed or they can be scrubbed (have all data removed using special software) to assure that no security breaches occur.

Information Technology Job Roles

Systems administrator, database administrator, network administrator and security administrator are the four IT positions that deal most directly with the security of the EHR installations. All networks regardless of size have a systems administrator who is responsible for adding and removing network users, software installation, data backup and other common administrative functions. Systems administrators have control over everything on the network and obviously a disgruntled systems administrator could do a lot of damage to an EHR installation. The systems administrator is not necessarily an IT professional (in some practices it might be the office manager or the head of medical records). Whatever the situation, care should be taken to assure that there is a second person who has access and can administer all resources on the network. This can be accomplished through outsourcing (have an outside company administer your network in conjunction with a practice employee) or designating a second employee as a part-time systems administrator. In any case, no practice should have a single systems administrator who has control over all resources.

When selecting IT employees always hire employees who are certified for the operating system that you are using and look for security training or experience.

Backups, Disaster Recovery, and Business Continuity

Backup/disaster recovery planning is probably one of the most neglected areas of information security. In many situations backup/disaster recovery planning is neglected due to cost or failure to appreciate the business value of good data security. However, once the potential business impact of a major data loss or security breach is grasped, resistance often quickly disappears. Unfortunately, the approach taken in managing backups and preventing data loss is usually fairly lackadaisical. Backups should be done based on the frequency that the stored data changes. Data intensive systems such as EHRs house data that changes frequently over the course of the day. A backup that is done at the end of business each day could potentially result in an entire day's loss if a major system failure occurs at three in the afternoon.

The most basic backup strategy is to make a copy of your data at the end of each business. This is not a good idea for an EHR. A more reasonable back up strategy for practices without significant IT staff would be to use an outside data security vendor that offers remote back-up services. In the simplest form of remote back up vendors take snapshots at various time points over the course of the day of your data. Continuous back-up (data is sent off site as it is stored on the local system) is also available and provides the highest level of data security. Practices that have more sophisticated IT resources and more money can invest in fault-tolerant servers, failover clusters, and other high-availability data protection solutions. Another common mistake is keeping copies of the backups at the same site where the system is located. Fires and natural disasters would then be able to destroy the main system and backups. The lesson here is always store backups offsite. Also, make sure that backups are secured (password-protected, encrypted and locked-up). "Best practices" for data protection are summarized in **Table 25-3**.

Disaster Recovery vs. Business Continuity

If a major system failure occurs either from a natural disaster, fire, or malicious act, often a backup alone is not sufficient to get you up and running again. You may need new servers, replacement of network components, new workstations, or replacement software in addition to a copy of stored data. Disaster recovery and business continuity are often used interchangeably. However, there is a difference between the two. Disaster recovery deals with the process of restoration or recovery of computer systems back to the state of business before the system failure

Table 25-3

DATA PROTECTION BEST PRACTICES

- Make multiple copies of your data: local copy and a remote, off-site copy
- Use a fault tolerant server (a server that has redundant components and duplicate copies of data)
- Encrypt all data
- Transmit data using secure protocols
- Hire a security consultant to look over your system

occurred. Business continuity includes disaster recovery along with the plan to get things back to "business as usual". Therefore, business continuity includes not only getting your computer systems back online, but also, restoration of your place of business. For example, if your practice were to be severely damaged in a tornado your disaster recovery plan would say how your server, computers, network, software and data would be restored to their previous condition. Your business continuity plan would add to this how your office is rebuilt and how you would obtain temporary office space in the meantime.

A Suggested Data Security Plan for Smaller Practices

First create a formal security policy and train all staff. Be sure to include HIPAA training as part of your security policies. If your practice has its own information technology staff then make sure that they are properly trained and certified for the operating systems that you use. Even if you have your own IT staff, you should consider having an outside group of networking specialists review your network configuration and backup plan.

Next, formalize your data protection and data security plan. If you are considering using a fault tolerant server or continuous on-line, remote backups there are number of vendors that can work with you or your IT staff to make sure that you have an appropriate backup strategy. Many of these vendors also offer disaster recovery services as part of their data security and data protection services. A disaster recovery strategy with continuous, remote backups and a local fault-tolerant server is definitely more expensive than doing a tape backup of your run-of-the-mill local server. However, if you ever suffer through a fire, burst pipe, hurricane, tornado or other disaster, you will consider it to be money well spent.

Be sure that your practice can recover quickly from a major disaster. Business continuity planning is somewhat more complicated because it involves more than simply assuring that your computer systems and network can be rapidly replaced. If your place of business is destroyed or severely damaged your choices are either find a temporary place to conduct business or wait until your site has been fully repaired and restored. A good first step in ensuring business continuity is having appropriate insurance for natural disasters. Also check to make sure that your business owner's policy covers business interruptions due to criminal acts by your own employees and others. It also helps to establish contacts with those who provide services that would be needed such as commercial real estate agents, bank loan officers, construction contractors, and other similar businesses.

Review the security provisions of your EHR with the vendor. Obtain a business associate agreement if the vendor's staff will have access to your patient data. Also, review data ownership and access clauses in your EHR contract to assure that the vendor does not have a right to access or resell your data.

Summary

Securing your data involves much more than simply having a backup. Dangers posed to your data come in many forms: malicious attacks, accidents, natural disasters, poor software design, network weaknesses, careless employees, uninformed information systems professionals, and many other ways. Protecting your data requires a well thought-out approach using policies and procedures, employee training and the involvement of competent information systems professional in preventing unauthorized access, and ensuring data safety and integrity through a sound backup plan that provides for disaster recovery and business continuity.

Resources

Off-site backup vendors:
- Iron Mountain - http://www.ironmountain.com/
- AmeriVault - http://www.amerivault.com/

Fault-tolerant servers:
- Stratus: http://www.stratus.com/products/

Appendix A: Glossary

Thompson M. Kuhn, Maria Rudolph,
Stephen Spadt, and Jerome H. Carter, MD

Computer-Based Patient Record (CPR) / Electronic Medical Record (EMR) / Electronic Health Record (EHR). These terms are, for all practical purposes, synonymous. EHR is the preferred term and is applied to systems regardless of origin (in-house, open source, or commercial products) or setting (inpatient or ambulatory) that have met the CCHIT criteria for certification.

* * *

AJAX

Asynchronous Javascript and XML, a programming technique that enables Web applications to move data between the server and client without reloading an entire page. Web applications that are built using this and related approaches are often called Rich Internet Applications (RIAs) because they offer users an experience that more closely resembles traditional desktop applications in terms of richness of functionality and responsiveness. The term Dynamic HTML (DHTML) is also used to describe this level of increased user interaction.

Application Service Provider (ASP)

A method for delivering a computer application over the Internet as opposed to running an application on local hardware. Some EHR software vendors offer an ASP option as an alternative.

Authentication

The process of verifying a user identity. User names and passwords are the most common type of authentication approach, although more secure techniques are increasingly being employed.

Authorization

A component of security, authorization is the ability to define not only a user's allowable functionality (e.g., look up a patient, create a clinical note, order a lab test) but also the type of data that may be viewed (e.g., all test results except HIV results, all clinical notes including psychotherapy notes).

Broadband

A network connection method that offers higher speed than standard telephone service, broadband services are offered by cable television and telephone services (*see* **Digitial Subscriber Line**). Broadband speeds vary based on a number of factors. There is no agreement on a definition for broadband speed.

Browser

An application that enables downloading and viewing of content from the Internet. Microsoft Internet Explorer and Mozilla Firefox are the most commonly used browsers in Windows environments.

Client/Server

A means for accessing information that resides on a central computer (server) by any number of connected computers (clients). This architecture, on which the Internet itself is based, continues to be the leading approach for most small- and medium-sized business applications. Traditionally the term *client-server* meant that the application, or some part of it, is installed on the workstation, in contrast to a *Web-based* system, in which the only thing needed on the workstation is a Web browser. Some client-server applications are "Web-enabled" which means some part of the functionality is available through a Web browser.

Clinical Data Repository (CDR)

The component of an EHR system that stores and manages patients' clinical information. CDRs are features of inpatient EHR systems

Clinical Decision Support (CDS) System (CDSS)

The component of an EHR system that analyzes clinical data and provides care recommendations.

Computerized Physician Order Entry (CPOE)

The component of an EHR system through which a clinician inputs requests for services such as diagnostic tests, procedures, and medications.

Controlled Vocabulary

A list of preferred terms for describing actions, concepts, and findings within a particular domain. In health care, a controlled vocabulary might be used to identify acceptable terms for encoding the progress note. Common vocabularies include ICD for encoding diseases and health conditions, CPT for services and procedures, SNOMED-CT for relatively broad use, LOINC for laboratory observations, and NDC for medications.

DBMS

Database Management System, an application that manages the creation, storage, and retrieval of data. The most common type of DBMS uses relational data models (tables of data related to other tables), but object-based data models are becoming more common.

DICOM

Digital Imaging and Communications in Medicine, the primary standard for exchanging images (e.g., X-rays, EKGs, ultrasounds).

Digital Subscriber Line (DSL)

A network connection method that offers higher speed than standard telephone service. DSL service is typically offered by telephone companies.

Disease Registry

An application that tracks clinical information relevant to the management of patients with chronic diseases. Disease registries may focus on a single disease or multiple diseases. Disease registries may be stand-alone applications or components of EHR systems.

Dynamic HTML (DHTML)

See **AJAX.**

Electronic Data Interchange (EDI)

EDI consists of rules and standards that typically allow businesses to use computers and networks to conduct business transactions. Health care billing systems often use EDI to exchange billing information with payers.

Electronic Document Management (EDM)

An application component that enables the storage, indexing, and retrieval of scanned paper documents (e.g., driver's license, insurance cards, faxed or photocopied reports).

Enterprise Master Person Index (EMPI)

The term *Enterprise Master Patient Index* is also used. An EMPI is a database that lives on the network of a healthcare enterprise and keeps track of relevant information about people who are of interest to the enterprise. The main functions of the EMPI are person/patient identification, matching, and reconciliation. EMPI keeps track of all the ways that different systems and applications identify the same patient and can locate information about a patient that is stored in another system or in multiple systems.

Firewall

Hardware or software that prevents harm from external systems by limiting access to a computer. Common firewall protections include anti-virus software, spam filters, spyware, and secured access (e.g., token-based **authentication**). Firewalls often form the first line of security for protecting computers and networks from unauthorized access.

Health Level 7 (HL7)

HL7 is one of the primary standards used to exchange information between different vendors' systems (e.g., between an EHR and LIS [Laboratory Information System]). The standard is message-based, meaning information is packaged and sent in defined message formats from system to system. HL7 version 2.x is the most prevalent version of the standard in use.

HTML

Hypertext Markup Language, the formatting code that is used to display content within a browser. HTML is the simplest technique for controlling formatting and layout of Web pages but is increasingly being replaced by richer, more robust techniques (e.g., AJAX).

Integration

Two computer applications are said to be integrated when they can exchange data in a form that each can understand and act upon. Generally, integration results when applications exchange data using standard formats and standard coded terminologies.

Interface

In information technology there are two uses for this term. One is to describe the way a user views and controls the operation of an application; this is often referred to as the GUI ("gooey", Graphical User Interface). Every computer application that is directly operated by a user must have a user interface. The other use of the term is to describe the method by which applications automatically exchange data with other applications; this type of interface is known as the API (Application Programming Interface). A user does not see this kind of interface, but it is critical for ensuring the exchange of data between applications. For example, an EHR system may have an application interface that is designed for receiving messages and reports from clinical laboratories.

Internet Service Provider (ISP)

Everyone who uses the Internet uses an ISP to connect to the Internet. The ISP charges for maintaining the user's connection and for passing data between the user and all of the sites on the Internet with whom the user interacts. An ISP may provide other services such as e-mail accounts, user Web pages, and online storage. An ISP may offer Internet connections via various technologies such as phone lines, DSL, and cable TV.

Javascript

A scripting language used largely to provide a richer user interface. Javascript is used primarily in the development of the Web front-end (i.e., what the user sees as the application screen). It is part of the AJAX standard. Note that Javascript is *not* equivalent to the Java programming language.

National Provider Identifier (NPI)

The NPI is a unique ten-digit identification number issued to health care providers in the United States by the Centers for Medicare and Medicaid Services (CMS). The NPI replaces the unique provider identification number (UPIN) as the required identifier for Medicare services and will be used by other payers, including commercial health care insurers.

Operating System (OS)

An operating system is software that controls the functioning of a computer. The various versions of Microsoft Windows (XP, 2000, Vista) Macintosh OS X, and Linux are operating systems. Computer applications must be written so that they can interact properly with the operating system. A single version of a computer application cannot operate on more than one type of operating system.

Optical Character Recognition (OCR)

With OCR a printed or hand-written document is scanned and a computer application attempts to determine what each letter in the document is intended to be. In this way the text of hard copy documents can be imported into an EHR. The accuracy of OCR is not perfect and depends on the quality of the document being scanned. Usually someone must review the results of a scan and make corrections.

Patient Portal

Some EHR systems offer clinicians the opportunity to provide their patients with a Web-based portal. This is a Web site where patients can look for educational information and links to other sources of information that are recommended by the clinician. Also, patients can use the portal to exchange secure structured messages with their clinicians and possibly perform activities such as scheduling appointments and ordering refills of prescriptions.

Personal Digital Assistant (PDA)

Small handheld devices capable of running relatively complex applications. PDAs are increasingly being equipped with wireless Internet access, enabling them to serve as gateways to Web applications, albeit with rather limited screen resolutions (typically less than 25% of full-size computer monitors). Smart phones are devices that converge mobile phones and PDA functionality into a single device.

Personal Health Record (PHR)

The PHR is a relatively new concept that describes a range of activities in which patients interact with health information. Development of PHR systems is moving in various directions, and there is no consensus on a definition. A PHR may include health information about a patient that is collected from clinical systems and/or entered directly by a patients or caregivers. PHRs may also offer services that allow patients to improve and monitor their health and to research and learn about their conditions.

Practice Management System (PMS)

A PMS is a computer application that assists clinicians and their staffs in managing the day-to-day operations of a practice. PMS applications typically manage patient demographics, appointments, insurance claims, billing, and payments. Although PMS and EHR applications may be separate, there are significant benefits if they are integrated.

Registry

See **Disease Registry.**

Rich Internet Applications (RIAs)

See **AJAX.**

Structured Data

Structured data are more easily understood and processed by computer systems than are **unstructured data.** Elements of structured data have been assigned codes from a standard controlled vocabulary or terminology such as ICD9-CM, CPT, or SNOMED CT.

Tablet PC

A mobile computer that is based on the notebook or laptop format but enables users to rotate the screen and position it over the keyboard such that the user interface becomes a large touchscreen. Although affording the advantages of a larger screen and more computing power than a PDA and greater mobility than a traditional notebook computer, tablet PCs have not been as popular as was originally expected. The prevalence of computing "carts" in many facilities, coupled with the disadvantage of their greater weight than PDAs, are likely contributing factors.

Template

Some EHR systems use templates in order to assist clinicians in collecting clinical information during an encounter. Using point-and-click widgets such as check boxes and drop-down lists, templates can speed data collection and offer reminders of possibly relevant additional questions to ask.

Unstructured Data

Free text that has not been coded with standard controlled vocabulary or terminology (*see* **Structured Data**).

Virtual Private Network (VPN)

VPNs provide a more secure way to communicate over the Internet. A VPN is like a tunnel that runs through the Internet but is shielded from it. Normal Internet communications can be spied upon relatively easily by unauthorized parties, whereas VPNs make such eavesdropping considerably more difficult. An example of VPN is the remote access of a corporate network by employees working from home.

Voice Recognition

An alternative input method to direct typing into an application. Voice recognition allows users to dictate, rather than use keyboard or mouse point-and-click techniques, to complete documentation. There is no additional transcription step. Voice recognition has improved in accuracy over the last few years, although the acceptability of remaining errors will vary by factors such as medical specialty and physical environment.

Wireless Local Area Network (WLAN; Wi-Fi)

A wireless version of a Local Area Network (LAN) that enables computers to communicate without network cabling. Wi-Fi, the common name for a family of 802-11 standards, is the most common form of WLAN; it is most often used to connect handheld or portable devices and other mobile computers.

Workflow-enabled

This growing area of functionality within EHRs provides the ability to automate aspects of practice workflow. In the simplest case, an event, such as arrival of a lab result, triggers an action, such as sending a notification message. Typically workflow is applied to end-to-end processes (e.g., initial appointment scheduling through billing), but it can also be used to manage certain aspects of practice (e.g., ordering a lab test through communication with the patient).

XML

Extensible Markup Language, a data representation language that is human-readable (i.e., is based on plain text) and the standard for formatting data that are exchanged or shared between systems (e.g., sending a lab result to the ordering provider). Because the data are human-readable and not routinely compressed, care must be taken to ensure that access to the data is protected with additional layers of security.

Appendix B: Resources

Electronic Health Records
Certification Commission for Healthcare Information Technology (CCHIT)—
organization charged with certifying the functionality of electronic health
records systems. They publish a list of all certified products that is updated
on a regular basis.

233 N. Michigan Avenue, 21st Floor
Chicago, IL 60601
Email: info@cchit.org
Telephone: (312) 233-1582
www.cchit.org

Magazines
The magazines and web sites listed below are good sources of information
concerning current issues in health care computing. Health Data Management, Healthcare Informatics, and Advance for Health Information Executives have annual issues devoted EHR products and reviews.

Advance for Health Care Executives	http://health-care-it.advanceweb.com/
Health Data Management	www.healthdatamanagement.com
Health Care Informatics	www.healthcare-informatics.com

News Services
News services are an excellent source of up-to-date information about
products, vendors and important trends in the marketplace. Subscriptions
to electronic newsletters are free.

Digital Health Care and Productivity   www.digitalhcp.com
eWeek/Health   www.eweek.com
Healthcare IT News   www.healthcareitnews.com/

Case Studies
The Davies Awards are given to organization that have successfully implemented electronic health records and demonstrated their impact. The case reports for awardees provide an excellent source of examples of solving complex implementation problems.
http://www.himss.org/ASP/davies_organizational.asp

Web Sites
The Providers Edge: EHRCentral—The best source of EHR information on the web includes links to books, consultants, articles, web sites, and events. This site has no ties to health information technology vendors.
http://www.providersedge.com/index.html

Computing for Clinicians—created by editor of this book. The site provides vendor/product lists, links to news articles, useful resources and contact information for the editor.
www.computingforclinicians.net

Organizations
These organizations provide educational materials as well as conferences that focus on electronic health records and related issues.

American Health Information Management Association
233 N. Michigan Avenue, 21st Floor
Chicago, IL 60601-5800
(312) 233-1100
www.ahima.org

Healthcare Information and Management Systems Society
230 East Ohio Street, Suite 500,
Chicago, IL 60611-3269
(312) 664-4467
www.himss.org

American Medical Informatics Associations
4915 St. Elmo Ave, #401
Bethesda, MD 20814
301-657-5918
www.amia.org

The Medical Records Institute is a for-profit organization that offers confer-ences and publications aimed at individuals and organizations trying to make the transition to computer-based patient records.

Medical Records Institute
567 Walnut St.
P.O. Box 600770
Newton, MA 02460
www.medrecinst.com

Quality Improvement

Doctors Office Quality—Information Technology

One of the more useful resources to begin to explore how EHRs are used for measuring quality is the DOQ-IT website. (**www.qualitynet.org**). It contains information regarding specific measures that are applicable to primary and preventive care settings. Most importantly, it provides the reader a resource for all the technical aspects of 1) definitions of the clinical measures, 2) tech-nical specification and conformance criteria for capturing, recording and re-porting of performance measures.

Doctors Office Quality—Information Technology
Phone: (866) 288-8912 (7 a.m.–7 p.m., CT Monday–Friday)
Fax: (888) 329-7377
E-mail: qnetsupport@ifmc.sdps.org

Medicare Quality Improvement Community

Another useful resource regarding quality improvement and the role of health information technology is the Medicare Quality Improvement Community (MedQIC—www.medqic.org)). Supported by the CMS, this website provides an extensive wealth of information regarding quality improvement and health IT adoption. A list of health IT vendors supporting QI activities may be found on the site.

Informatics Standards Groups

Health Level 7 (HL-7)	www.HL7.org/ehr	EHR functional, legal and interoperability models
Digital imaging and com-munications (DICOM)	http://medical.nema.org/	Images
Health Information Tech-nology Standards Panel (HITSP)	www.ansi.org/hitsp	Interoperability
International Classification of Diseases (ICD)	www.who.int/classifications/icd/en/	Disease/diagnosis
Current Procedural Terminology (CPT)	www.ama-assn.org/ama/pub/category/3113.html	Procedures

Systematized Nomenclature of Medicine (SNOMED)	www.snomed.org/	Terminology/vocabulary
RxNorm	http://www.nlm.nih.gov/ research/umls/rxnorm/ index.html	Medications
MEDCIN	www.medicomp.com	Terminology/vocabulary
Logical Observation Identifiers Names and Codes (LOINC)	http://www.regenstrief.org/ medinformatics/loinc/	Laboratory and clinical

General Hardware & Technology Resources

Below are sites that provide timely information on the latest technology. Most offer in-depth product reviews and analysis of trends and issues. They also offer searchable archives of past product reviews and articles, white papers and tutorials.

Computerworld	www.computerworld.com
Infoworld	www.infoworld.com/
Government Computer News	www.gcn.com/
ZiffDavis	www.zdnet.com/
PC Magazine	http://www.pcmag.com/
PC World	www.pcworld.com/

Books

The following books are aimed at beginners and provide good introductions to their respective fields.

Project Management
Absolute Beginner's Guide to Project Management, Greg Horine, 2005.
ISBN13: 9780789731975

Foundations of Project Management, James P Lewis, 2006.
ISBN-13: 978-0814408797

Process Analysis
Process Mastering, Ray Wilson, Paul Harsin, 1998.
ISBN 0527763446

Business Process Improvement Workbook: Documentation, Analysis, Design, and Management of Business Process Improvement, H. James Harrington, K. C. Esseling, and Van Nimwegen, 1997.
ISBN-10: 0070267790
ISBN-13: 978-0070267794

Appendix C: Using the EHR Evaluation Checklist

The sample EHR checklist contains a broad range of EHR features that you may find useful in creating an RFP or evaluation materials for site visits and demonstrations. Of course it should be altered to fit you particular situation. Aside from the listing of product features, three additional columns are present. The first, "Present/Absent", provides a simple means for noting which features are available in the product. This is a good way to do a "first cut" of evaluated products. Next, determine which features are absolutely essential to meet your needs (i.e., features that if missing automatically eliminates the product from further consideration). Comparing the "Present/Absent" column to the "Essential" column provides a quick way to assess the potential value of products under consideration. The nice thing about this approach is that it makes it easy for those who did not enter the data (i.e., other committee members) to rapidly review products and assess their relative suitability. Also you may use "Essential" to indicate a "priority score" by entering a value between 0 and 1 to indicate how important a feature is (0, not required; 1, must be present). The final column, "Point Value", is used to record the quality of the implementation of a feature. For example, if the feature under consideration is "Allergy List", then a product that provides for easy list updates in two steps and alerts the user during prescription writing may be deemed superior to one that requires a four-step list update process and requires the user to remember to look up the patient's allergy history. The former product may be given a score of 1 for "Allergy List", while the latter only 0.7. Using this approach, fine differences between close competitors can be made more objective and analyzable. Of course, the rules for assigning points to various feature components must be determined by those performing the evaluation. Ideally, point assignments are made based upon information gleaned from process analyses.

Table C-1

EHR FEATURE CHECKLIST 2008

Product Name: _____

Company: _____

Evaluation Date: _____

Chart Features	Present/ Absent	Essential?	Point Value (quality if present)
Medication Features			
Long-term			
Per episode			
Active/inactive			
Failed after trial			
Allergy list			
Automatic allergy warning			
Prescription writer			
e-mail or FAX to pharmacy			
maintains Rx history			
Maintains formulary information			
by insurance plan			
Drug interactions			
multiple drug-drug adjustable			
Practitioner-specific medication list			
Drug information			
side effects			
adverse reactions			
overdose			
dosages			
forms supplied			
Reports by			
Patient			
Medication			
Provider			
Laboratory/X-ray/Pathology Features			
Maintains test history			
By Patient			
By Provider			
Permits automatic data download			
from outside facilities			
Permits uploading of orders to			
other facilities (ex: lab orders)			
Maintains profile of available tests and			
indications			
Flags abnormal results			
Permits tracking of abnormal lab			
follow up			
Permits creation of panels			
Disease-specific			
Patient-specific			
Population-specific			
Alerts for redundant testing			
Guideline-aware order entry			

continued on next page

Table C-1

EHR FEATURE CHECKLIST 2008 (*CONT'D*)

Chart Features	Present/ Absent	Essential?	Point Value (quality if present)

Laboratory/X-ray/Pathology Features (*cont'd*)
   Reports by
      Patient
      Test
      Provider

Telephone Call Features
Maintains call history
   Patient
   Site
   Provider
   Number called from
   Automatic dialing
   Captures call reason and action
      taken
   Provides alerts and reminders for
      required follow-up
   Report by
      Patient
      Provider
      Call reason
      Call action

Diagnosis Features
   Problem list
   Long-term
   Per episode
   Guideline-based advice
   Access to knowledge resources
      Internet
      Practice Guidelines
   Report by
      Patient
      Provider
      Diagnosis

Referral Features
Maintains list of referral sites/providers by
   Specialty
   Reason for referral
   Location
Maintains referral history
   Patient
   Provider
   Site
   Reason/Diagnosis
Maintains list of approved
   providers/sites by
      Insurance plan
      Provider preference

continued on next page

Table C-1

EHR FEATURE CHECKLIST 2008 (CONT'D)

Chart Features	Present/ Absent	Essential?	Point Value (quality if present)
Referral Features (*cont'd*)			
Report by			
Patient			
Provider			
Reason/Diagnosis			
Referral Site/Provider			
Reports by email			
Store and forward for images			
Preventive Medicine Features			
Maintains patient intervention history			
Permits design of intervention			
protocols by			
Sex			
Age			
Disease state			
Insurance Plan			
Permits guideline-based protocols			
Provides user-defined alerts			
Report by			
Patient population			
Patient			
Provider			
Diagnosis			
Protocol			
Clinical Encounter			
Progress note			
Plain text			
Encoded and searchable			
Vital signs			
Clinical findings			
E&M Templates			
Defined by en d-user			
Specialty specific			
Disease based guidelines/protocols			
Defined by end-user			
Specialty-specific			
Patient Education Features			
User definable			
Preloaded			
Updated regularly (quarterly)			
Web access to educational materials			
Population Health Management			
Provider profiles			
Medications			
Labs			
Referrals			
Preventive health			

continued on next page

Table C-1

EHR FEATURE CHECKLIST 2008 (*CONT'D*)

Chart Features	Present/ Absent	Essential?	Point Value (quality if present)
Population Health Management (*cont'd*)			
Site profiles			
Medications			
Labs			
Referrals			
Preventive health			
Reports by			
Guideline/Protocol			
Provider			
Disease			
Site			
Pre-defined reports			
HEDIS			
JCAHO			
Disease Registry			
Health Status reports			
SF-36			
Data Exchange and Reporting			
Create P4P Data sets			
Quality Improvement Reports			
Communications and Infrastructure			
Communications			
Remote access			
FAX support or linkage			
Word processor support or linkage			
Spreadsheet support or linkage			
Provides e-mail support or linkage			
Internet			
Web-enabled version			
Decision Support			
Statistical Analysis (internal)			
Knowledge Resources (access from within EHR)			
MEDLINE			
Internet resources			
Electronic textbooks			
Data Storage and File Formats			
Permits Data Export			
ASCII			
Support for Clinical Data Repository			
Data warehouse			
Statistical analysis packages			
Permits Data Import			
ASCII			
Relational Database files			
Application Programming Interface			

continued on next page

Table C-1

EHR FEATURE CHECKLIST 2008 (*CONT'D*)

Chart Features	Present/ Absent	Essential?	Point Value (quality if present)
Data Storage and File Formats (*cont'd*)			
Supports varied data types			
Sound			
Video			
Graphics			
Standards Supported			
HL-7			
SNOMED CT			
ICD			
CPT			
MEDCIN			
LOINC for lab data			
Interface Options			
Pen			
Voice			
Keyboard			
Graphical			
User modifiable			
Security Features			
Audit trail			
Permits audit trail analysis			
Automatic activation			
Passwords			
Text/Numeric			
Biometric			
Face			
Voice			
Fingerprint			
Electronic Signatures			
Role-based Access			
Data validation			
Back-up process			
Encryption			
Operating Systems			
Unix			
Macintosh OS X			
Windows 2003			
.Net Framework			
Internet-Based (ASP)			
Client/Server			
Technology			
Database			
Relational			
Object-oriented			
Servers			
Fault-tolerant			
Clustering			
virtualization			

continued on next page

Table C-1

EHR FEATURE CHECKLIST 2008 (CONT'D)

Chart Features	Present/ Absent	Essential?	Point Value (quality if present)
Total desired features present			_____
Total Number of essential features			_____
Total quality points			_____

Evaluation Computation suggestion:

Step 1: Narrow product field to no more than 4 packages

Step 2: Add up "Total desired features present". Eliminate low ranking products.

Step 3: Add up "Total Number of essential features". Eliminate low ranking products.

Step 4: For all remaining products determine the quality of the implementation for all features in each product.

Index